Situational Leadership® in
NURSING

D1315586

Situational Leadership in NURSING

Paul Hersey, Ed.D., M.B.A.
Chairman of the Board and Founder
Leadership Studies, Inc.
President and Chairman of the Board
California American University
Escondido, California

Bonnie Weaver Duldt, Ph.D., R.N.
Professor
School of Nursing
East Carolina University
Greenville, North Carolina

APPLETON & LANGE
Norwalk, Connecticut/San Mateo, California

0-8385-8553-1

Notice: The authors and publisher of this volume have taken care that
the information and recommendations contained herein are accurate and
compatible with the standards generally accepted at the time of publication.

89 90 91 92 93 / 10 9 8 7 6 5 4 3 2 1

Prentice-Hall International (UK) Limited, *London*
Prentice-Hall of Australia Pty. Limited, *Sydney*
Prentice-Hall Canada, Inc., *Toronto*
Prentice-Hall Hispanoamericana, S.A., *Mexico*
Prentice-Hall of India Private Limited, *New Delhi*
Prentice-Hall of Japan, Inc., *Tokyo*
Simon & Schuster Asia Pte. Ltd., Singapore
Editora Prentice-Hall do Brasil Ltda., *Rio de Janeiro*
Prentice-Hall, *Englewood Cliffs, New Jersey*

Hersey, Paul.
    Situational leadership in nursing.

    Includes index.
    1. Nursing services—Administration. 2. Leadership.
I. Duldt, Bonnie Weaver. II. Title. [DNLM:
1. Leadership. 2. Nursing, Supervisory. WY 105 H572s]
RT89.H48 1988   362.1'73'068   88-7604
ISBN 0-8385-8553-1

Production Editor: Susan T. Meiman
Designer: Kathleen Peters Ceconi
Cover: Michael Kelly

PRINTED IN THE UNITED STATES OF AMERICA

REVIEWERS

CONTENTS

PREFACE

For the past few years, the nursing profession has been moving toward a more explicit and carefully defined humanistic and holistic orientation. With the advent of this philosophical stance, we are concerned with the incongruence and disharmony of nursing's philosophical orientation against the backdrop of leadership in a highly structured, task-oriented health care delivery system. Our health care delivery system has become complex and often seems fragmented; it also often seems dehumanizing to both clients and nurses.

Many nurses who function as leaders in first-level management positions need assistance, not only in preparing for this role, but also in moving toward a humanistic and holistic perspective of the leadership role. Introductory leadership courses designed to prepare the graduate for such first-level leadership positions are offered in baccalaureate nursing programs, in-house staff development, and continuing education. This text, designed for use in such courses, is an attempt to extend the profession's humanistic and holistic philosophical perspectives into roles of leadership in nursing. Problems and approaches to team building and organizational development in nursing are presented within a dual theoretical framework: Dr. Paul Hersey's Situational Leadership theory and Dr. Bonnie Duldt's theory of Humanistic Nursing Communication.

Situational Leadership theory is described in Chapter 1. This organizational communication theory has been used by leaders in business, industry, government, religious, and education arenas, providing practical guidance founded on extensive research. Successful and effective leaders adapt their own behavior to meet the leadership and management problems in each specific situation.

In Chapter 2, the theory of Humanistic Nursing Communication is presented. This theory summarizes and organizes relevant communication theory and research within a nursing context. It emphasizes a range of attitudes and interaction patterns (skills) that nurses may deliberately choose to use to meet interpersonal communication demands with clients, peers, and colleagues. As with Situational Leadership theory, the focus of this approach is on diagnosing and adapting one's communication to meet interpersonal problems or objectives in relating with clients, peers, and colleagues in clinical nursing practice. Together, these two theories represent the theoretical core of this text, which can provide the nurse-leader with a practical perspective to assist in the appropriate and discriminating application of each theory.

For a nurse, the care of the client is clear. For a nurse-leader, care of one's followers is similar to care of clients, but there are distinctions that require the nurse to adapt behavior to the situation unique to nursing leadership. Chapter 3 presents a description of these unique distinctions along with relevant requirements and expectations of nursing leadership in contemporary situations.

Leadership is generally defined as an interpersonal communication process that influences the task group members to achieve task goals and maintain relationships. The purpose of this text is to serve as a reference about managing *relationships* among task group members as well as managing the *task*. The concept of leadership, then, is viewed as consisting of two major elements: people and task.

The element of people management is comprised of a subset of elements: communicating, motivating, initiating, integrating, and facilitating. These elements are discussed in Chapters 4 through 8. The element of task management is comprised of a subset of elements, too: planning, organizing, staffing, directing, and controlling. These elements are discussed in Chapters 9 through 15. Other concepts relevant to leadership are included in these chapters: status, power, change, conformity, cohesiveness, commitment, conflict resolution, value clarification, alienation, prejudice, job satisfaction, and productivity. This, then, composes our conceptual approach to leadership offered in this text.

There are certain unique aspects of this nursing leadership text. First, of course, is the philosophical perspective of humanistic and holistic leadership. Second, a positive approach is taken in emphasizing the development of good leader–follower relationships through interpersonal communication. Third, because leadership is defined as influencing people, we have included the process of persuasion and public speaking, as well as the development of a speech designed to influence a specific type of audience, including a hostile audience. Fourth, many special concerns of nursing leadership are considered in detailed, with practical suggestions for handling them; these include distrust, motivation, budgets, legal aspects, and disciplinary interventions. Finally, in most of the chapters, we provide statements of principle that summarize and emphasize the preceding discussions. These statements are intended to serve as the basis of thoughtful discussion rather than as "truth." These principles are offered as guides for your consideration. We believe these statements represent the best information currently available as derived from theory, research, and practice. We are concerned with the application of theory and research as the foundation for our readers' understanding and for improving the practice of nursing leadership.

ACKNOWLEDGMENTS

We wish to acknowledge the contribution of many nursing clinicians, workshop participants, students, and faculty, who have contributed ideas and examples to this text.

Acknowledgments should be given also to our spouses, Suzanne and John for their continuous support and encouragement; to the numerous nursing colleagues and students for their interest and contributions, particularly those at East Carolina University; to Sylvene Spickerman, R.N., M.S.N., Associate Professor, School of Nursing, East Carolina University, who carefully read the manuscript and offered her suggestions and encouragement; to Judy Wojcik and her staff of reference librarians at the East Carolina University Health Sciences Library for their persistence in locating sources and citations; to Nancy K. Mayberry, Ph.D., Professor, Foreign Languages and Literature, East Carolina University, who proofed our galley sheets, to Anna Donoghue, Ph.D., Vice-President for Graduate Studies, California American University, who served as our West Coast anchor, advisory, and collaborating colleague; to Mary Heindel, Paul's secretary, who helped us keep in touch; to Jamie Mount Sokol, former assistant to the Editor and now assistant Editor in her own right, for her timely and uniquely forthright approach to motivating authors; and last but not least, to Marion Kalstein-Welch, our editor, for her continuous enthusiasm and support in this effort. With sincere appreciation, Paul Hersey and Bonnie Duldt.

I

INTRODUCTION: THE STATE OF THE ART: NURSING LEADERSHIP

Most leaders in top management positions call in consultants to assist in solving leadership problems; first-line managers and supervisors tend not to have this support. In nursing, directors or vice-presidents of nursing service often have funds available for consultation services regarding staffing problems, budget development, interpreting accreditation criteria, resolving conflicts with unions, and so on. Nurses in top management positions in health agencies often are encouraged, and even expected, to attend and participate in meetings, seminars, workshops, and programs that focus on leadership approaches to problems and situations. The staff nurse, however, who is promoted to a first-level leadership position such as that of assistant head nurse or head nurse seldom has such opportunities to learn about leadership roles and expectations. Nurses who are assistant head nurses and head nurses often have no one to whom they can turn for guidance except a supervisor, one who has *survived* long enough to be promoted. Nursing supervisors very often have been promoted merely because the predecessor resigned, not necessarily because of their own outstanding successes as head nurses or knowledge of the leadership role. Betty Donaho, Corporate Director of Nursing at Sisters of Mercy Health Corporation in Farmington Hills, Michigan, reports statistics about the qualifications of *upper*-level nursing managers:

> Looking at the type of positions nurses are filling across the country in relation to their education, some inferences can be drawn. We know that roughly 60,000 nurses hold administrator and assistant administrator positions. Among them the following is true:
> 9.4% are associate degree graduates
> 47% are diploma graduates
> 23% are baccalaureate graduates
> 18% have master's degrees
> 1.4% have doctorates.
> Without question, the education of nursing management is not adequate to provide the kind of leadership that is needed.[1]

If this is true of upper-level nursing managers, then middle management or the first-line managers in nursing, the head nurses and the supervisors, need even greater support and guidance. It is this group to whom we direct this book: staff nurses, head nurses, and supervisors. While experience in any endeavor is useful and necessary, learning by experience alone can be a difficult and disheartening process. Experience within a philosophical and theoretical perspective provides one with a broader and sounder basis for career development as a leader in any area; we believe this to be particularly true in nursing.

Most organizations and agencies provide general guidance to first-line managers through in-house training programs or by sending a few promising people to leadership training programs—management "charm schools." In the health care system, a great number of hospitals are quite small. It is difficult for such agencies to provide extensive and sophisticated in-house leadership development programs for a small number of nurse–leaders. Nurses in larger agencies or in the armed services are more fortunate.

Whether the agency is large or small, however, research shows it is *not* advisable to send a few people to leadership training programs. When the individuals return, resistance to change on the part of peers and colleagues often negates implementation of the ideas learned at the training program. The best approach has been found to be the introduction of a new approach at the top management level, implementing it progressively downward according to the organization chart or chain of delegated authority and responsibility.[2,3]

Many agencies make no effort to provide guidance to professional staff who assume leadership roles within the organizational structure. Professional competency is assumed to predict or to be correlated with leadership success. This may be a false assumption, particularly in nursing. Competency in clinical nursing may be based on experience in one-to-one relationships with clients, as in the case of intensive care units. It may also be based on experiences with small groups of clients who are very ill, as in general medical–surgical units. The most leadership experience a staff nurse obtains comes as "relief-charge," that is, being the only nurse in the area during the evening, night, or weekend periods. This temporary position is generally without delegated authority and power. Although responsibility and accountability are usually emphasized to the individual nurses, any "real" leadership or management problems are turned over to the "official" head nurse to be resolved during "regular" business hours.

Thus while most organizations provide some guidance through educational efforts, the nurse seeking a leadership position in nursing seldom has the benefit of long-term career planning for education and experience, as is the case in formal management training programs developed for individuals in banks or large organizations in industry and business. Administrators of health agencies tend just to promote professional nursing staff, expecting the nurses to know how to behave as leaders and managers. As a consequence, some nurses are successful leaders, and others are not. Knowledge, skills, and attitudes as leaders often develop serendipitously rather than by design.

Instead of allowing one's potential as a successful leader to develop by chance, we propose that it is better to have a clear definition of a successful leader and of what elements are important in developing one's own leadership potential. Careful consideration of the leadership definition and its elements contributes to self-assessment and the development of one's self image in the leadership role. For those already in nursing leadership roles, self-assessment and self-evaluation processes are helpful in identifying strengths and weaknesses. Observation and assessment of one's own leader and others in leadership roles help in identifying role models and perhaps even a mentor.

Historically, nurses having clinical expertise have been urged, pressured, and even coerced into accepting leadership roles and responsibilities for which they often felt ill prepared. Modern nurses can avoid allowing themselves to be put into such a situation, which often proves distressing to the nurses. Health care delivery systems today are too complex for Pollyanna attitudes toward leadership preparation to be successful. Modern nurses seek educational and experiential preparation for leadership positions in nursing.

We propose that one element is crucial to successful leadership; that element is *communication*—specifically, that communication occurring in the superior–subordinate or leader–follower relationship. One classical definition of leadership is *followership:* without followers, one is not a leader. This is a fundamental truth. Peter Drucker has stated that one of the scarcest resources in our world is effective leaders. Paul Hersey observes further, that, while this is true, he believes the scarcest resources of all are *effective followers.* Unless people understand the leadership role and agree to follow a leader, to comply with the leader's guidance, direction, and counsel in regard to achieving interdependent organizational and personal goals, the task group's goals (and individual members' goals as well) have a high probability of remaining beyond the reach of all. Research has shown that communication occurring between leader and followers is at the core of effective leadership, and of follow-ership as well.[4] Thus whether one chooses to be a leader or follower in nursing, one's effective-ness in either role necessitates knowing about the leader–follower relationship. We believe effective leader–follower relationships make a significant, positive impact upon the quality of nursing care provided.

We present an integrated perspective of our two communication theories. One focuses on communication in leadership: the Situational Leadership theory of Hersey.[5] The other focuses on communication in nursing: the Humanistic Nursing Communication theory of Duldt.[6,7]

Situational Leadership, providing a perspective of leader communication behaviors adapted to behaviors of followers, is the result of integrating the field of applied behavioral sciences with management discipline. Humanistic Nursing Communication provides a philo-sophical perspective of humanism and holism as developed and expressed in nursing as a discipline and a practice profession, and as developed from the speech communication disci-pline. This theory is applied not only to nurse–client relationships, but also to peer and collegial relationships. Here unique distinctions are made between the nurse–client and the nurse-leader–follower relationship. Together, we believe the two theories provide practical guides to contemporary nurses who want to be effective and successful leaders in nursing.

REFERENCES

1. Donaho, B. *Survival of the fittest.* Pub. No. 52–1904. New York: National League for Nursing, pp. 2–3, 1982.
2. Bavelas, A. Communication patterns in task-oriented groups. *Journal of the Acoustical Society of America,* 1950, *22,* 725–730.
3. Cartwright, D., & Zander, A. (Eds.), *Group dynamics.* New York: Harper & Row, 1968, pp. 503–511.
4. Pincus, J. D. Communication: Key contributor to effectiveness—the research. *Journal of Nursing Administration,* 1986, *16* (9), 19–25.
5. Hersey, P., & Blanchard, K. *Management of organizational behavior: Utilizing human resources* (4th ed.). Englewood Cliffs, N.J.: Prentice-Hall, 1982.
6. Duldt, B. W., Giffin, K., & Patton, B. R. *Interpersonal communication in nursing.* Philadelphia: Davis, 1984.
7. Duldt, B. W., & Giffin, K. *Theoretical perspectives of nursing.* Boston: Little, Brown, 1985.

1

SITUATIONAL LEADERSHIP®
THEORY

INTRODUCTION

During this century, those individuals concerned about the role of leaders have focused on identifying one best leadership approach. Extensive research reveals, however, that different approaches can be successful in different situations. Situational Leadership theory is based on the modern assumption that there is no one, singularly successful leadership style, but that leaders need to have a variety of styles that can be adapted to the unique combination of variables present in each situation. Theorists and researchers of leadership have also studied extensively the many variables occurring in leadership situations, believing that first one, then another, has a key effect upon leadership. Of all the variables studied, research tends to show that the most important variable in leadership is the communication that occurs between the leader and follower(s).[1] It is this variable—communication—that is central to Situational Leadership theory. These two factors—using multiple leadership styles and focusing on communication as a significant variable—above all others combine to make Situational Leadership theory a most significant theory today. Thus it is important that this theory be brought to the attention of nurses and others involved in health care professions and services.

Situational Leadership theory is an example of the symbolic interactionists' theoretical model. In this model, the human being is described rather explicitly as a logical (and illogical) symbol user (and misuser) who seeks hierarchy within society, is aware of symbolic negatives (rules, laws, and nonexistence), and is aware of the unattainable perfect. Man (in the generic sense, meaning both men and women) is both active and reactive, can influence the environment, and be influenced by it. The objective of communication is to bring about unity among people by agreeing on categories of more or less ambiguity in order to transcend conflict. Language reveals reality, and it is through a *term*inistic screen that one sees reality, as if through a fog of symbols. Motivation lies in words; people can be aroused to achieve goals through the influence of words. Meaning, however, resides within people; symbolic interactions among people develop and sustain the self or the self-system, and meaning arises out of relationships. The symbolic interactionists' model presupposes a dynamic relationship in which both speaker and receiver have shared responsibility for the interpersonal communication occurring between them, and this model has potential for providing a holistic view of people, synthesizing body, mind, and spirit.[2]

In this chapter, an analysis is presented of Situational Leadership theory according to its assumptions, concepts, and relationship statements and evaluation. See Appendix C for a summary of the theory to which the reader may refer while reading this chapter.

ASSUMPTIONS

Assumptions are theoretical statements that are accepted as truth or reality and are not questioned. These premises or presumptions are not tested, but provide a framework within which a theory is developed. Assumptions often include statements about philosophical stances the theorist takes. In addition, each discipline tends to have a particular set of concepts that comprise a primary paradigm for that discipline, and these concepts are often the topics or issues about which theoretical assumptions are made. In management of organizations, the major concepts include the human being (as follower and leader), communication, change, power, and productivity. Assumptions about these things are posed in Situational Leadership, and these assumptions are presented in this section.

Human Beings

The human being is viewed as having classical humanistic and holistic characteristics in several respects. First, we assume a process or systems model of reality in that many variables interact and influence one another. The reality in which leaders function is seen as having multiple variables, which have unique influences upon the leader, the follower, and the organizational processes. Thus it is also assumed that even the best leader cannot depend upon one particular set of behaviors or attributes to work in all circumstances, since the followers and the organizational situation change continually. Rather, the effective leader is able to adapt his or her own behaviors to the needs of followers or of the situation.

Human beings, both leaders and followers, are characterized by being adaptable, capable of making choices, and responsible for their own actions. Each human being, both leader and follower, views the situation from a unique perspective relative to his or her own role and position within an organizational setting and develops values and attitudes according to this unique perspective. Both leaders and followers develop values and attitudes that are reflected in the behaviors displayed by them. This theory focuses on the leader's observation of follower behaviors relative to task performance, such as productivity, demonstrated commitment to organizational goals, and expressions of cohesiveness among the task group. While some theorists give paper-and-pencil tests to determine attitudes and try to predict behavior from these attitudes, we believe that one can do a better job of predicting future job-related values and attitudes from present behavior. "If you want to know a person's heart, look at what that person does. Look at the person's behavior."[3] Thus if one wants to know the values and attitudes of the older nursing supervisor toward the new, young graduate, one observes how the supervisor behaves toward this newly graduated nurse.

Human beings are also seen as being adaptable and thus open to influence. We posit that leaders have considerable influence upon their followers. Behaviors, and ultimately attitudes and values, of followers can be influenced by interpersonal communication with leaders. The implication of this assumption is that the leader is responsible for the development of the followers in task-relevant behaviors, such as competence and commitment. The leader can influence the internal states of the followers in such a manner that the followers can become more motivated and willing to perform tasks well. The opposite can happen, too. The impact of leadership behavior can result in the followers choosing not to follow the leader's directives. Hersey and Blanchard state, "We have found that if the follower decides not to follow, it really doesn't matter what the boss thinks, what the nature of the work is, how much time is involved, or what the other situational variables are."[4] The interpersonal communication between the leader and the follower is assumed to be the key factor in effective leadership. It is the follower who decides whether or not leadership happens.

Communication

One particularly unique characteristic of human beings is the ability to communicate. When human beings band together to form an organization and seek to accomplish some task that no individual would be capable of achieving alone, it is the network of communication that holds the organizational system together. Hersey assumes the organizational situation in which leadership functions is an "open social system," subject to all general assumptions and behaviors of a systems model. The implications of this assumption are described by him as follows: ". . . all aspects of an organization are interrelated; a change in any part of an organization may have an impact on other parts of, or on the organization itself."[5] Thus the leadership behavior of a director or vice-president of nursing services can be expected to have an impact on the assistants, on the supervisors, and ultimately on the staff nurses and non-nursing staff. A ripple or domino effect occurs, and it may occur both downward and upward along the formal organizational lines of authority.

We also posit that there is a need for a system of common understandings and language between and among leaders and their followers: Communication congruency is believed to help people function well together to achieve unity. Having a common language enables two things to happen. First, feedback can be given in a rational, logical manner with minimal emotional overtone. (See the discussion of feedback on pages 111 and 115.) Second, the follower can learn that it is one's own behavior that determines how the leader will be responding to the follower. For example, if Mary Jones, a staff nurse, wants to be closely observed and have the head nurse hovering over her, she just needs to make a few medication errors, toss out a specimen or two, and make errors in changing dressings or giving instructions to patients. Mary's irresponsible behavior will "call out" reciprocal behavior in her head nurse.[6*]

Change

In accordance with the process view of the human being, we assume that change is a key characteristic of all life. Modern organizations are seen as changing daily, and we suggest further that it is the effective leader who is able to develop strategies to plan, direct, and control change. Thus the ideal leader is seen as one who is very skilled in observing and analyzing change, a key characteristic of all life.[7] The leader is also seen as being *proactive,* that is, capable of having an impact upon the environment and controlling it rather than being *reactive,* or capable only of responding to the environment and being controlled by it.

The ultimate objective of effective leadership is to support the holistic development (change) of the followers or employees. Situational Leadership theory is believed to be a vehicle by which people learn to be active, responsible, and mature, self-motivated individuals; it is a means whereby both leader and follower are enabled to become all that they can become as human beings.[8]

---

*Duldt & Giffin, *Theoretical perspectives of nursing.* See Chapter 5, regarding the DASH paradigm in interpersonal relationships.

Power

Power is assumed to be a major resource of leadership. It is the means whereby a leader is able to influence followers to change behavior in the direction chosen by the leader.[9] Thus we acknowledge a perceived hierarchy among human beings; there is a natural tendency for people to seek some order or pattern in relationships. While all may be equal, some are more equal than others.[10] Power is the factor that determines whether or not a follower will comply with the leader's attempts to influence. The logic we use is this: If many factors in the situation change, and if the communication of the leader is to influence the follower to comply in the situation, then one needs to assume that multiple characteristics or sources of power will be appropriate. The implications of this assumption are that the theory will focus on analysis of sources of power available to a leader within a situation and development of wisdom regarding its use. It is further assumed that the actual usefulness power has is based on the leader's potential power being perceived by the follower. Thus a leader's power, working with communication, is believed to be an important element in effective leadership.

Productivity

Many assume that productivity refers primarily to the number of units of some commodity put out or services provided in a given time. We believe, however, that productivity is not limited to output or completing the function of the organization. We believe productivity involves output of goods and services *plus* development of human potential.

> Managers need to devote time to nurture the leadership potential, motivation, morale, climate, commitment to objectives, and the decision-making, communication, and problem-solving of their people. Thus, an important role for managers is the development of the task-relevant maturity of their followers.[11]

Thus Situational Leadership theory assumes the scope of a leader is task productivity and task readiness of the follower.

Explicit and implicit assumptions deemed relevant to nursing and upon which Situational Leadership is based have been presented. Specific statements of these assumptions are to be presented in Appendix A. Having set this theoretical stage, the major concepts of Situational Leadership theory will be presented.

CONCEPTS

Concepts represent the building blocks of a theory. When reading a theory, one needs to give careful attention to the way each theorist defines terms, because the definition has implications for the way concepts work together in theoretical relationship statements. Conceptual definitions function like characters in a novel: the characters are extensively introduced and "defined" before the novelist begins to tell how the characters relate in the story.

> A concept is a term or word used to describe, classify or designate a specific set of phenomenon or a set of conceptions. It is a timeless, abstract, impersonal idea that serves as a norm. A set of concepts provides the necessary elements of theories and may have definitions unique and specific to particular theories.[12]

One needs to give particular attention to the defining of concepts in theories of leadership; there are numerous theories of leadership, and the distinctions among them may seem rather minute to some.

The task of defining the concepts of Situational Leadership theory is approached in a very practical way; the definitions make sense for pragmatic and research purposes. The major concepts of this theory include the following: leadership, leadership style, and leader expectations; task behavior; relationship behavior; readiness; the developmental and regressive cycles; power; and change. Several of the concepts have important subsets, which are discussed in this section. For convenience, succinct definitions of these terms are found in Appendix A.

Leadership

Leadership is defined as "a process of influencing the activities of an individual or a group in efforts toward goal achievement in a given situation."[13] We make several important distinctions with this definition. First, the leadership phenomenon is seen as being a process in nature; we describe the leadership context as being one of flux and change. Second, the definition is inclusive of all leadership contexts and organizational settings. This is a very desirable characteristic of a theoretical definition, facilitating practical applications and concept operationalization in research efforts to validate theoretical statements. Finally, while leader and follower are mentioned, this definition is not limited to a boss–employee relationship. Rather, it is to be interpreted as describing a "potential" leader seeking to influence a "potential" follower. This means the leadership role does not necessarily remain with the person having the official title, such as director or supervisor; the function of leadership can move to other members of a task group. Again, it is the potential follower who finally decides whether or not to *be* a follower, resulting in the potential leader in fact becoming a leader.

Leadership Style

A *style* is a pattern of behavior that is consistent as perceived by others. Leadership style, then, is: ". . . the consistent behavior patterns they [leaders] use when they are working with and through other people as perceived by those people."[14] The followers can come to know the leader well enough that they can predict how the leader will behave in particular situations. Style may be considered as synonymous with "personality."

In Situational Leadership theory, leadership styles refer primarily to a set of four patterns of communication the leader may choose to use in talking to the follower: telling, selling, participating, and delegating. (See Fig. 1–1.) These differ in the following ways. First, telling and are both leader-oriented and primarily monological or one-directional communications; telling involves low socioemotional support, and involves high support. The leader makes the decisions about the task. Second, participating and delegating are both follower-oriented and primarily dialogical or two-directional communications. There is a high degree of socioemotional involvement on the part of the leader in participating; in delegating, support and involvement decreases. The followers make task-related decisions. Thus these labels categorize leadership styles into four basic patterns of communicating, which are useful in a practical sense for the leader in making "on-the-run" diagnostic judgments.

Leader Expectations

The concept of *expectations* generally refers to that behavior deemed appropriate to a particular role or position within a group or organization as perceived by members of the group. The

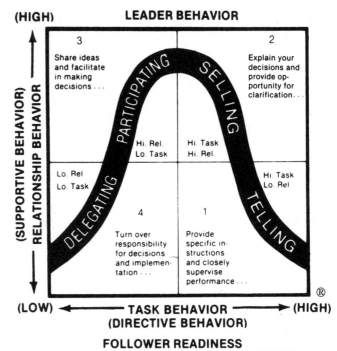

Figure 1–1. The Situational Leadership Model. (*From Hersey, P. The situational leader. New York: Warner Books, 1984, p. 63.*)

degree to which expectations are compatible means there is agreement among all concerning how one is to behave when fulfilling a particular role in the group or organization. In Situational Leadership theory, the concept of *leader expectations* refers primarily to the expected behavior of the leader as perceived by others, especially the followers.[15] Expectations range from highly restrictive, predetermined, detailed supervisory behaviors to ambiguous behavioral expectations allowing freedom to express the leader's own personality or style. The behavior of the followers and their expectations of the leader need to be congruent with the leadership style. "Followers in any situation are vital, not only because individually they accept or reject the leader but because as a group they determine whatever personal power that leader will have."[16] It is on the basis of observed follower behavior that the leader wisely selects the appropriate leadership style: that style most compatible with perceived leadership expectations of the followers.

Task Behavior

The leader's communications are primarily one-way or monological and concern the structuring of the job or task. The leader lets the followers know what is expected of them; this involves explaining what each follower is to do, when, where, and how.[17]

Relationship Behavior

The leader's communications are primarily two-way or dialogical and supportive in nature, concern socioemotional support and psychological "strokes," and facilitating interactions among people.[18]

Readiness

Readiness refers to the follower, and it consists of two elements: ability and willingness. Readiness in Situational Leadership does not refer to age or educational background. It refers to how well one is able to do the task and whether or not the person is willing to do it when asked. Ability is divided into a continuum that indicates the degree of necessary knowledge and skill the individual possesses:

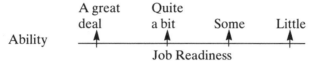

Willingness is also presented in a continuum that indicates the degree of confidence and commitment an individual possesses:

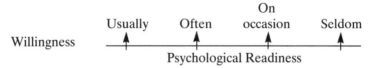

It is important to note that the readiness refers to a dimension of the follower, not the leader. Readiness also involves the education and experience (or both) of the follower, and it involves the capacity to set *high* but *attainable* goals for an individual or a group. Effective leaders provide an environment in which appropriate goals (incentives outside people) are available for motivation. Motivation involves those things, such as needs, wants, drives, and impulses, that provide the "whys" of behavior. Behavior is basically goal-directed, and activity is a fundamental unit of behavior.

A function of the leader is to set organizational goals and develop "work maps" to show how the goals can be accomplished. In the leader–follower relationship, goals need to be set (management by objectives) in order to arouse and maintain activity and to determine the direction of behavior. (See pp. 293–298 for a more complete discussion of management by objectives.) Goals need to be moderately difficult but potentially achievable with a moderate degree of risk. Goals set too high or too low tend to be either frustrating and too risky or too easy and uninteresting. Achievement-motivated followers respond favorably to task-relevant education and feedback; they want to know the score. The need for achievement is a distinct human motive, and this motive can be developed. Chronological age and formal education are not issues. Rather, the concern of Situational Leadership theory is the here-and-now (existential) psychological state of the follower. The job-ready follower is capable of performing tasks without direction, and the psychologically ready follower possesses self-confidence and motivation to feel good about performing the task.[19] The ready follower is able and willing.

Developmental and Regressive Cycles

The concept of developmental and regressive cycles focuses on the leader's responsibility to develop and maintain human resources of the group. The developmental cycle is initiated after the leader diagnoses the readiness level of the follower. The leader designs and implements a plan of intervention in order to increase the readiness level of the follower or group regarding some aspect of the task.[20] The regressive cycle occurs when the followers begin to behave in a less ready manner than previously. In response, the effective leader diagnoses the regressive behavior and designs and implements a plan of interventions to halt the regression in readiness, turning the trend around.[21]

Style Range and Adaptability

According to Situational Leadership theory, the leader can communicate in four basic leadership styles: telling, selling, participating, and delegating, with varying emphasis on directive and supportive behavior. The extent to which a leader is able to vary the style of communicating is called the *style range*. *Style adaptability* refers to the degree in which a leader is able to change the style of communicating to be congruent with the situation.[22] Most individuals tend to have at least two leadership styles in their style profile, and, with education and practice, are able to increase the range of styles available to them.

Power

In Situational Leadership theory, power is defined as a leader's influence potential. Power is the means whereby a leader persuades followers to conform or comply. There are a number of ways a leader can accumulate power or develop power bases from which to draw sources of influence. One is through fear, or *coercive* power. Through one's own skill and knowledge, one can have *expert* power. *Legitimate* power is based on position or title within an organization. *Reward* power is based on the leader's ability to obtain the rewards the followers like. Some leaders are so charming and attractive interpersonally that people naturally follow; this is *referent* power. *Information* power is based on the leader's possession or access to information valued by the followers. When a leader knows people who are perceived by the followers to be influential or important inside or outside the organization, the leader is said to have *connection* power.[23] Knowledge of one's bases of power is a necessary factor to consider in selecting the appropriate leadership style for influencing followers in a particular situation.

Change

Change is an inevitable fact of life in organizations and society at large. A large portion of change is unplanned; however, according to Situational Leadership theory, it is considered the leader's function to plan change. Change, in Situational Leadership theory, occurs in a sequential developmental pattern in people and in an organization. Knowledge comes first, then attitudes; next, individual behaviors are affected, and finally the total group changes. Knowing this pattern of change, effective leaders can use a plan of *change process*. This plan consists of three sequential elements or stages: *unfreezing, changing,* and *refreezing*. First, current (or old) patterns of behaving and thinking are broken down in the unfreezing stage in order to motivate the followers for accepting change. Second, the followers identify and internalize the changes, following the leader's influence (changing). Finally, refreezing occurs as the new patterns of performance become a part of the follower's attitudes, behavior, and personality.

Directed or coercive change tends to be destructive and resisted by followers. Until the people involved recognize the problem as their own, it is going to be much more difficult to produce change in their behavior.[24]*

In this section, concepts of Situational Leadership theory have been defined. The next step in the theoretical analysis is to describe the relationships between and among the concepts.

THEORETICAL RELATIONSHIP STATEMENTS

Theoretical statements that describe the way two or more concepts interact or relate are called *relationship statements* and are the heart of a theory. These statements function like scripts for actors in a play: scripts describe in detail the actions and interactions of each character with and among one another in such a way that a sequential pattern or story emerges. Plays and novels are usually fictional; theoretical relationship statements can be considered fictional patterns of reality until tested through research. In the degree to which relations between concepts are found to agree with the real world, to that degree a theory tends to be considered a reasonably safe guide to action.

In this section, the theoretical relationship statements of Situational Leadership theory are presented. For the readers' convenience, an abbreviated summary of these statements is presented in Appendix D.

Primary and Derived Relationship Statements

In many theories, one can identify one or two major relationship statements from which all other statements are derived. Such is the case in Situational Leadership theory:

1. If a leader is to be an effective manager of change, then the leader must be able to analyze the demands of their environment, and then diagnose and adapt leadership style to fit these demands and develop means to change some or all of the other situational variables.[25]

Of all the variables in a changing environment, research has shown that the leader–follower relationship, the follower's behavior, attitudes, and values regarding the leader, are the most critical. There are many important variables. For example, the leader's boss or the leader's leader is one. If the leader's boss is in close geographic proximity, the leader will tend to receive more direction about how to get the task group to produce than if the boss is located at some distance. The leader's peer group, that is, other supervisors or managers, has an influence in that the leader will tend to conform to the expectations of peers. Organizational history or personality and job demands will also influence the leader, particularly the selection of this leader. Even the amount of time available for making a decision has some influence upon a leader's effectiveness. Sanford has found, however, that the most important variable in leadership effectiveness is the interface between leader and follower.[26] If this relationship does not work out, the relative strength of the other variables makes no difference.

A second primary theoretical relationship statement of Situational Leadership focuses upon the interface of the leader and follower:

---

*This aspect of Situational Leadership incorporates Kurt Lewin's Change theory.

2. The appropriate leadership style (communicating by telling, selling, facilitating, or delegating) for given levels of follower readiness is in a curvilinear functional relation to the directive and supportive behaviors.[27,28]

Each of the four leadership communication styles—*telling, selling, participating,* and *delegating*—is a combination of task, or directive, and relationship, or supportive, behavior. *Task behavior* is the extent to which a leader provides direction for people: telling them what to do, when to do it, where to do it, and how to do it. It means setting goals for them and defining their roles. *Relationship behavior* is the extent to which a leader engages in two-way communication with people: providing support, encouragement, psychological strokes, and facilitating behaviors. It means actively listening to people and supporting their efforts. The readiness of followers is a question of degree. As can be seen in Figure 1–1, some benchmarks of readiness are provided for determining the appropriate leadership style by dividing the readiness continuum below the leadership model into four levels: low (R1), low to moderate (R2), moderate to high (R3), and high (R4). The appropriate leadership style for each of the four readiness levels includes the right combination of task behavior and relationship behavior.

We can now identify two derived theoretical relationship statements concerning directive versus supportive behaviors, as follows:

2.1   As the level of readiness of the follower increases in terms of accomplishing a specific task, the leader should begin to reduce task and increase relationship behavior.[29]

2.2   As the readiness level of the follower moves into an above-average level, the leader should decrease task behavior and relationship behavior.[30]

Now, a composite description of the four leadership styles can be described in more detail.

Telling Is for Low Readiness

People who are both *unable and unwilling* (R1) to take responsibility to do something are not competent or confident. In many cases, their unwillingness is a result of their insecurity regarding the necessary task. Thus a directing "telling" style (S1) that provides clear, specific directions and supervision has the highest probability of being effective with individuals at this readiness level. This style is called "telling" because it is characterized by the leader's defining roles and telling people what, how, when, and where to do various tasks. It emphasizes directive behavior. Too much supportive behavior with people at this readiness level may be seen as permissive, easy and, most importantly, as rewarding of poor performance. This style involves high task behavior and low relationship behavior.

Selling Is for Low to Moderate Readiness

People who are *unable but willing* (R2) to take responsibility are confident but lack skills at this time. Thus the "selling" style (S2) that provides directive behavior, because of their lack of ability, but also supportive behavior to reinforce their willingness and enthusiasm appears to be most appropriate with individuals at this readiness level. This style is called "selling" because most of the direction is still provided by the leader. Through some two-way communication and explanation, however, the leader tries to get the followers psychologically to "buy into" desired behaviors. Followers at this readiness level will usually go along with a decision if they understand the reason for the decision and if their leader also offers some help and direction. This style involves high task behavior and high relationship behavior.

Participating Is for Moderate to High Readiness

People at this readiness level are *able but unwilling* (R3) to do what the leader wants. Their unwillingness is often a function of their lack of confidence or of insecurity. If, however, they are competent but unwilling, their reluctance to perform is more of a motivational problem than a problem of insecurity. In either case, the leader needs to open the door (two-way communication and active listening) to support the follower's efforts to use the ability he or she already has. Thus a supportive, nondirective, "participating" style (S3) has the highest probability of being effective with individuals at this readiness level. This style is called "participating" because the leader and follower share in decision making, with the main role of the leader being facilitating and communicating. This style involves high relationship behavior and low task behavior.

Delegating Is for High Readiness

People at this readiness level are both *able and willing* (R4), or competent and confident, to take responsibility. Thus a low-profile "delegating" style (S4), which provides little direction or support, has the highest probability of being effective with individuals at this readiness level. Even though the leader may still identify the problem, the responsibility for carrying out plans is given to these task-ready followers. They are permitted to run the show and decide on how, when, and where to do the task. At the same time, they are psychologically ready and therefore do not need above-average amounts of two-way communication or supportive behavior. This style involves low relationship behavior and low task behavior.

Thus we can now condense the above discussion in the form of four additional derived theoretical relationship statements.

2.21. If the follower's readiness level is low (R1), unable and unwilling, then the appropriate leadership style is "telling," or high task and low relationship behavior.

2.22. If the follower's readiness level is low to moderate (R2), unable but willing, then the appropriate leadership style is "selling," or high task and high relationship behavior.

2.23. If the follower's readiness level is moderate to high (R3), able but unwilling or insecure, then the appropriate leadership style is "participating," or high relationship and low task behavior.

2.24. If the follower's readiness level is high (R4), able and willing, then the appropriate leadership communication style is "delegating," low relationship and low task behavior.[31]

The key to applying Situational Leadership theory is accurate diagnosis of the follower's readiness. Once this is identified, the descriptive leadership style of communication behavior is relatively easily applied. See Figure 1–2 for instructions in using the model.

Style Range and Adaptability

An instrument has been developed that provides individuals with information about the style they most commonly use. This instrument, the "LEAD-Self," and its companion instrument, "LEAD-Other," to be completed by the follower, provides information about how the leader is perceived by others. Similar instruments have been developed to identify the readiness level

FIRST   Determine what you want to accomplish through your followers. ASK: "What is the task or goal?"

SECOND   Determine the readiness level of the follower or group that is relevant to the task. Readiness is:
          Achievement Motivation
          "Is the individual or group able to set high but realistic goals?"
          Responsibility
          "Willingness to assume responsibility?"
          "Ability to assume responsibility?"
          Education/Experience
          "Does the individual or group have the education and/or experience that is necessary to accomplish the task?"
          Mark the Readiness Level of the Follower or Group
          R1?. . . . R2?. . . . R3?. . . . R4?. . . .

THIRD   Draw a line from the readiness level up to the leadership style curve. The point where the lines hit is the MOST EFFECTIVE LEADERSHIP STYLE that is appropriate for that follower or group.
          S1?. . . . S2?. . . . S3?. . . . S4?. . . .
          Give the follower or group the appropriate combination of directive (task) behavior and supportive (relationship) behavior.

          Directive Behavior is:
          The extent that a leader engages in spelling out the role of an individual or group. The extent that a leader tells an individual or group what, when, where, and how to do the task.

          Supportive Behavior is:
          The extent that a leader engages in two-way communication, listening, supporting, facilitating, and giving psychological strokes.

Key Words for Appropriate Leadership Styles
          Telling: high directive/low support
          Selling: high directive/high support
          Participating: high support/low directive
          Delegating: low support/low directive

Figure 1–2. How to use the Situational Leadership model. (*From Hersey, P., & Blanchard, K.,* Situational Leadership Model, Center for Leadership Studies, 1977.)

of the follower. Now we can state two more derived theoretical relationship statements about the leader's *style range* and *style adaptability* as follows:

2.3. If a leader has a wide style range, then effectiveness in leadership has a high level of probability, when appropriately applied in a given situation.[32]

2.4. Style adapatability tends to increase the probability of leadership successfulness and effectiveness.[33]

In short, the more leadership styles a leader learns to use, the more effective the leader will tend to be. Most individuals have one or two styles that they commonly use; with training, people can learn to use three and perhaps all four styles.

Since leadership is the process of trying to influence others, and power is the means whereby the leader can induce compliance and conformity in followers, the two concepts are inseparable. There are one primary and several derived theoretical relationship statements relative to the concept of power that we can now identify.

Power Bases and Style

3. If the power bases available to the leader are consistent with the leadership style(s) appropriate to the readiness level of the followers, then the leader will tend to be successful and effective.[34]

3.1. To the degree that others perceive a leader's power, the leader is enabled to induce compliance or to influence behavior of others.[35]

3.2. If a leader is to avoid an eroding power base and to increase the chances of successfully influencing others' behavior, then the leader needs information about the sources of power he or she is perceived by others as having.[36]

3.3. If a leader communicates the power he or she possesses, then others will tend to perceive it.[37]

Instruments are available that provide individual feedback regarding power: "Power Perception Profile—Perception of Other," and "Power Perception Profile—Perception of Self."

3.4 As the readiness level of the follower increases from low (R1) to high (R4), the follower tends to respond to leader influence based on different types of power.[38]

3.41. Low readiness (R1) tends to be influenced by perceived power based on *coercion* and *connection.*

3.42. Low to moderate readiness (R2) tends to be influenced by perceived power based on *legitimate, connection,* and *reward.*

3.43. Moderate to high readiness (R3) tends to be influenced by perceived power based on *legitimate, referent,* and *information.*

3.44. High readiness (R4) tends to be influenced by perceived power based on *information* and *expertise.*

Thus it is not just leadership style of communicating that determines whether or not a leader is maximizing effectiveness. This also depends upon whether or not the power bases available to the leader are consistent with the readiness level of the individuals or groups the leader is attempting to influence.

Cycles and Style

The concepts of leadership and change are also inseparable, since it is the leader's role to try to anticipate and control change. In Situational Leadership, the focus is on the followers' behavior. The leader is to be continually attentive to developmental and regressive cycles in followers' behavior. The following primary and derived theoretical relationship statements refer to these cycles.

4.   If a leader is to break the ineffective cycle and increase task-relevant readiness of followers, then the leader must increase gradually the responsibility delegated to the followers, with a reasonable degree of risk.[39]

4.1   If the leader increases socioemotional support or relationship behavior too rapidly, then the followers may view the leader as becoming a "soft touch."

4.2   If the leader rewards as quickly as possible the slightest appropriate behavior exhibited by the individual, then the individual's performance will come closer and closer to the leader's expectations.[40]

Before intervening in the regressive cycle, however, the leader needs to analyze the follower's behavior and the situation to determine who "owns" the problem and therefore is responsible for making the needed change.

5.   If the follower begins to behave in a less ready manner for whatever reason, then the leader must intervene to correct inappropriate behaviors with appropriate timing and at the appropriate level on the regressive cycle at a lower emotional level (i.e., without anger).[41]

5.1   If the behavior is unacceptable to the leader, then the leader needs to make the follower aware of the problem and the follower ultimately is to solve the problem. This requires extensive, temporary intervention by the leader.

5.2   If the behavior is unacceptable to both leader and follower, the follower ultimately is to solve the problem after a period of shared responsibility with the leader. This requires temporary intervention by the leader.

5.3   If the follower's behavior is acceptable to the leader but not to the follower, then the leader needs to be supportive of the follower's efforts to solve his or her own problem. This requires minimal intervention by the leader.

5.4   If the follower's behavior is acceptable and no problem exists, then no intervention on the part of the leader is necessary.[42]

These then, are the theoretical relationship statements between the major concepts in Situational Leadership theory.

EVALUATION

In evaluating any theory, one needs to select certain criteria to serve as a framework of analysis. The criteria we have selected are presented here, together with our critique of Situational Leadership.

Clearly Stated

This theory is presented in logical sequence, and the assumptions are stated in such a manner that the reader can identify the philosophical perspective of the theorists. The concepts are clearly defined, and many already have been operationalized for research purposes. The relationship statements are readily adaptable to research and applicable to practice.

Scope
Situational Leadership theory is narrow in scope in that it seeks to describe, explain, predict, and control the communication between leader and follower, essentially two people in a superior–subordinate relationship. Its primary focus is within an organizational context. This theory is also broad in scope in that it is to be applied to small task groups as well as to total organizations. For example, one large business includes this theory in the orientation program of all employees, and the president and all managers use it. This provides a common basis for communication among all.

Applicability
Situational Leadership can be applied to many contexts in which relationships analogous to that of leader–follower exist. For example, it is being used in parent–child relationships.[43] Teachers and principals in public and private elementary and high schools are using this theory, and a number of graduate students have based their advanced doctoral research on this theory. People attending the Situational Leadership workshops come from many areas of society, such as the armed services, government service, and religious groups. Workshop participants have reported using the theory in helping alienated teenagers and young people with drug problems.

Research Support
Gumpert and Hambleton studied 65 managers in the Xerox Corporation to determine whether managers who used the Situational Leadership theory correctly in their communications with employees are more effective than managers who did not use it.[44] The findings show that highly effective managers had a greater knowledge of Situational Leadership and used it more than noneffective managers. The data also show that when Situational Leadership was correctly applied, employee job performance tended to be rated higher and to improve more than when Situational Leadership was not used.[45] In other studies, research is progressing on the validity of interpretation of the job-readiness and psychological-readiness scales. Preliminary results provide considerable support for these scales.[46] Work on diagnostic tools such as "LEAD-Self" and "LEAD-Other" is continuing. Norms, reliability, and validity have been established for many of these instruments so that they can be used not only for research purposes but also for consultation and management training programs.

Generalizability and Agreement with Known Data
This theory has been derived from early work in leadership and management by such notable scholars as Skinner (Behaviorist theory), Maslow (Motivation theory), Feidler (Contingency theory), French and Raven (Power), Lewin (Force Field Change theory), Blake and Mouton (Managerial Grid theory), and many others. Hersey and Blanchard present a reanalysis of data and perspectives of these and numerous other theories and research, applying these to the Situational Leadership theory. The analysis is quite remarkable in that Hersey and Blanchard demonstrate the theory's applicability to many contexts and theoretical perspectives. In fact, we believe it is no longer a theory, but a model based on tested methodologies and outcomes. A model is a pattern of already existing phenomena. Situational Leadership is the culmination and synthesis of the best knowledge available to us through research and practice regarding leader–follower communication and organizational management.[47]

Importance to the Discipline and Profession of Nursing
We propose that Situational Leadership is of considerable value and applicability to nursing, not only in the area of leadership and management, but also in nursing education and clinical

practice. In leadership and management, it seems that nursing leaders have not demonstrated a particular preference for any leadership theory. There is a conspicuous lack of nursing leadership theory, and a tendency to accept the perspectives of hospital administrators. In nursing education programs, nurses are taught to include health teaching as a major nursing intervention in nursing care plans for individual clients. There is, however, usually little emphasis on how to teach, or on educational theories and practice generally, below the master's degree level. While some students may select electives, nursing courses of necessity focus on nursing content; this is appropriate. Since Situational Leadership has been applied to teacher–student relationships, it would seem effective and efficient to teach this theory early in the nursing curriculum to provide a framework for students learning how to teach patients how to care for themselves. This theoretical perspective could also be applicable later in the curriculum in teaching psychiatric nursing, community mental health, and parent–child nursing, as well as nursing leadership.

Situational Leadership could provide a means of developing nursing students' sensitivity to the individual client and skill in adapting communication styles to clients' behaviors or readiness in an appropriate fashion. We believe the client would feel increasingly comfortable within the nurse–client relationship, would relax, rest, and consequently tend to improve in health status. We believe this theory has potential for increasing the holistic and humanistic elements inherent in nursing.

SUMMARY

In this chapter, the assumptions have been presented, the major concepts defined, and the theoretical relationship statements of Situational Leadership theory listed. Little discussion has been presented regarding the research support of this theory; this is to be presented in later chapters, interwoven with discussions of clinical nursing situations in which the theory is applied. The purpose of this chapter is to introduce the theoretical perspective regarding leadership. In the next chapter, a theoretical perspective about communicating in nursing is presented, Bonnie Duldt's theory of Humanistic Nursing Communication.

REFERENCES

1. Sanford, F. H. *Authoritarianism and leadership*. Philadelphia: Institute for Research in Human Relations, 1950.
2. Duldt, B. W., & Giffin, K. *Theoretical perspectives of nursing*. Boston: Little, Brown, 1985.
3. Hersey, P., & Blanchard, K. *Management of organizational behavior: Utilizing human resources* (5th ed.). Englewood Cliffs, N.J.: Prentice-Hall, 1988, p. 123.
4. Ibid., 166.
5. Ibid., 361.
6. Leary, T. Theory and measurement methodology of interpersonal communication, *Psychiatry*, 1955, *16*, 153–156.
7. Hersey & Blanchard, *Management*, 333.
8. Ibid., 447.
9. Ibid., 202.
10. Orwell, G. *Animal farm*. New York: Harcourt Brace Jovanovich, 1946.
11. Hersey & Blanchard, *Management*, 229.

12. Duldt & Giffin, *Theoretical perspectives of nursing,* 95.
13. Hersey & Blanchard, *Management,* 86.
14. Ibid., 146.
15. Ibid., 149.
16. Ibid., 151.
17. Ibid., 189.
18. Ibid.
19. Ibid., 4, 44–47, 64–66, 183–186.
20. Ibid., 234.
21. Ibid., 249–250.
22. Ibid., 271, 273.
23. Ibid., 202–211.
24. Ibid., 347–353.
25. Remarks by Paul Hersey. Situational Leadership Workshop, New Orleans, December, 1981.
26. Sanford, *Authoritarianism and leadership.*
27. Hersey & Blanchard, *Management,* 142.
28. Korman, A. K. Consideration, initiating structure, and organizational criteria—A review. *Personnel Psychology: A Journal of Applied Research,* 1966, *19* (4), 349.
29. Ibid., 177–181.
30. Ibid.
31. Ibid.
32. Ibid., 102.
33. Ibid., 169, 286.
34. Ibid., 213.
35. Ibid., 219–220.
36. Ibid., 220–221.
37. Ibid., 220–223.
38. Ibid., 214–217.
39. Ibid., 230–233.
40. Ibid., 239–241.
41. Ibid., 249–250.
42. Ibid., 262–263.
43. Hersey, P., & Blanchard, K. H. *The family game: A situational approach to effective parenting.* Reading, Mass.: Addison-Wesley, 1978.
44. Gumpert, R. A., & Hambleton, R. K. Situational leadership: How Xerox managers fine-tune managerial styles to employee maturity and task needs. *Management Review,* December 1979, 8–12.
45. Ibid., 11.
46. Hersey, P., Blanchard, K. H., & Hambleton, R. K. *Contracting for leadership style: A process and instrumentation for building effective work relationships.* Escondido, Calif.: Center for Leadership Studies, 1977, p. 12.
47. Hersey & Blanchard, *Management,* 170.

2

HUMANISTIC NURSING COMMUNICATION THEORY

INTRODUCTION

One of the hallmarks of this century, along with atomic energy and computerization, is the resurgence of concern for the manner in which human beings are treated. Expressions of this concern extend from the issue of those servicemen missing in action (MIAs) after Vietnam, the plight of the boat people fleeing Cuba and Southeast Asia, and the increasing international concern for treatment of prisoners and hostages. On a more mundane level, business and industry have become aware of the need to treat employees, as well as clients and customers, in a more humane manner, as evidenced by the development of Situational Leadership theory and similar theories of leadership and management. In the health care field, administrators and professionals are also concerned about the way clients or patients are treated; patients' rights and informed consent are salient issues. As the health industry grows in size and complexity, it is becoming imperative that human resources, necessary for delivery of health care services, not only be appropriately qualified and effectively utilized, but also be given consideration in regard to human values. We believe that if health care personnel are treated humanely, then the personnel will tend to treat clients and patients in a similar manner; this is the belief and expectation. This seems particularly applicable in the delivery of nursing services. Nurses comprise over 50 percent of all health care personnel. According to the Institute of Medicine committee report to Congress on nursing and nursing education, nursing represents the one largest professional group of health care providers in the United States; this represents almost 10 percent of the gross national product.[1] This committee recommends future support of graduate-level preparation of nurse-administrators.[2]

In the evolving discipline and practice profession of nursing, numerous theories are being developed about nursing practice, and most involve communication as a significant concept or element. None of the theories of nursing, however, deal with client as well as nonclient communications, such as those between nurse and peer, nurse and supervisor, and nurse and colleague (other health professionals). As in Situational Leadership, we believe there needs to be a theory of nursing in which this explicit assumption is made: that there is no one way to communicate effectively with clients or with other nurses (peers and superiors) and colleagues. Rather, it seems important that nurses be intellectually aware of and sensitive to the wide range of humanizing and dehumanizing attitudes from which one can choose to apply selected patterns of interaction according to situational variables. While research has shown the communication variable to be most significant in effective leader–follower relationships, we believe that communication is also a significant variable in the nurse–client, nurse–peer, nurse–supervisor, and nurse–colleague relationships. There is considerable pressure for these interpersonal communication relationships to work. This pressure arises from the task, the delivery of effective, quality nursing care; it arises from the number of people seeking care; and it arises from the need for cost containment. In contemporary nursing practice, the nurse needs to be able to communicate effectively not only with clients, but also with subordinates, other nurses, superiors in the nursing administrative organization, and physicians, physical therapists, nutritionists, pharmacists, and other colleagues.

We propose that Humanistic Nursing Communication theory can be applied to this interpersonal communications for all these areas of nursing practice.[3] Like Situational Leadership, this theory is based on the symbolic interactionists' model[4] described in Chapter 1. In this chapter, an analysis of Humanistic Nursing Communication theory is presented broken down into assumptions, concepts, relationship statements, and evaluation.

ASSUMPTIONS

The primary paradigm for the discipline of nursing consists of the following set of concepts: client, nurse, environment, and health. The *client* is generally seen as a human being existing in a particular environment and having a health problem that requires the unique and specific knowledge and skills of a nurse. The nurse intervenes to influence some aspect of the paradigm in such a manner that the health of the client improves. Nursing theories are generally concerned with how the nurse effects this change so that one has a description of the process. Fundamental questions of the discipline and practice profession are answered by nursing theories, such as: explanations of how the nurse effects change; how the nurse can control what, when, where, and how often this change occurs; and how the nurse can predict outcomes of a specific situation to which the theory is applied. Since nursing is not only a discipline but also a practice profession, theories provide a guide to actions and inventions. In applying Humanistic Nursing Communication theory to the nursing leadership context, we focus upon the attitudes and patterns of communications occurring among and between nurses as one nurse–leader attempts to influence the group of nurses, and also the effect of these messages upon the delivery of nursing care and, ultimately, the health of clients.

The following assumptions of Humanistic Nursing Communication theory are derived from a study of philosophy, particularly humanistic and existential thought. First, human beings are believed to exist in a here-and-now existential context from which there is no escape. Each being is bound to a body occupying a particular position in time and space. Second, human beings are continually faced with a common core of existentialist elements: being, becoming, choice, freedom, responsibility, solitude, loneliness, pain, struggle, tragedy, meaning, dread, uncertainty, despair, and death. Third, it is also assumed that all of these elements of existential living and the imperative need to communicate are salient issues with which one must cope in critical life situations—situations that pose a threat to one's existence. Fourth, growth and change are believed to arise from within the individual and, to a considerable degree, are dependent upon the choices one makes. The decision whether or not to grow and change lies with the individual by design or by default. Fifth, while the focus of the nursing paradigm usually is upon the client and his or her health, the nurse shares with the client all characteristics of being human: they are equals. The implications of this for leadership are that, just as the nurse focuses on the health of the client, so the nursing leaders are believed inherently responsible for promoting the well-being and existence of the nurse-employee-practitioners under their direction. The nursing leader and follower also share all human characteristics and in this sense are equals.

There are assumptions of Humanistic Nursing Communication theory that reflect the influence of communication discipline. First, the need to communicate is believed to be an innate characteristic for human beings—an imperative that must be met. To communicate is as natural as breathing. Second, survival of the individual is dependent upon ability to communicate with others in order to share feelings and facts about the environment and to learn how to cope and survive. Third, the environment is seen as a "booming, buzzing" world of strange sensations that must be sorted out, categorized, and evaluated to determine which are important. This sorting and prioritizing process is achieved through communication with other human beings. Fourth, humans are also innately fallible, using and misusing all capabilities, especially the ability to communicate. People, intentionally or unintentionally, send distorted, incomplete messages, and often receive messages as if they included something more, less, or different than the sender intended. Fifth, the manner in which one communicates determines what one becomes. The way one communicates is reflected in the communicative responses of receivers, as if responses were a mirror image for the speaker: the "I see you seeing me seeing you" effect. Sixth, interpersonal communication is a significant humanizing factor among human beings. It is an innate element of the nursing process (assessment, planning, implementation, and evaluation)[5] and of the communication that occurs between nurses and clients, peers, superiors, and colleagues. Finally, evaluation of one's own communication skills is subjective. There are only general guidelines and few specific directions. Each individual is responsible for personal decisions and choices about communication behaviors. Each one can choose to change, depending upon ability to utilize feedback requested, shared, or mirrored in others' responses.

The following assumptions are derived from the discipline and practice profession of nursing. First, the goal or purpose of nursing is to support, maintain, and augment the client's state of health. All processes of nursing are intended to intervene to this end. Second, human beings are viewed as unique, whole (holistic) living systems responding openly to the environment. Generally, all the assumptions and beliefs about systems seem applicable to human life and death processes. While there may be other implicit assumptions, these are the primary assumptions that are relevant to nursing and nursing leadership contexts.

In addition to assumptions derived from areas of study, there are some assumptions that, while relative to the client's health status, are particularly relevant to application of the theory to the context of nursing leadership. First, it is believed that health, satisfaction, and sense of success in one's life and work, or one's state of being, is derived principally from one's feeling human. Second, due to the bureaucracy and complexity of the present health care delivery system, there is a tendency for clients, and professionals as well, to be treated in a dehumanizing manner and to relate to one another in a dehumanizing manner. It is difficult at times for nurses to feel a sense of satisfaction, success, and well-being about their nursing practice. Third, it is also believed that humanizing attitudes and patterns of communicating can be learned so that it is possible to increase the nurse-leader's awareness and sensitivity to followers' and others' state of being and of becoming. Fourth, the goal of the humanistic nurse is to break the communication cycle of dehumanizing attitudes and interaction patterns, and to replace these with communicative attitudes and patterns that tend to humanize. Finally, it is assumed that interpersonal communication is the means whereby the nurse becomes increasingly sensitive and aware of others' humanity.

The statements just made are assumed to be true and are not tested as such. The assumptions of the theory of Humanistic Nursing Communication presented provide a framework within which leadership in the nursing context can be studied. See Appendix D for a list of the statements of assumption. Preparatory to this study, the concepts of the theory need to be defined; this follows in the next section.

CONCEPTS

Concepts are the "leap of faith" between a word or group of utterances and some event or phenomenon that human beings experience or sense. In a theory, concepts need to be carefully defined, and the definitions to a considerable degree dictate how valid and reliable the theory can become. Concepts that are clearly defined and measurable contribute more to scientific progress than concepts that are vague and elude measurement. The concepts in the theory of Humanistic Nursing Communication include the human being (the client, nurse, peer, or colleague), health, environment, critical life situation, nursing, and communication. These concepts are briefly defined in this section and are related to the nursing leadership context; complete definitions of the concepts are available in an earlier publication.[6]

The Human Being

The human being is defined as an existentialist being composed of an interacting set of characteristics: living, communicating, negativing, inventing, ordering, dreaming, choosing, and self-reflecting. This set of elements composes the complex wholeness (holiness) of man, meaning both male and female. While not all are unique to the species, these characteristics are of particular concern to nursing as a discipline and to leadership occurring within the discipline as well. These elements are described from the perspective of the leader–follower relationship.

Living

Living refers to the ability of humans (leaders and followers) to function biologically and physiologically as animated, viable entities. This biological dimension is shared with other life forms and includes all bodily, life-sustaining processes. Susceptible to injury, infection, malfunction, and ultimately death, man reacts and interacts as a holistic being with the environmental stimuli, external or internal. Humans display orderly, sequential processes of growth and development (and aging), which are influenced to some degree by life-style and environment. Human existence depends upon interactions with other members of the human species. Psychological responses to stimuli, such as fight or flight responses to danger or attack, are also shared with other life forms. The human being tends to share with other life forms a sign system of nonverbal communication indicating status, territoriality, rejection, and acceptance. People bring these characteristics to the leader–follower relationship and roles in organizations.

Communicating

Communicating refers to the ability of humans to label things and to talk about them when not present. Humans are "symbol using, mis-using" beings.[7] As a consequence, humans as leaders or followers are able to build upon learnings, logic, and perceptions of predecessors and contemporaries through the written and spoken use of language. Using symbols enables one to think abstractly, to use logic and argumentation, to solve problems, and to learn as well as communicate perceptions regarding phenomena observed about the physical environment, about one's self, and about relationships with others. Humans are particularly capable of expressing feelings arising from within as a response to perceptions. Generally, humans tend to develop and demonstrate patterns of communicating that are colored by attitudes, varying the meanings conveyed. Humans as leaders or followers can influence each others' perception, motivation, and evaluation of people or of situations by the way they communicate with one another.

Negativing

Negativing refers to the ability of humans to perceive and talk about the symbolic negative (-1), no, none, not, nonexistence, not happening. Humans are able to develop moral codes, rules of conduct, and laws governing relationships and functions of individuals or of the environment. Directives, policies, and orders are the rule in organizations. One can be aware of one's own nonexistence, even death, and plan for the implications inherent in this fact. One can be aware of not being a leader or of not having a job. One does develop certain expectations of what can happen in the future. One can be aware of potential outcomes and plan interventions to change or influence outcomes. Being aware of actual and potential symbolic negatives has significant implications and expectations for the leader–follower relationship and roles.

Inventing

Inventing refers to the ability of humans to develop tools that separate the self from the immediate environment. Human beings can behave contrary to natural laws of the environment and contrary to restrictions inherent in other life forms. While a pet kitten or puppy can perceive only a restricted area about itself, humans extend physical capabilities through the use of tools in transportation (airplanes), communications (radio and television), chemistry (food additives and plastics), technology (computers), and so on. With electronic equipment, humans can hear a voice around the world, far out into space, and even into the future via tape recordings. Often it is through effective leader–follower relationships and roles that these advances are made possible. A human being, however, risks dangerous side effects from these inventions (for example, insecticides, drugs, and air pollution) in the quest of potential benefits in changing health, ability to function, and relationship with the social and physical environment. Use of technology influences communication behaviors among people, particularly leaders and followers, thus changing "who says *what* through *what channels* to *whom* with *what effect*."[8] The technology humans are capable of producing represents a significant influence not only upon the leader–follower relationship but also the task, time, distance, and leadership context generally.

Ordering

Ordering refers to the ability of human beings to develop categories and hierarchies according to some value or theme. People give structure and system to the environment and tend to organize life, relationships, and the environment according to a particular perspective, goal, or criterion. This is classic of organizational behavior and of leader–follower relationships. People tend to practice one-upmanship in relationships, and tend to seek power and status through control of others, of resources, of environment, or all of these. This sense of hierarchy tends to result in conflict, particularly when leadership roles are developing or declining in effectiveness and in the leader–follower communication.

Dreaming

Dreaming refers to the ability of humans to consider how things could be if all were perfect. Leaders individually and as groups can have hopes, expectations, and dreams for the future. They are able to think, plan, and work to increase the probability that goals and dreams become reality. Human beings are continually experiencing frustration and disappointment as dreams become unattainable. Absolute control is rarely possible beyond brief periods for fallible humans, and perfection is illusionary and elusive. Often a leader's effectiveness is measured in terms of a portion or percentage of success in achieving goals and making dreams come true.

Choosing

Choosing refers to the ability of humans—leaders and followers—to consider numerous alternatives, compare implications for the future, and select one of the alternatives that seems to be most desirable according to values and criteria. Thus leaders and followers are able to make choices and try to control events, particularly in their job-related lives. They can be highly motivated to achieve short-term as well as long-term goals, even lifelong goals. In choosing what to do, when to do it, where to go, and whether to lead or follow, there is also responsibility and accountability for the implications and results. These factors add a dimension of risk to the right of choosing.

Self-reflecting

Self-reflecting refers to the ability of a human being to think and talk about one's self, one's behaviors, and one's life situation. Self-reflecting often involves the existentialist elements: being, becoming, choice, freedom, responsibility, solitude, loneliness, pain, struggle, tragedy, meaning, dread, uncertainty, despair, and death. Self-reflecting typically becomes salient during critical life situations. Implications for this in the nurse–client relationship are focused on the client's health status being in jeopardy: in the leader–follower relationship, the focus is on the follower's job status being in potential jeopardy.

Roles and Functions

A significant factor about Duldt's theory of Humanistic Nursing Communication is that we believe this definition of human being is applicable not only to the client–nurse but also to the leader–follower relationship. All are human beings first. Each possesses, given individual variances, all the characteristics of elements of being human. In this very real sense, all are equal, yet each is unique in the individual expression of these characteristics. One of these characteristics is the position fulfilled within an organizational context. We need to define more specifically the set of human beings involved in nursing contexts according to role and function.

Nurse

The *nurse* is a human being who practices nursing, intervening through the application of the nursing process to develop a plan of nursing care for a specific client. The nurse possesses special educational and licensure credentials to qualify for practice of nursing according to the dictates of the society in which the nurse practices.

Client

The *client* is also a human being who is experiencing a health-related critical life situation, potential or actual. This human being has a need for the special services of the nurse, and this person is the focus of the nursing process. The client as a concept is intended to be one individual and also the family or individual(s) providing the social support system for the client; all are to be considered in the nursing process.

Peer
A *peer* of the nurse is defined as one who has equal standing in the same discipline and profession—for example, another registered nurse. Role and function within an organization designates which peer is a leader and which a follower.

Colleague
A *colleague* is defined as a member of another health care discipline or profession, particularly those professionals with whom nurses communicate to coordinate, consult, and sometimes to collaborate in the practice of nursing. Examples of colleagues of nurses include physicians, social workers, religious advisors, administrators, and other health providers and therapists.

This, then, completes the definition of man or the human being with emphasis on leader–follower communication. Having defined the human being, the other concepts in Humanistic Nursing Communication theory need to be defined. These are health, environment, critical life situation, and nursing.

Health
One's *health* is one's state of being, of becoming, and of self-awareness. It is indicative of one's adaptation to the environment. While many view health as a continuum, existing from illness to wellness, Duldt views health as a free-flowing, existential state. The health of the client, moving from illness to wellness, is the focus of nursing practice; in the practice of nursing leadership, however, the focus is upon the health of one's followers, that is, movement toward maximizing potential and developing job-relevant capabilities.

Environment
The point of one's time-space-relationship intersection is one's *environment*. Each human being exists in a particular time span in relation to the totality of the time continuum from past to future. Each human being also exists in a particular point in space on the universe; one cannot be in two places at once. Given this time-space intersection, each develops a particular network of interpersonal communication or relationships with other human beings. This existential intersecting point of time-space-relationship state of being moves forward through time and provides each person with a unique orientation, perspective, and experience. Just as nurses consider the function of the client's environment in planning care, so the nursing leader needs to consider the function of the time-space-relationship perspective of the follower in management and administrative planning.

Critical Life Situation
Nursing theory, by definition, requires the inclusion of a client's health. The concept of *critical life situation* functions primarily to describe the client's perceived, jeopardized state of existential being, becoming, and self-awareness. In applying this concept in the leader–follower relationship, the leader views his or her own and the follower's job situation as being in jeopardy. Problems, concerns, and disruptions in the work setting are known to have potential adverse effects upon productivity, health, personal relationships, and the general quality of life. The nurse-leader has a responsibility to develop and maintain followers' task-relationship

orientations in such a manner that the work setting does not develop into a critical job situation.

Nursing

In Humanistic Nursing Communication, the concept of *nursing* is defined as follows: "Nursing is the art and science of positive, humanistic intervention in changing health states of human beings interacting in the environment of potential or actual critical life situations."[9] *Humanistic* nursing denotes the kinds of communicative patterns and attitudes with which interventions are operationalized. Humanizing nursing is communicating and relating interpersonally to clients in such a manner that the client senses warmth and acceptance and reports feeling good about the care received. Humanistic nursing happens *between* people.

Nursing Leadership

> We believe the notion of humanistic nursing can be applied to leadership, and we offer the following definition: process of interpersonal communication which influences team members (followers) to achieve task goals and to maintain relationships.[10]

The humanistic nurse seeks to communicate and relate interpersonally with clients so that the client often senses warmth and acceptance and often comments on feeling good about the care given. The humanistic nursing leader seeks to communicate in a similar manner with followers, but in slightly different fashion: sharing equally with followers the common bond of human existential being: respecting one another; and showing a concern for others' individual feelings, needs, worth, and responsibility. The subset of elements for nursing is communicating, caring, and coaching, all providing a unique health service to the client. The subset of elements for the humanistic nursing leader recognizes the independence and interdependence of the leader–follower relationship and assumes significantly more contributions, accountability, and responsibility from the follower than the nurse expects from a client. These nursing leadership elements are (1) people- or relationship-oriented, that is, communicating, motivating, initiating, facilitating, and integrating, and (2) task-oriented, that is, planning, organizing, staffing, directing, and controlling. These elements are examined in later chapters.

To this point, we have defined all of the concepts in the Humanistic Nursing Communication theory except that of communication, the major concept of the theory. We propose it is this concept that provides the humanizing factor, the heart of this theory.

Communication

Communication is defined as a dynamic process involving continued adaptation and adjustment between two or more human beings engaged in face-to-face interactions during which each person is continually aware of the other(s). It is the exchange of a message between human beings. This ability to communicate enables the nurse to use the nursing process— assessing, planning, implementing, and evaluating—as a systematic approach to nursing practice.

Message

The message consists of facts and feelings, and it is conveyed in a manner involving attitudes and patterns of communicative behaviors.

Continuum of Attitudes

An *attitude* is defined as a mental position toward a person, fact, or state: it is one's demeanor or predilection toward something. An attitude can be humanizing or dehumanizing in nature. To communicate with a humanizing attitude generally means to be aware of the eight characteristics of a human being as defined previously. To dehumanize is to ignore these characteristics. Thus these two types of attitudes can be thought of as occurring on a continuum (Fig. 2–1). These gradations of attitudinal dimensions of communication are believed to reflect the best available research and knowledge about how people interact and communicate generally, in nursing practice, and particularly in the leader–follower relationship. These dimensions represent an attempt to identify humanizing attitudes of communication wherein people are treated as people, not as things. (A more extensive discussion of these attitudes is presented in Appendix B.) These, then, are the elements for operationalizing Humanistic Nursing Communication theory in leadership.

Patterson and Zderad state the following about humanistic nursing practice:

> In terms of actual practice, then, it is more realistic to think of humanistic nursing as occurring in various degrees. It may be far more useful, in fact, to consider humanistic nursing as a goal worth striving for; or an attitude that strengthens one's perseverance toward attaining the difficult goal; or fundamentally, a major value shaping one's nursing practice.[12]

We propose that this statement is analogous to the application of Humanistic Nursing Communication theory in most nursing leadership contexts. While one may find these elements attrac-

HUMANIZING   DEHUMANIZING

ATTITUDES

HUMANIZING	DEHUMANIZING
DIALOGICAL	MONOLOGICAL
INDIVIDUAL	CATEGORIES
HOLISTIC	PARTS
CHOICE	DIRECTIVE
EQUALITY	DEGRADATION
POSITIVE REGARD	DISREGARD
ACCEPTANCE	JUDGMENT
EMPATHY	TOLERANCE
AUTHENTICITY (of feelings)	ROLE PLAYING
CARING	CARELESSNESS
IRREPLACEABILITY	EXPENDABILITY
INTIMACY	ISOLATION
COPING	HELPLESSNESS
POWER	POWERLESSNESS

Figure 2–1. The continuum of attitudes. (*Reproduced with permission from Duldt, B. W., & Giffin.* Theoretical perspectives for nursing. *Boston: Little, Brown, 1985.*)

tive and congruent with hopes and desires, real-life experiences in being a leader, a follower, or both are usually quite variable. In fact, there may be situations in which communicating in a dehumanizing mode may be very prudent and appropriate. So, while one may value and strive to establish and maintain humanizing communication attitudes, it is important to recognize that one has options all along the humanizing-dehumanizing continuum. Each person chooses the degree of humanizing or dehumanizing attitude to use in communicating interpersonally in specific situations.

Patterns of Interaction

A second set of communication elements are specific skills or *interaction patterns* of interpersonal behaviors—the sequencing and structuring of the message one communicates. These patterns include communing, asserting, confronting, conflicting (resolution), and separating. Each of these patterns will be defined in the following paragraphs.

Communing

Communing refers to dialogical, intimate, humanizing communication that occurs between two or more people involved in nursing. It is a subjective event that happens between people, involving each being aware of the other person's presence. It is "being there" and "being with." Dialogical communing is the element that makes nursing humanistic; if monological communication is used, nursing becomes dehumanizing. Typically, those involved are the nurse and client, but communing also involves the nurse communing with peers and with colleagues in other professions. Communing, the core of humanistic communication, consists of three elements: trust, self-disclosure, and feedback, the tripod and heart of communing.

TRUST

Trust is one person relying on another, risking potential loss in attempting to achieve a goal when the outcome is uncertain and the potential for loss is greater than the potential for gain if the trust is violated.[13] The trustworthy person is *reliable,* that is, will perform as promised. The trustworthy person is an *expert,* who has the knowledge and ability to perform. The trustworthy person is *dynamic,* that is, open and frank. Research has shown these three elements are essential to the development of trust in interpersonal communication.[14,15]

SELF-DISCLOSURE

Self-disclosure is risking rejection in telling what one feels, thinks, likes, wants, and so on, regarding here-and-now events. Self-disclosure invites involvement interpersonally, and if it is authentic, it tends to create intimacy. It is not abandonment of autonomy; it is cherishing one's privacy without rejecting others. Too little self-disclosure may lead to intrapersonal distress and diminished mental health, while too much self-disclosure is seen as a weakness. The over-discloser is not trusted because of the lack of discrimination; the under-discloser does not trust others and seeks to be self-sufficient. The reticent person, the social chit-chatter, and the "historian" (the one who repeatedly tells about the trip to Europe or the big fish that got away) all avoid the here and now. Discrete, timely, appropriate self-disclosure serves as a bridge between people, not a barrier. One prudently self-discloses to those individuals whom one trusts.[16]

FEEDBACK

Feedback is revealing how one sees another; it is *describing* another's behavior plus *evaluating,* or telling how one feels about the behavior. It enables people to learn how they appear to others, and what impact they have interpersonally. It is the way one person validates and confirms another, or invalidates and disconfirms. Direct and owned feedback that is specific in nature and scope is most helpful: "I feel uncomfortable when you say that, because . . .". Indirect feedback is ambiguous, global, and suspect: "Some of us here feel that you . . .". According to Giffin, maturity in interpersonal communication is a process of relating to others by self-disclosing and *seeking* feedback and changing one's behavior as necessary and appropriate.[17]

THE HUMANIZING TRIPOD

Trust, self-disclosure, and feedback characterize communing, the heart of a humanizing relationship. These three elements are seen as necessary to the development of a relationship in which each person is *understood, cooperative,* and *satisfied.* The relationship is valued by each person, and humanizing communication behaviors tend to occur to a significant degree.

Asserting

Assertiveness is expressing one's needs, thoughts, feelings, or beliefs in a direct, honest, confident manner while being respectful of others' thoughts, feelings, or beliefs. If humanistic in nature, it "is asserting with authenticity."

Confronting

Confrontation is providing feedback about another plus requesting a change in another's behavior. It occurs when one person, a leader, deliberately or inadvertently does something that influences another, a follower, to think about, examine, question, and possibly change some aspect of behavior, such as actions, inaction, attitudes, or moods. It includes only salient, timely, here-and-now behaviors. It is to be done with concern for the confrontee, and the vehemence of confrontation and the behavior confronted are to be in proportion to the needs, sensitivity, and capabilities of the confrontee. It is not "telling someone off," "wolf-packing," or being concerned about unchangeable characteristics (skin color, handicaps, disfigurements, and so on). Confronting is "calling one's game," and withholding social support. It is a powerful force for interpersonal growth.

Confronting is operationalized in five steps. First, in a face-to-face interaction, the confronter gets the *attention* of the confrontee: "I have something important to tell you." Eye contact is important here, and the impact is enhanced if the sentence is almost whispered. Second, the confronter states the behavioral *facts:* "This is how you have been behaving . . ." or "This is what you said . . .". Third, the confronter describes how he or she *feels* about this behavior: "It annoys me, and it's distracting my attention from my work when you do this: I don't like it!" Fourth, (and optional step), the confronter may give an interpretation or *hypothesis* regarding what the perceived behavior means: "It almost seems as if you want to prevent me from doing my work." This is unrequested feedback for the confrontee, and there is a risk of antagonizing the confrontee. To propose an alienating interpretation of the confrontee's behavior may therefore hinder progrss toward a resolution of the situation. One may be well advised to omit this step. Finally, the confronter asks the confrontee to *change* behavior: "I just wish you would stop doing this!" Certainly, this encounter is to be conducted in privacy, face to face, with considerable eye contact.

Reactions to the confrontation may be acceptance of the confronter's concerns and a promise to change. The confrontee, however, may become defensive[18] and counterattack. The confronter then has to decide how to respond to this information. There is choice. There is risk. In any event, the confrontation is to be avoided if the confrontee has too many other problems with which to cope, or states, "I am not ready for this now" (perhaps later), or just is not interested.[19,20] If humanistic in nature, confrontation is "confronting with caring."

Conflicting

Conflict calls for a decision over an issue to which there is risk of loss as well as possible gain, in which there are two or more alternatives from which to choose, in which one's values are involved, and in which some degree of cooperation is required. It often involves some blockage in achieving a goal, and the people involved can estimate the outcomes. In conflict, some people can behave in a dehumanizing, disruptive manner by arguing, quarreling, and name-calling, becoming competitive and uncooperative. Some may become frozen in their opinions, and the focus may slide from the goal(s) to personal attacks. Other behaviors include aggressiveness, withdrawal, and scapegoating. On the other hand, conflict can be humanizing and constructive. If one expects to encounter conflict within a group, one can consciously try to engage in humanizing behaviors and to disagree in a productive, problem-solving manner. When there are differing viewpoints, an interpersonal climate of cooperative exploration of the issues can occur through dialogue. This requires each member to seek to understand the other positions and to give careful, respectful consideration to each idea. All views need to be heard in order to reach consensus on the most workable option(s) available to the group in goal achievement. While dehumanizing, destructive conflict narrows perception and increases defensiveness, humanizing and constructive conflict broadens understanding, allows exploration of more alternatives, and promotes positive interpersonal involvement and commitment. Conflict can be a healthy, satisfying experience. If humanistic in nature, it is "conflicting with dialogue."

Separating

Separating occurs at the end of a relationship. It may be due to change, choice, or commitments outside the relationship. For example, a client may move to another area of the hospital or be discharged. The nurse may accept a promotion or move away. One leader may be transferred; a new leader is assigned to the group of followers or employees. There usually is a change in proximity, so that face-to-face interactions decrease or cease. In a dehumanizing situation or relationship, one may choose to break up a relationship, as in the case of alcoholism, verbal abuse, and sexual harassment in personal or professional relationships. This may be a wise thing to do if the relationship is destructive. One may have such a positive relationship with another that communing occurs consistently and the experience is quite satisfying, yet, other choices or events may dictate separation. In such a humanistic relationship, the individuals will probably be able to resume the relationship easily, almost as if whatever time, distance, or circumstance causing the separation had not even occurred, should they meet again at a future time. If humanistic in nature, this is "separating with communing."

All of the concepts of humanistic nursing communication theory have been defined. For the reader's convenience, an outline or hierarchical arrangement of the concepts is presented in Table 2–1. Also for the reader's convenience, a summary of the definitions of all concepts highlighted in Humanistic Nursing Communication theory can be found in Appendix D.

THEORETICAL RELATIONSHIP STATEMENTS

Relationship statements of a theory describe how concepts of a theory interact. By way of analogy, if the assumptions set the stage and the concepts are the actors, the relationship

TABLE 2–1. HIERARCHY OF CONCEPTS AND SETS OF ELEMENTS

Human Being (Man)
A. Characteristic
1. Living
2. Communicating
3. Negativing
4. Inventing
5. Ordering
6. Dreaming
7. Choosing
8. Self-reflecting

B. Role
1. Nurse
2. Client
3. Peer
4. Colleague

Health

Environment

Critical Life Situation

Nursing
a. Communicating
b. Caring
c. Coaching

Nursing Leadership
A. People
1. Communicating
2. Motivating
3. Initiating
4. Facilitating
5. Integrating

B. Task
Planning
Organizing
Staffing
Directing
Controlling

Communication
A. Message
1. Facts
2. Feelings
B. Attitudes
1. Humanizing (dialogue, individuality, holistic, choice, equality, positive regard, acceptance, empathy, authenticity, caring, irreplaceability, intimacy, coping, and power.)
2. Dehumanizing (monologue, categories, parts, directive, degradation, judgment, tolerance, role playing, carelessness, expendability, isolation, helplessness, and powerlessness.)
C. Interaction Patterns
1. Communing (Trust, self-disclosure, and feedback)
2. Asserting
3. Confronting
4. Conflicting
5. Separating

statements function similarly to the script of a play. The actors follow the script. As in scriptwriting and acting, sometimes the script does not do justice to the acting; so a theory may not organize, explain, and predict an event as it is experienced in reality. This is the crucial test for any theory: How well does the theory match the reality of nurses' experience in communication interpersonally with clients, peers, and professional colleagues? In the paragraphs to follow, the theoretical relationship statements or hypotheses and a model of Humanistic Nursing Communication theory are presented.

The major relationship statement is this: to the same degree to which one chooses to communicate with humanizing attitudes and interaction patterns, one will tend to operationalize humanistic nursing communication. More specific statements of relationship are as follows:

1. To the same degree that one receives humanizing communication from others, one will tend to feel recognized and accepted as a human being.
   a. While applying the nursing process, to the same degree that a nurse is able to use humanizing communication, the client, peer, or colleague will tend to feel recognized and accepted as a human being.
   b. In a given environment, if a critical life situation develops for a client, to the same degree the nurse uses humanizing communication attitudes and patterns while applying the nursing process, the health of the client will tend to move in a positive direction.
2. To the same degree a nurse (leader or follower) uses humanizing elements to communicate, that nurse will tend to receive humanizing communication from peers, colleagues, followers, and superiors.

The attitudes with which one communicates are used with the interaction patterns of communication. A model is presented in Figure 2–2 showing the specific patterns of interaction within varying levels of closeness in a relationship. Trust, self-disclosure, and feedback represent the heart of humanistic communications, or communing. These three elements tend to interrelate: increase trust, and self-disclosure tends to increase, as well as feedback. Decrease any one of these three elements, and the others tend to decrease also. Thus the following relationship statement can be made:

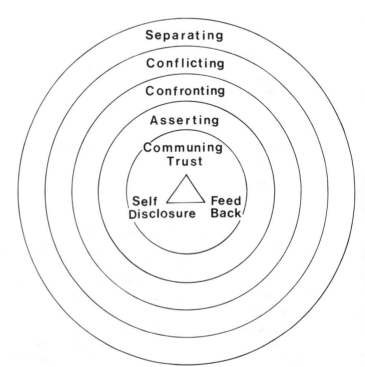

Figure 2–2. The communication patterns of interaction. (*Reproduced with permission from Duldt, B. W., & Giffin, K. Theoretical perspectives for nursing. Boston: Little, Brown, 1985.*)

3. To the same degree that trust, self-disclosure, and feedback occur, humanizing communication or communing also occurs.
4. In the event one tends to experience dehumanizing communication (monological rather than dialogical, categorical rather than individualistic, and so on), one tends to move outward on the model to the next pattern of interaction.

One tends to feel the need to express needs, thoughts, feelings, or beliefs with a little more definiteness and clearness in the hope of moving the relationship back toward the center, to trust, self-disclosure, and feedback, to understanding, cooperation, and satisfaction. The following relationship statement can be made:

5. In a communing relationship of trust, self-disclosure, and feedback, to the same degree that dehumanizing communicative attitudes are expressed by another, one tends to use assertiveness as a pattern of interaction.

In the event use of assertiveness fails to move the interpersonal relationship toward the center and the dehumanizing attitudes continue to be expressed, one tends to move to confronting or even to conflicting as an effective communication pattern. The following relationship statements can be made:

6. To the same degree that assertiveness tends not to reestablish communing (trust, self-disclosure, and feedback), and that dehumanizing communication attitudes continue to be expressed by another, one tends to use confrontation as a pattern of communication.
7. To the same degree that confrontation tends not to reestablish communing (trust, self-disclosure, and feedback), and that dehumanizing communication attitudes continue to be expressed by another, one tends to use conflict resolution as a pattern of communication.

Conflict situations may involve verbalization of polarization in regard to beliefs, values, and opinions. Cooperation may not be forthcoming, and dialogue may not happen. All involved may be so dissatisfied with the relationship that one or more choose to terminate it. Thus the following relationship statement can be made regarding separation of individuals in the relationship:

8. To the same degree that conflict tends not to reestablish communing (trust, self-disclosure, and feedback), and that dehumanizing communication attitudes continue to be expressed by another, one tends to terminate the relationship by separation.

Although separation occurs, however, it may not be the end of the relationship. Consider the following relationship statement:

9. To the same degree that humanizing communication attitudes occur in a relationship, in the event of separation, the relationship can be resumed to the same degree of closeness regardless of the separation.

Individuals often speak of feeling so close to another that, although separated by distance and time, it seems as if they had only been apart for a few minutes upon reuniting. Apparently individuals can feel so close to one another that mutually each is able to pick up their conversations almost as if the separation had not occurred. Separation need not dictate termination of a relationship. Separation sometimes increases the value of a humanizing relationship.

Generally, as one moves away from the center of the model and away from the tripod of humanizing communication elements—trust, self-disclosure and feedback—dehumanizing patterns of communication tend to occur. It must be noted however that in each of these circles the interaction pattern can be either humanizing or dehumanizing. One can behave in a manner that generates the feeling of trust in others for the purpose of deceiving or manipulating. One can be assertive in an aggressive, disrespectful manner. One can confront in a punishing, hostile way. One can initiate conflict in a vicious manner. One can separate from another in a way that terminates the relationship. Consequently, we can view the humanistic communication model in its totality as the dimensions of (1) attitudes and (2) interaction patterns (Figure 2–3). One has choice. One may use all of the interaction patterns with varying degrees of humanizing or dehumanizing attitudes. There is a wide range for each dimension. The assumption here is that the nurse-leader will choose to use the patterns of interaction in a humanizing mode, particularly when communicating with followers.

The usual response, however, is to communicate to another in the same manner in which the other communicates. The principle of reciprocity rules. Consider the following relationship statement:

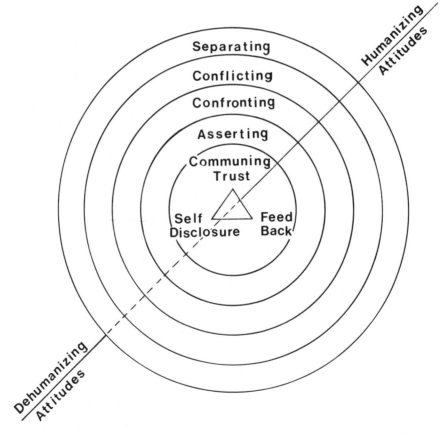

Figure 2–3. The humanistic model of the interacting continuum of attitudes and patterns of interaction. (*Reproduced with permission from Duldt, B. W., & Giffin, K. Theoretical perspectives for nursing. Boston: Little, Brown, 1985.*)

10. The same degree that a nurse uses humanizing communication, humanizing communication will be received from others—clients, peers, colleagues, followers, and superiors.

When one nurse approaches another in a respectful, considerate manner, the other nurse will tend to respond in a similar fashion. The opposite is also true; when one speaks with anger, abruptness, and disrespect, the other usually responds with anger, abruptness, and disrespect.

One has choice, however. Each person is responsible for at least half of whatever is going on in a relationship between self and other. The choices one makes are closely related to one's motives and expectations of the relationship. With the knowledge of the dimensions of interaction patterns and attitudes, it is proposed that nurses take greater control of relationships. Instead of randomly using interaction patterns and attitudes, the nurse can choose to communicate by design to meet personal and professional motives and goals. Thus the following relationship statement can be made:

11. To the same degree that one is aware of one's own choices about interaction patterns and attitudes, one is able to develop communication behaviors that tend to have predictable results in establishing, maintaining, and terminating interpersonal relationships.

It seems reasonable to propose that nurses who tend deliberately to choose humanizing attitudes in situations which, in their judgment, require assertiveness, confrontation, conflict resolution, or separation, will tend to establish, maintain, and possibly end interpersonal relationships in a humanistic way. Movement on the model (Figure 2–2) from the center to the outer circles may not necessarily be sequential. In fact, nonsequential movement may be more typical of reality. For example, in an evaluation conference, a nurse-leader may recognize a situation in which assertiveness is needed in discussing an aspect of a follower's task performance. Once assertiveness has been used, the interpersonal relationship can be expected to change. Conflict resolution with bargaining and negotiating processes may become the next appropriate interaction pattern in order to resolve differences of opinion and arrive at a decision regarding the follower's evaluation. To learn one pattern only, such as assertiveness, although helpful to some degree, tends not to be sufficient. It is believed nurses need to be able to recognize, categorize, and apply the appropriate interaction pattern as well as attitude in the complex, random, and multiple situations that arise in a typical day of nursing practice.

It is also proposed that dehumanizing messages of facts and feelings from others can be effectively handled by nurse-leaders through the use of these few interaction patterns. Dehumanizing attitudes are expressed in messages of defensiveness, communication denial, verbal abuse, anger, and sexual harassment; these present special problems for nurses. For example, the feeling of anger may be expressed in any interaction pattern of the model (Fig. 2–3), and it can be expressed in destructive (dehumanizing) or maintenance (humanizing) modes.[21-25]

Use of trust, self-disclosure, and feedback is the basis of the *maintenance mode* of expressing anger. This is the recommended way to receive another's anger expressions, which are usually in the *destructive mode*. The maintenance mode is a helpful mode for expressing one's own anger, too. It is often necessary, however, to use the other patterns. Defensiveness, communication denial, verbal abuse,[26] and sexual harassment[27] also tend to require assertiveness, confrontation, conflict resolution, and separation rather than communing. In some relationships, communing may not be preferred or desirable in the leader's perspective, given expectations, leader styles, readiness of the follower, power, and change.

A nurse-leader may very wisely choose a dehumanizing attitude in talking to some individuals. For example, a young woman as a nurse-leader may choose to use dehumanizing attitudes and a confronting interaction pattern to discourage a potential sexual harasser. If one chooses to terminate a relationship, dehumanizing attitudes and the conflict interaction pattern will probably hasten the process toward separation. Nevertheless, in those contexts and relationships that are particularly relevant to providing care to clients, use of the humanizing attitudes with interaction patterns seem generally to be a preferable combination to achieve unity. Overall, it is important that the nurse be aware of the range of choices available. (See Fig. 2–4.)

In summary, we propose humanizing and dehumanizing sets of attitudes which, when used with a set of interaction patterns, can provide a considerable measure of control and predictability in leader-follower interpersonal relationships, as described in Situational Leadership. While human behavior is to a great extent unpredictable because human beings have choice, it is through informed choice that the unpredictability can be decreased for nurse-leaders who communicate in a manner each deems appropriate for the task situation and the leader–follower relationship.

These, then, are the theoretical relationship statements of relationship. It is believed a humanistic manner of communicating is preferable in most situations. This will not always work: there are no guarantees. Application of this theory of Humanistic Nursing Communication will tend to result in outcomes that are predictable. Again, for the readers' convenience, a summary of these relationship statements is found in Appendix D.

The operationalization of Humanistic Nursing Communication is not seen as all sweetness, love, and laughter. The nurse-leader who uses this theory most effectively is the one who displays a wide range of attitudes, both humanizing and dehumanizing, and who displays skill in all of the interaction patterns. The nurse-leader need not be controlled by others' communications because of instinctively responding in like manner to others. The humanistic nurse-leader is the thinking, planning, and choosing person who can deliberately select the attitude

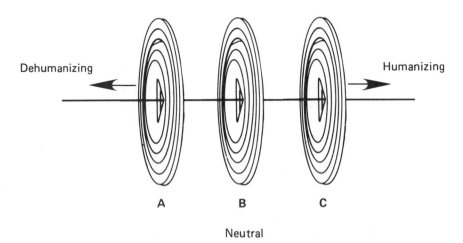

Interaction Patterns

Dehumanizing   Humanizing

A   B   C

Neutral

Figure 2–4. The Humanistic Nursing Communication model. Interaction patterns move to points A, B, or C on the attitude dimensions continuum according to one's choice. (*Reproduced with permission from Duldt, B. W., & Giffin, K. Theoretical perspectives for nursing. Boston: Little, Brown, 1985 p. 226.*)

and interaction pattern most appropriate to the message content (facts and feelings), to be communicated in specific situations, for needs, for motives, and for relationships.*

EVALUATION

In evaluating the theory of Humanistic Nursing Communication, we use the same criteria used earlier to evaluate Situational Leadership theory.

Clearly Stated

Often students of nursing have difficulty analyzing theories because the assumptions, definitions of concepts, relationship statements, and general discussions of each are all blended together, making it easy to become lost. In contrast, we believe Duldt's theory is presented in an organized, logical sequence, so that all might readily understand it.

Duldt's statements of assumption describe the human being as an active (rather than reactive), process-oriented, symbolizing being who is capable of being influenced by communication events in the existential here and now. These concepts are extensively defined so that operationalization and measurement are facilitated for future research purposes. The relationships between the concepts are stated in classic correlational, logical, deterministic, or probabilistic forms so that research hypotheses, designs, and statistical tools can readily be developed and applied. Thus we believe that this theory will be readily adapted to research to test its validity.

Scope

Duldt's theory is intended to be applicable to nurse–client, nurse–peer, and nurse–colleague interpersonal communication occurring in all areas of nursing practice. It is a traditional paradigm variation that, according to Reynolds, is a continuation of currently accepted theoretical perspectives, but with a change proposed to make the theory more useful and realistic.[28] It is a paradigm variation of Martin Buber's "I-Thou" theory of communication.[29] The main distinction Buber makes is that human beings communicate differently with things ("I-It") than with people ("I-Thou"). Duldt's theory is also a paradigm variation of Patterson and Zderad's theory of humanistic nursing practice, which is itself a variation of the "I-Thou" theory.[30] We believe that Duldt's Humanistic Communication Theory differs from both of these in that:

1. It defines the human being in a manner most relevant to the realities of nursing practice and consistent with the holistic perspective of nursing as a discipline.
2. It provides clearly stated assumptions, concepts, and relationship statements that are readily testable.
3. It provides a cohesive perspective of specific attitudes and interaction patterns that can be taught in schools of nursing as basic communication skills.
4. It provides a theory of nursing requiring qualitative research methods and designs, a relatively new direction for contemporary nursing research approaches.

Indeed, much of the theory is probably being taught currently in nursing curricula in America, albeit in a fragmented manner.

---

*For additional discussion of Humanistic Nursing Communication theory, see also Duldt & Giffin, *Theoretical Perspectives for Nursing, 181*.

Applicability, Generalizability, and Agreement with Known Data

Duldt's Humanistic Nursing Communication theory is based on a wide range of theory and research, which we believe represents the best information currently available about interpersonal communication.[31] It is based on ways in which normal people tend to communicate and miscommunicate with one another. Moving from this broad base, it is focused on the interpersonal communication occurring in the professional role for nurses and has been extensively developed in selected areas of concern. These areas of concern include the leadership role. Again, for the reader's convenience, a summary of these relationship statements are found in Appendix D.

This theory also has rather broad application. Duldt has applied it to a broad spectrum of personal and occupational relationships. In the public presentations of an anger-dismay workshop, for instance, some of the problem relationships presented by the participants include parent–child, salesperson–customer, teacher–student, leader–follower, and, in particular, the hospital cashier and the discharged consumer of health services.

We propose that all interpersonal communication can potentially be helpful if it tends to be humanistic, as we have defined humanistic attitudes. To become therapeutic, a few additional patterns of communication are needed, such as those suggested by Carkhuff.[32,33] These also need to reflect humanistic attitudes in order to be effective.

The theory of Humanistic Nursing Communication gives unique recognition to all the negative, alienating, and dehumanizing encounters nurses experience with peers and colleagues. It provides a structure for thinking of ways to cope with negative aspects of nursing practice, not just the "ought to," "should," and "must" some theorists inappropriately tend to impose on nurses' professional behavior. A review of most nursing theories shows that communication is included in them but is not developed extensively. It is thus anticipated that this theory of nursing communication can be used in association with other nursing theories to provide more specific guides to action—that is, to the selection of patterns and attitudes to use in interpersonal relationships. It is for this very reason that we are using this theory in association with Situational Leadership; it provides additional dimensions to the leadership style in communicating in the task and relationship modes.

Research Support

Duldt has proposed a three-dimensional research design for testing her theory. (See Fig. 2–5.) Currently, research testing this theory is limited. Dehumanizing communications such as verbal abuse, anger, and sexual harassment have been studied.[34–40] The area that is the focus of Duldt's investigations is the message consisting of feelings of anger and facts of task criticism in relation to the continuum of attitudes and the patterns of interaction. In a descriptive correlational study using a convenience sample of 118 RNs, Jones found an inverse correlation between the number of angry messages received and the nurses' job satisfaction. The investigator suggests that lowering the number of angry messages received (Herzberg's extrinsic factor) merely decreases dissatisfaction, and in order to increase satisfaction, nursing leaders need to increase recognition and improve communication (intrinsic factors).[41] Using random sampling, Currin found no significant differences between the modes of handling anger in the families of an experimental group of 23 teen-age schizophrenic boys and their mothers in comparison with the control group of 26 "normal" teen-age boys and their mothers.[42]

Equating Blake and Mouton's "people orientation" and "task orientation" with the humanizing and dehumanizing attitudes of Humanistic Nursing Communication theory, findings by Duldt and Doland suggest that nurses who practice in various areas of nursing may have

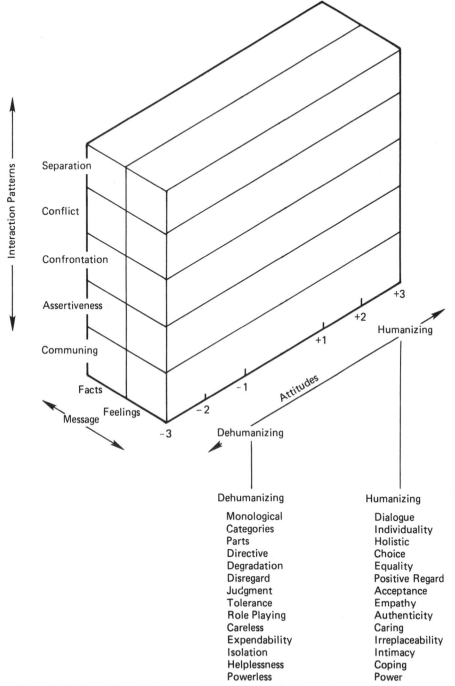

Figure 2–5. Three-dimensional research design for humanistic nursing communication. (*Reproduced with permission from Duldt, B. W., & Giffin, K. Theoretical perspectives for nursing. Boston: Little, Brown, 1985, p. 228.*)

perspectives appropriate to the area. Intensive care nurses were found to be people-oriented,[43] while rehabilitation nurses were found to be task-oriented.[44]

Salyer and Stuart have demonstrated reciprocity in communications between intensive care nurses and patients on mechanical ventilators.[45] Their findings show that if the patient initiated a negative message, none of the nurses responded positively. This tends to support the assumption that there is a lack of sensitivity and individualized communication between nurses and patients in a critical life situation, especially if the patients are unable to communicate verbally. Replicating the Salyer and Stuart study, Longest reports not only finding reciprocity of humanizing and dehumanizing communications between nurses and patients; she also found more humanizing communicative behavior occurring between nurses and patients being weaned from mechanical ventilation than between nurses and patients supported by the machines.[46] Perkins reported the perceptions of patients and nurses differed significantly concerning the problematic aspects of the ventilator care situation. Nurses who paid too much attention to the mechanical ventilator equipment were perceived as dehumanizing.[47]

Other clinical studies include one by Boyd in which a tool was developed to identify specific nursing behaviors that tend to increase patients' reported trust of nurses. A convenience sample of nine spinal cord injury patients responded to the questionnaire. While touching might be interpreted as humanizing, Boyd found the nurses who touched the subjects on neurologically "dead" areas of the body were perceived as unaware of and insensitive to the patient's spinal cord injury and life situation; these nurses were not trusted.[48] Replicating the study, Eberhardt used the questinnaire to identify behaviors of hospice nurses that enable the hospice patient's primary care giver to trust the nurse.[49] In both studies, listening was vital.

Finally, Rodri observed the communication occurring between nurses and expectant mothers in obstetrical labor rooms. A new communication observation tool was used to classify the messages of both nurse and client as humanizing or dehumanizing during 30-minute observation periods. Predominantly humanizing reciprocal communication behaviors were observed. Although facts and feelings were noted in the messages of both, the nurses tended to communicate facts while the clients tended to communicate feelings. All of the clients were on continuous electronic fetal monitoring. A humanizing nurse focused her attention on the expectant mother, while the dehumanizing nurse paid attention to the monitoring equipment.[50] Work continues on refining and developing the original tool; it is now the Nursing Communication Observation Tool (NCOT). Patterned after the Interaction Process Analysis tool developed by Robert Bales,[51] it includes all elements of the continuum of attitudes and the patterns of interaction of Humanistic Nursing Communication theory.

Importance to the Discipline and Profession of Nursing

With variations, numerous nursing scholars and leaders tend to support the idea of humanistic nursing. For example, Pilette describes the nurse as a "humanistic artist" in an existential philosophical context, and identifies the "nurse–client relationship as the cornerstone of the art of humanistic nursing."[52] She further states that:

> Art, our most basic birthright, can be traced to the Biblical character Phoebe and her charitable manner of ministering to the Romans. This early intuitive art meant no more or less than comforting and caring for another human being. . . . In this humanistic era, it is fitting that nursing has reclaimed and updated its birthright. . . . The art of nursing has its deepest roots in the human care transaction and is confirmed in the dialogical process or "I-Thou" relationship.[53]

She further states however that dialogue does not require special techniques.[54] We propose that there is considerable evidence to support the opposite position. First, Carkhuff and Truax have found that didactic and experimental group training programs for professionals have resulted in increased levels of empathy, respect, and genuineness—all concepts that are included in Duldt's proposed theory.[55] Numerous special techniques or communication behavior patterns have also been described and classified by Carkhuff and Truax as either promoting or destroying an interpersonal relationship—in other words, as either humanizing or dehumanizing. We have focused particularly on those communication patterns that seem to be most relevant to the current practice of nursing—that is, communing, assertiveness, confrontation, conflict resolution, and separation.

Second, LaMonica specifically identifies positive attitudes as determinants of behavior congruent with humanizing rather than dehumanizing attitudes as an essential factor in humanistic communication in nursing.[56] This inherently humanistic quality of nursing has been described and discussed not only by LaMonica but also by Flynn, Blattner, and Watson.[57-60] King and Gerwig also draw on humanistic education and the psychology of humanistic nursing education when they state that:

> Somewhere amidst all that equipment, behind all that SOAP charting, among all those nursing care plans, there is a human being—the patient. Have we become so involved in keeping up with the fast-paced technology and science of nursing and the hospital organizational routines, that we have lost sight of the art, the caring *humanistic* side of nursing? . . . It would appear that nursing is in need of a humanistic revolution, a return to the caring function of the nurse. It is our belief that a society weary of technology wants to put a stop to loss of identity and dehumanization, and that within our own profession, our patients desire a humane system of care that recognizes the humanity of us all as nursing priority number one.[61]

Many of the nursing authors identified above described the nurse and nursing as being inherently humanistic. King and Gerwig even state that nursing educators have the responsibility of establishing models of humanistic education and learning so that this philosophy will ultimately permeate nursing practice.[62]

Thus we believe it is inherently important for a humanistic discipline and profession such as nursing to have a theory that focuses on the very process of humanizing, interpersonal communication. Duldt's theory has potential heuristic and practical value in application to research, education, and practice contexts. It is not intended to stand alone, but to augment and enhance the use of other theories such as Situational Leadership, developing the concept of humanistic communication. The description of the human being can be seen as a refinement of humanistic and holistic perspectives of the client that are compatible with historic and modern nursing, that is, being sensitive to the needs of the client. We propose that a preferred future direction for the profession is toward humanistic and holistic nursing leadership, that is, being sensitive to the needs and goals of one's followers.

SUMMARY

This chapter presented Duldt's theory of Humanistic Nursing Communication. The assumptions have been discussed, and the academic discipline from which each is derived was identified. The definitions of the concepts and relationships between these concepts have been presented, with emphasis on the leadership context. The theory has been evaluated according to selected criteria. Although limited due to small sample size or lack of randomization, the research seems to support the theory. Future research needs to expand and replicate the clinical studies. Research of nursing leadership is needed, which is the contextual focus of the next chapter.

REFERENCES

1. Division of Health Care Services, Institute of Medicine. *Nursing and nursing education: Public policies and private actions* (A Committee Report to Congress). Washington, DC: National Academy Press, 1983, p. 1.
2. Ibid., 9.
3. Duldt, B. W., & Giffin, K. *Theoretical perspectives for nursing.* Boston: Little, Brown, 1985, p. 181.
4. Ibid., 181–186.
5. Yura, H., & Walsh, M. B. *The nursing process: Assessing, planning, implementing and evaluating* (2nd ed.). New York: Appleton-Century-Crofts, 1973.
6. Duldt & Giffin, *Theoretical Perspectives,* pp. 302–333.
7. Burke, K. *Language as symbolic action.* Los Angeles: University of California Press, 1968, pp. 3–24.
8. Lasswell, H. D. The structure and function of communication in society. In Bryson, L. (Ed.), *The communication of ideas.* New York: Harper & Brothers, 1948, pp. 37–51.
9. Duldt, B. W., Giffin, K., & Patton, B. R. *Interpersonal communication in nursing.* Philadelphia: Davis, 1984, p. 6.
10. Duldt, B. W., & Doland, P. R. *Alienation of super sensitive ICU nurses.* Unpublished research report: Memphis, Tenn.
11. Duldt, Giffin, & Patton. *Interpersonal Communication in Nursing,* 259–274.
12. Patterson, J. G., & Zderad, L. T. *Humanistic nursing.* New York: Wiley, 1976.
13. Giffin, K. The contribution of studies of source credibility to a theory of interpersonal trust in the communication process. *Psychological Bulletin,* 1967, *68,* 104–120.
14. Giffin, K. Interaction variables in interpersonal trust. *Humanities,* 1973, *9,* (3), 297.
15. Giffin, K. Interpersonal trust in the helping professions. *The American Journal of Nursing,* 1969, *69* (7), 1491–1492.
16. Egan, G. *Encounter: Group processes for interpersonal growth.* Belmont, Calif.: Brooks/Cole, 1970, pp. 190–245.
17. Giffin, K., & Patton, B. R. *Personal communication in human relations.* Columbus, Ohio: Merrill, 1974, pp. 138–139.
18. Gibb, J. R. Defensive communication. *Journal of Communication,* 1961, 11, 141–148.
19. Carkhuff, R. R., & Berenson, B. G. In search of an honest experience: Confrontation in counseling and life. In G. Egan (Ed.), *Encounter groups: Basic readings.* Belmont, Calif.: Brooks/Cole, 1971, pp. 288–298.
20. Egan, G. *Encounter: Group processes for interpersonal growth.* Belmont, Calif.: Brooks/Cole, 1970, pp. 287–335.
21. Giffin & Patton. *Personal communication,* 138.
22. Duldt, B. W. Anger: An occupational hazard for nurses. *Nursing Outlook,* 1981, *29* (9), 510–518.
23. Duldt, B. W. Anger: An alienating communication hazard for nurses. *Nursing Outlook,* 1981, *29* (11), 640–644.
24. Duldt, B. W. Helping nurses to cope with the anger-dismay syndrome. *Nursing Outlook,* 1982, *30* (3), 168–175.
25. Duldt, B. W. Commentary—about anger. *Nursing Outlook,* 1982, *30* (2), 84–85.

26. Duldt, Giffin, & Patton. *Interpersonal communication in nursing,* 234–238.
27. Duldt, B. W. Sexual harassment in nursing. *Nursing Outlook,* 1982, *30* (6), 168; see also Letters (to the editor), *Nursing Outlook,* 1982, *30* (9), 493–498.
28. Reynolds, P. D. *A primer in theory construction.* Indianapolis: Bobbs-Merrill, 1971.
29. Buber, M. *I-Thou.* W. Kaufmann, trans. New York: Scribners, 1970.
30. Patterson & Zderad. *Humanistic nursing.*
31. Duldt, Giffin, & Patton, *Interpersonal communication in nursing.*
32. Carkhuff, R. *Helping and human relations: A primer for lay and professional helpers* (Vol. I. *Selection and training*). New York: Holt, Rinehart and Winston, 1969.
33. Carkhuff, R. R., Helping and human relations: A primer for lay and professional helpers (Vol. II, *Practice and research*). New York: Holt, Rinehart and Winston, 1969.
34. Duldt, B. W. Anger: An occupational hazard, 510–518.
35. Duldt, B. W. Anger: An alienating communication, 640–644.
36. Commentary: About anger, 84–85.
37. Duldt, B. W. Helping cope with anger-dismay, 168.
38. Duldt, B. W. Sexual harassment in nursing, 336.
39. Duldt, B. W. "Anger and trust: Are nurses different than non-nurses? [x] Yes [ ] No. Mimeographed paper available from author, 1984.
40. Duldt, B. W., & the Community Education Department Staff. *Anger: An occupational hazard for nurses: theory, research and applications* (A workshop participant's manual). Minneapolis: Metropolitan Medical Center Foundation, 1983.
41. Jones, S. K. Job satisfaction and expressed anger. Master's degree research project report, 1985. Greenville, North Carolina: School of Nursing, East Carolina University.
42. Currin, C. T. Modes of coping with anger in individuals with schizophrenia. Thesis, East Carolina University, 1987.
43. Duldt, B. W., & Doland, P. Alienation of the super sensitive ICU nurses. Mimeographed research report, 1983. Memphis, Tennessee.
44. Dorland, P. Leadership styles in rehabilitation nursing. Mimeographed research report. Memphis, Tennessee.
45. Salyer, J., & Stuart, B. J. A description of the content of the interaction between nurses and patients requiring mechanical ventilation. Mimeographed research report, University of Alabama School of Nursing, Birmingham, Alabama, 1975.
46. Longest, R. P. An analysis of nonverbal communicative behaviors between nurses and patients on mechanical ventilation. Thesis, East Carolina University, 1986.
47. Perkins, A. Communicating with the patient requiring mechanical ventilation. Thesis, East Carolina University, 1986.
48. Boyd, B. The relationship of nursing behavior and trust. Master's Degree research project report, 1986. Greenville, North Carolina: School of Nursing, East Carolina University.
49. Eberhardt, G. The relationship of hospice nurses' behavior and primary caregivers' trust. Masters degree research project report, 1987. Greenville, North Carolina: School of Nursing, East Carolina University.
50. Rodri, J. A. A descriptive study of the communication occurring between nurses and laboring clients on continuous electronic fetal monitoring. Master's degree research project report, 1986. Greenville, North Carolina: School of Nursing, East Carolina University.
51. Bales, R. *Interaction process analysis: A method for study of small groups.* Boston: Addison-Wesley, 1950.
52. Pilette, P. C. The nurse as a humanistic artist. In A. B. Saperstein & M. A. Frazier (Eds.): *Introduction to nursing practice.* Philadelphia: Davis, 1980, p. 232.
53. Ibid., 233.
54. Ibid., 237.

55. Carkhuff, R. R., & Truax, C. Training in counseling and psychotherapy: An evaluation of an integrated didactic and experimental approach. *Journal of Consulting Psychology,* 1965, *29,* 333–366.
56. LaMonica, E. L. *The nursing process: A humanistic approach.* Menlo Park, Calif.: Addison-Wesley, 1979, p. 465.
57. Flynn, P. A. R. *Holistic health: The art and science of care.* Bowie, Md.: Robert J. Brady, 1980.
58. Flynn, P. A. R. (Ed.). *The healing continuum: Journeys in the philosophy of holistic health.* Bowie, Md.: Brady, 1980.
59. Blattner, B. *Holistic nursing.* Englewood Cliffs, N.J.: Prentice-Hall, 1981.
60. Watson, J. The philosophy and science of caring; Curative factors in nursing," In P. A. R. Flynn (Ed.): *The healing continuum,* pp. 109–112.
61. King, V. G., & Gerwig, N. A. *Humanizing nursing education: A confluent approach through group process.* Wakefield, Mass.: Nursing Resources, 1981, p. 19.
62. Ibid., 32–33.

3

NURSING LEADERSHIP: MANAGEMENT OF PEOPLE AND TASKS

INTRODUCTION

To become a leader in nursing requires a change in perspective: one must change from being responsible for clients having health problems and needing help to being responsible for people who are capable of caring for themselves and others as well. Clients generally are dependent, powerless, isolated, and helpless to varying degrees. Nurses "look after" these people. When these clients are unable to provide for themselves, nurses perform those necessary activities. They expect to "do for" others in ways that are often intimate and personal. Legally nurses are directly accountable to the client for the services they provide. Nurse-leaders, however, become responsible for another group of people, followers, who are very capable of managing their own personal care, health, finances, family, and many obligations and commitments. Nurse-leaders do not "look after" or "do for" followers in the same manner in which nurses do for clients. Instead, the nurse-leaders "oversee" or "watch over" the tasks which nurses perform. They "see to" the entire task situation—the physical environment, personnel policies, and the interpersonal climate of the work setting. Nurse-leaders become "trustees," responsible to management. As trustees in nursing, they are commissioned not only to continue indirectly taking care of an even larger number of clients than before, but also to oversee and manage the nursing staff who provide the nursing care. As nursing leaders, they are not expected to become involved in providing direct, hands-on nursing care, but to provide direct, hands-on administration of nursing practice in a unit within a health care organization. Former ways of being successful now need to be replaced with new perspectives and behaviors.

What are these new perspectives and behaviors? New perspectives are derived from (1) a well-defined description of the nursing leader role and (2) individual philosophical and theoretical choices. New behaviors can be identified, observed, studied, and learned. In this chapter, a description is presented of the clinical nurse-specialist, a relatively new role, and the function of this clinician-leader is described. Second, the Joint Commission for Accreditation of Hospitals criteria and the American Nurses' Association Guidelines for nursing administration are presented to establish the task-management expectations of nursing leadership. To establish the people-management expectations, we have used the continuum of attitudes from Humanistic Nursing Communication theory to describe the unique characteristics of the way nurses communicate with clients versus the way nurse-leaders communicate with their followers. These statements are proposed to serve as guidelines in operationalizing nursing leadership in any clinical practice setting. Finally, a set of elements is presented that includes both management of task and of people and that comprises the typical job description of first-level management in most clinical nursing practice settings.

THE CLINICAL NURSE-SPECIALIST AS A LEADER

We define the nursing leader as the *clinical nurse-specialist,* a role described in current nursing literature and identified as appropriate for clinician-leader roles by the National League for Nursing.[1-9] Formal preparation for this emerging role occurs at the master's level in nursing educational programs. A limited number of other nursing educational programs are designed to prepare nurse clinicians for *executive nurse-administrator* roles, that is, for upper-level administrative positions without the clinical component.[10]* We recognize that many readers may not become involved in graduate programs in nursing. We believe, however, the discussions that follow will be of assistance to all nurses, irrespective of experience and education, who are involved in nursing leadership roles generally.

In our review of the literature, we have derived certain key concepts that seem to differentiate the clinical nurse specialist role from that of a generalist. The first concept is *autonomy.* The clinical nurse specialist possesses a sense of self-discipline, freedom, and accountability in the practice of nursing that is greater and broader in scope than that of the generalist. The specialist functions autonomously in all settings of nursing practice, even private practice.

The second concept is *provider* of expert nursing care. This includes taking health histories and performing physical examinations; noting symptoms and evaluating the implications of abnormal findings, recording the clinical data base, and identifying the client's coping and adaptation resources and support systems and general knowledge of the health care problem.[11] The specialist applies the nursing process to populations or communities at risk or to a case load of selected clients in any setting. The expert provider develops theory- and research-based nursing care plans to reflect social health needs.

The third concept is *colleague.* The clinical nurse specialist participates with nursing peers and representatives of other health care professions in planning, providing, and evaluating health care programs for individuals, groups, and communities. Through inter- and intraprofessional collaboration, expert health care can be provided to target at-risk groups, and long-term health care plans can be developed for future implementation. Since professional roles and functions tend to overlap, an important aspect of developing collegial relationships is clarifying and defining one's role. Erickson et al suggest some distinctions between clinical medicine and clinical nursing, a particularly important area for role clarification.[12] The clinical nurse specialist can develop ways for interfacing with other professionals to provide optimal health care to the public.

The fourth concept is *consultant.* The clinical nurse specialist is able to provide specialized expertise by responding to requests for guidance and leadership in specific situations. This advisory role may be provided for individuals, complex client situations, or to unique target groups in a large community or region. It may also involve consultation with nursing staff by making rounds, evaluating new procedures, or serving on committees of an organizational nursing staff.

A *scholar* is the fifth concept. The clinical nurse specialist is knowledgeable about nursing

---

*Note: An executive nurse-leadership program without the clinical component is offered at the University of Iowa and the Medical College of Virginia/Virginia Commonwealth University. These programs are sponsored by the Commonwealth Fund.

theories and research as well as other disciplines' theories and research relevant and applicable to the practice and administration of nursing. This scholar regularly identifies critical issues and questions to be studied through research. This professional nurse may become involved in writing grants, conducting research to test nursing theories, and, as a consequence, expanding the knowledge base of the discipline of nursing.

Finally, the last key concept is that of *leader.* As a leader, the clinical nurse-specialist attempts to influence the quality of nursing care and its knowledge base through theory- or research-based practice, teaching, and administration. This professional is knowledgeable about organizational management theories, research, and practice and is able to apply this knowledge appropriately to specific situations requiring change. The clinical nurse specialist as a leader is able to analyze the organization of an area of health care delivery and participate in setting administrative policies. In order to have the greatest influence upon nursing and health care, we advocate the placement of the clinical nurse specialist within the administrative structure of health agencies.[13] With administrative authorization and title, this clinician-leader is able to provide a unique combination of expertise in nursing care as well as the administrative power and authority to make things happen.

TASK MANAGEMENT EXPECTATIONS

As is true in many fields, a significant influence upon expectations for the task management of health agencies is the standards set up by national accrediting agencies. The major accrediting agency of hospitals and similar health institutions is the Joint Commission for the Accreditation of Hospitals (JCAH).[14] (See Table 3–1 for the JCAH standards for nursing service.) Participation in this accreditation process is "voluntary" in that it is not necessarily required, but accreditation by the JCAH is an important means of helping consumers of health care to identify sources of safe and reasonably regulated services. There are other groups setting standards that are required, such as state licensing and accrediting agencies, as well as city or county codes and laws; these standards must be met. Often the standards are overlapping; if one set is met, there is a high probability that similar criteria required of another certifying or accrediting group will be met also. Of particular interest to nursing leaders are the criteria for nursing services set out by the American Nurses' Association (ANA).[15] These voluntary standards are unique in that they reflect the optimum level to be achieved; other standards usually reflect the minimum level considered acceptable. (See Appendix A–1 for a complete statement of the ANA criteria.) As a nursing leader, one can expect to function within the parameters of these statements when associated with health agencies subscribing to accreditation standards, and one can use these statements as a guide to initiating and implementing improvements in nursing service administration and management.

PEOPLE MANAGEMENT EXPECTATIONS

Drawing from humanistic and holistic philosophical perspectives of nursing and from Humanistic Nursing Communication theory, we have reprinted in Appendix B a set of statements that describes how nurses communicate with clients.[16,17]

We have developed a second set of statements about the leader–follower relationship to reveal what we believe are important distinctions and unique communication behaviors for

TABLE 3–1. JOINT COMMISSION FOR THE ACCREDITATION OF HOSPITALS STANDARDS FOR NURSING SERVICE.

Principle

The hospital shall maintain an organized nursing staff to provide high-quality nursing care for the needs of the patients, and to be responsible to the hospital for the professional performance of its members.

Standard I.

The nursing service shall be under the direction of a legally and profession-ally qualified registered nurse. There shall be a sufficient number of duly licensed registered nurses on duty at all times to plan, assign, supervise, and evaluate nursing care, as well as give patients the nursing care that requires the judgment and specialized skills of a registered nurse.

Standard II.

The nursing service shall have a current written organizational plan that delineates its functional structure and its mechanisms for cooperative planning and decision making.

Standard III.

Written nursing care and administrative policies and procedures shall be developed to provide the nursing staff with acceptable methods of meet-ing its responsibilities and achieving projected goals.

Standard IV.

There shall be evidence established that the nursing service provides safe, efficient, and therapeutically effective nursing care through the planning of each patient's care and the effective implementation of the plans.

Standard V.

There shall be continuing training programs and educational opportunities for the development of nursing personnel.

From Joint Commission for the Accreditation of Hospitals, Accreditation Manual for Hospitals, 1979. Chicago: JCHH, 1986, with permission.

nurse-leaders. We propose these statements to serve as a basis of discussion rather than to be viewed as facts to be accepted without question. We believe these statements also uniquely capture (1) the best available research and knowledge about how people communicate interpersonally, and (2) the essence of sound leadership theory as well. Using Humanistic Nursing Communication as our theoretical base, we propose it is primarily the attitude with which the leader communicates that determines whether or not the leadership will be perceived as being humanizing by the follower. Using Situational Leadership as our theoretical base, we propose it is the leader's use of appropriate communication behaviors perceived by the follower that determines whether or not the leadership will be effective.

PULLING IT ALL TOGETHER

What do you really DO as a head nurse or supervisor that is different from what you did as a staff nurse? It is important to know about the educational expectations of clinical nursing leaders, and the accreditation criteria and professional guidelines are helpful, but a closer view is needed of what is expected of the staff nurse and the first-level nursing manager in order to identify similarities and differences between the two positions. In order to change behaviors, one needs to know how duties of staff nurses are different from those of head nurses or supervisors.

The four major types of duties required of nurses in the "real" work situation, identified by Kramer, are technical, administrative, organizational, and educative.[18] In this section, the duties included in a typical staff nurse job description are discussed and compared with those frequently included in a typical head nurse's or supervisor's job description.[19]

Technical

The technical duties of the staff nurse are centered about application of the nursing process: assessment, planning, implementation, and evaluation. Health assessment skills are necessary for obtaining a data base for the nursing care plan for each client or patient. Planning and implementing the nursing care includes all of those duties associated with procedures, medications, and life support systems. The staff nurse is also expected to maintain a written plan of care for each client or patient.

At the head nurse and supervisor level, nurses are expected to be able to carry out or participate in the technical duties of the staff nurse. Considerable effective experience at the staff nurse level is usually expected and necessary for promotion to first-level management positions. The amount of time, however, devoted to the technical duties of the staff is limited to that necessary for setting an example, for providing direction, instruction or orientation, and for emergency purposes. New skills to be learned include making out time schedules, developing budgets, and setting long-term goals.

Organizational

The duties of the staff nurse include participating in and attending all unit or departmental meetings. As a group, staff nurses are expected to cooperate in planning for nursing care of all clients or patients assigned to them, including health education, referrals, and discharge planning. Together they are responsible for fire and disaster planning and prevention, cost containment in using equipment and supplies, and infection control. The staff gives and accepts professional recommendations to maintain quality nursing care of all patients. The nurses need to know and adhere to the health agency or hospital's policies and procedures, and each nurse needs to support and maintain the morale of the group.

The organizational duties of the head nurse or supervisor are similar to those of the staff nurse, but broader in scope. For example, the head nurse may occasionally make rounds with physicians, but typically will be interviewing and selecting nursing staff, assigning and scheduling staff for 24-hour coverage, and writing reports. This first-line manager is expected to plan, to set goals, to lead departmental staff meetings, and to represent the administration to the nursing staff. For example, when one staff nurse complains about something, the head nurse might say, "Well, I ordered that a long time ago, and I don't know why they didn't get it for us yet." What this accomplishes is destruction of the staff nurses' confidence in the hospital organization and management. This is not a good thing to do. Rather, she might say, "Oh yes, that order will be here soon. I'll check it out." The head nurse is expected to build confidence in the hospital management, not wreck it.

In representing administration, the head nurse or supervisor is expected to appropriately interpret and apply policies and procedures under which the agency is to operate. While these may be viewed as restrictive by some, when uniformly applied, policies and procedures prevent many problems and grievances. Orders are similar in that it is the responsibility of the first-line manager to follow orders and get things done, so, it is also this nurse-leader's responsibility to plan how to carry out these orders as efficiently and economically as possible. Regardless of how well one develops plan A, it is important to have alternative plans B and C in the event problems develop. Often difficulties develop, and adjustments need to be made. This is one of the basic reasons why supervisors are needed. If upper management's plans were always workable, there would be no need for first-line managers. In interpreting policies and procedures, in carrying out orders, and in planning, the head nurse or supervisor needs to consider the budget and to contain costs of all resources, human as well as material.

Upper management expects the first-line manager to serve as a channel of communication. This involves dialogue or downward–upward communication. The head nurse and supervisor need to have the personal respect, admiration, and support of the nursing staff in order to function as a representative of upper management and talk about policies and orders. Downward communication flows relatively easily and frequently, but the upward communications of the nursing staff can easily be eliminated from the communication channel by an inconsiderate leader. It is the first-line manager's responsibility to listen closely to what the nursing staff is saying. The professional recommendations or personal complaints of nursing staff are to be accepted and acted upon as appropriate; these are not to be filed and forgotten. Just taking time to talk things out is often enough to settle an issue and solve the problem at the unit or department level. When something can be changed, it is the head nurse's or supervisor's job to take appropriate action. This, too, is a part of maintaining and building the morale of the staff.

Education

The duties of the staff nurse in relation to education have a dual focus. The first is the education of the client or patient. Most staff nurse job descriptions include assisting in the development, implementation, and evaluation of health teaching plans for specific clients or groups of at-risk clients. The second involves the staff nurse's own education; staff nurses are expected to attend and participate in in-service educational programs designed to orient, update, and develop job-relevant nursing knowledge and skills.

The educational duties of the head nurse or supervisor focus on three areas: on the orientation, education, and development of nursing staff. The leader participates in planning and implementing orientation programs for all new staff in cooperation with total agency orientation programs. It is the head nurse's or supervisor's job to be sure each nursing staff member knows how to perform nursing care procedures or emergency codes, and perhaps require a return demonstration, even if the staff member has had considerable experience in another agency. Time for this indoctrination to the total agency as well as to specific tasks needs to be provided within the regular staffing schedule. This includes information about personnel policies, promotion opportunities, and routine information about parking stickers, lunch hours, and lockers.

In addition, the first-line manager is responsible for developing, implementing, and evaluating in-service education programs for the unit or departmental staff in order to maintain and update nursing knowledge and skills; this also involves identifying new information the staff needs to know in order to adapt to new equipment, procedures, or nursing interventions.

A major responsibility of the first-line nursing manager is the identification of nursing staff members who have potential for promotion. It is always a wise leader who has someone ready to fill his or her position in the event of the leader's own promotion. Mentor relationships can establish important professional support systems for both individuals. Upon his or her own promotion, the mentoring nurse can then anticipate the support, cooperation, and good will of the mentored nurse. This is an effective way to build cohesive management teams.

Administrative

The administrative duties of the staff nurse focus on nursing care. First, the staff nurse is expected to prioritize and organize his or her own work, coordinating it with other staff members' work as appropriate. Accurate recording of all nursing care is also required. The staff nurse serves as a member of agency nursing committees as a departmental representative, ready to speak out as an advocate of clients or patients; often staff nurses serve on personnel policy committees as representatives of nursing staff. Certainly the staff nurse is expected to know and implement appropriately the legal responsibilities associated with nursing practice within the health agency, being equally aware of limitations and restrictions associated with the staff nurse position. Finally, the staff nurse is expected to report patient care problems, unusual events, and high-risk situations to the head nurse, the physician, and others as appropriate.

The administrative responsibilities of the head nurse or supervisor include patient care and care of the nursing staff as well. As representative of administration, the first-line manager has the responsibility to plan, prioritize, and organize all nursing staff assigned to the unit or department. He or she is responsible for solving problems as these arise, and referring problems upward if these cannot be resolved at this first-line level. The head nurse or supervisor serves as the administrative channel of downward communication regarding policies, procedures, and orders. Serving as a channel of upward communication, this first-line nursing manager functions as an advocate of professional and personal recommendations of the nursing staff to upper management.

One major duty of the first-line manager consists of evaluating the job performance of nursing staff. This is a continuous process, and is closely tied to staff development and morale building. Accurate, concurrent feedback is necessary for staff to appropriately alter and adjust their behavior and to achieve quality job performance. This works two ways, like it or not. The nursing staff are continually evaluating the head nurse or supervisor, too. It may not be a conscious process, but if the nursing staff evaluates their leader highly, this is reflected in positive attitudes, group cohesiveness, and enthusiasm about nursing practice.

THE MANAGEMENT PROCESS

Leadership and management are often considered synonymous, but we propose that there is an important difference. We define management as *working with and through individuals and groups to accomplish organizational goals*. Leadership is a broader concept; it occurs any time one attempts to *influence the behavior* of an individual or group, regardless of the reason. The goals may or may not be in harmony with organizational goals. Leadership requires interpersonal communication skills. The achievement of organizational goals through leadership is management. Thus management is to be considered a special form of leadership in which achievement of organizational goals is paramount.

The management process involves the fundamental functions of planning, organizing, staffing, directing, and controlling. Leadership, in order to influence the behavior of others, involves communicating, motivating, initiating, facilitating, and integrating. All of these functions, both of management and of leadership, are relevant, regardless of the type of organization and level of management with which one is concerned.

There are at least three areas of skill identified by Katz as necessary for carrying out the process of management: technical, human, and conceptual. Technical skill is defined as the ability to use knowledge, methods, techniques, and equipment necessary for the performance of specific tasks acquired from experience, education, and training. Human skill is the ability and judgment in working with and through people, including an understanding of motivation and an application of effective leadership. Conceptual skill is the ability to understand the complexities of the total organization and where one's own operation fits into the organization. This knowledge permits one to act according to the objectives of the total organization rather than only on the basis of the goals and needs of one's own immediate group.[20] Generally, as one advances from lower to higher levels within an organization, less technical skill tends to be needed, but more conceptual skill is necessary. Certainly one needs to know how all functions are interrelated to accomplish the goals of the total organization of health care agency. The common denominator that appears to be crucial at all levels is human skill.[21]

SUMMARY

In this chapter, several perspectives are presented of the new behaviors a staff nurse needs to acquire in order to move into first-line management or leadership positions in nursing. The educational preparation for nursing leadership is being developed in baccalaureate programs in nursing and is being refined in master's programs in nursing. Hospital accreditation criteria and professional standards offer another perspective of the staff nurse and head nurse or supervisor roles. We have identified what we believe are unique characteristics of the nurse–client versus the leader–follower relationship to highlight the different ways attitudes are used in communicating in each relationship. The duties commonly found in the job descriptions of the staff nurse and the head nurse or supervisor were described, identifying further the differences between the two. Finally, leadership in the management process was defined as it applies to any organization, including health care institutions, noting the importance of human skill at all levels of management. In the sections and chapters that follow, each of the functions of the leadership process will be explored.

REFERENCES

1. McMullan, D. *Preparation of the nurse specialist.* (Publication #14-1678), New York: National League for Nursing, 1977.
2. McMullan, D. *Characteristics of graduate education in nursing leading to a master's degree.* (Publication #15-1759), New York: National League for Nursing, 1979.
3. McMullan, D. *Nursing: A social policy statement.* (Publication #NP-63 20m 9/82R), Kansas City: American Nurses' Association, 1980, pp. 21–29.
4. Ozimek, D. *The nurse practitioner, the current situation and implications for curricular change.* (Publication #15-1607), New York: National League for Nursing, 1976.
5. Ozimek, D. *Developing the functional role in master's education in nursing.* (Publication #15-1840), New York: National League for Nursing, 1980.
6. Ozimek, D. *Curriculum in graduate education in nursing. Part I: Factors influencing curriculum in graduate education in nursing.* (Publication #15-1596), New York: National League for Nursing, 1975. A collection of papers presented at a series of workshops.
7. Ozimek, D. *Curriculum in graduate education in nursing. Part II: Components in the curriculum*

development process. (Publication #15-1632), New York: National League for Nursing, 1976. A collection of papers presented at a second series of workshops.

8. Ozimek, D. *Curriculum in graduate education in nursing. Part III: Development and improvement of graduate education in nursing.* (Publication #15-1679), New York: National League for Nursing, 1977. A collection of papers presented at a third series of workshops.

9. Ozimek, D. *Criteria for the evaluation of baccalaureate and higher degree programs in nursing,* (5th ed.). (Publication #15-1251), New York: National League for Nursing, 1983. The criteria state: "V. Curriculum for the First Professional Degree: #27. The curriculum provides for the development of skills in leadership and management for beginning professional practice."

10. Maszkiewicz, R. C., Yesko, J. M., & Kirilloff, L. H. The clinical specialist role. In D. Ozimek, *Developing the functional role in master's education in nursing.* (Publication #15-1840), New York: National League for Nursing, 1980, pp. 13–23.

11. Ibid.

12. Erickson, H., Tomlin, E. M., & Swain, M. A. P. *Modeling and role modeling: A theory and paradigm for nursing.* Englewood Cliffs, N.J.: Prentice-Hall, 1983, pp. 51–53.

13. Wallace, M. A., & Corey, L. J. The clinical specialist as manager: Myth versus realities. *Journal of Nursing Administration,* 1983, *13* (6), 13.

14. Joint Commission for the Accreditation of Hospitals. *Accreditation Manual for Hospitals,* 1986. Chicago: JCAH.

15. *Standards for Nursing Service.* (Publication no. #NS-1), American Nurses' Association Commission on Nursing Service. Kansas City: American Nurses' Association, 1982.

16. Duldt, B. W., Giffin, K., & Patton, B. R. *Interpersonal communication in nursing.* Philadelphia: Davis, 1983, pp. 262–271.

17. Duldt, B. W., & Giffin, K. *Theoretical perspectives for nursing.* Boston: Little, Brown, 1985, pp. 195–197.

18. Kramer, M. *Reality shock: Why nurses leave nursing.* St. Louis: Mosby, 1974, p. 21.

19. Beaman, A. L. What do first-line nursing managers do? *Journal of Nursing Administration,* 1986, *16* (5), 6.

20. Katz, R. L. Skills of an effective administrator. *Harvard Business Review,* January–February 1955, *33* (1), 33–42.

21. Hersey, P., & Blanchard, K. *Management of Organizational Behavior: Utilizing Human Resources* (5th ed.). Englewood Cliffs, N.J.: Prentice-Hall, 1988. p. 8.

II

MANAGEMENT OF PEOPLE

The behavioral sciences, organizational theory, and research of the past half century have provided important information about human relationships in the work setting. If the people who are doing a job are qualified and know what they are doing, as in the case of professional nurses, then why worry about how people get along with one another? "Just leave 'em alone, let 'em do their work, and don't worry about how they get along together!" was the advice one experienced supervisor gave a newly promoted head nurse. Unfortunately, this has been the view of too many managers and leaders in nursing. Important findings of research in the behavioral sciences indicate that the accomplishment of tasks tends to suffer when people do not get along. For example, research by Deutsch indicates there is decreased productivity and increased personal insecurity when members of a group are competitive rather than cooperative. Generally, competitiveness is destructive in a task group.[1] According to research by Schachter, if one member consistently expresses an opinion that disagrees with established group norms and beliefs (in other words, is a group deviate), this tends to lead to that member's rejection by the group.[2] The early research of Festinger,[3] Heider,[4] Asch,[5] and Newcomb[6] support the notion that the way people receive and integrate information, or communicate about their social world, influences their behavior. Festinger and Heider found that, when conflicting information is received, cognitive dissonance or unbalance occurs. Newcomb's experiments showed friendships are predictable from similarity of attitudes on important issues; the more disagreement in expressed opinions, the less likely friendships are prone to develop. Asch's experiments demonstrate that some people will go along with the group opinion, even when their own senses tell them it is inaccurate. Grant found that criticisms about how a task is performed, when expressed in an angry manner, decreases members' desire to remain with the group.[7] The implications of these studies are that disagreements, uncooperativeness, unfriendliness, criticisms, and anger consume group energy and resources; as a practical matter, such distractions from task performance reduce productivity.

There are many other factors in a job setting that Hersey has identified as having significant influence on whether or not the task is accomplished and how well it is done.[8] First, association among leaders has an influence on the attitudes and values of both leaders and followers. How well the group of leaders within an agency are able to work together is important to task accomplishment by followers; if all of the head nurses are able to work well together, then task accomplishment benefits. This is also true of the leader's leader group—that is, the degree to which the head nurses work well together also has an influence on the head nurses.

Second, the proximity of the leader to the followers also makes a difference. For example, whether the head nurse is continually in the presence of the nursing staff or frequently out of the area will determine how often that nurse will be able to directly view the nursing staff functioning in the working situation. Generally, the more opportunity for face-to-face interactions between the head nurse and the nursing staff, the more potential for the head nurse as a leader to influence the staff and be influenced by them; the less proximity, the less influence. The implications of proximity in relation to power, control, conformity, and commitment are inherent.

Third, as a unit within society, the organization or health care agency develops a personality of its own, which also influences human behavior. For example, over time, attitudes and beliefs influence how people as employees are handled within the organization. This may be found in written statements of philosophy or personnel policies, but how these are implemented reflects more accurately the true attitudes and beliefs about people. For example, employees notice how one of their number is received by managers when there is an error in clinical judgment, a drug-dependency problem, or a request for vacation days.

Fourth, the demands of the task itself make a difference in how people work together, too. The degree to which the task is structured determines to considerable degree the opportunities for creativity and innovation on the part of the employees. In nursing, to some degree the structure is high in regard to procedures and policies, but clients' responses are often very ambiguous in regard to outcomes of nursing interventions. Commitment to professional values and beliefs interacts with task expectations, and outcomes (positive changes in the client's health status) are dependent on multiple factors, many out of human control. How job "enrichment" or "enlargement" is defined and operationalized also has an influence. Is "enrichment" truly making a job more challenging and stimulating, or is it merely adding on tasks and territory to the point of staff disillusionment and burnout? These and similar job demands also have a significant influence in how well people work together.

Fifth, "decision time" makes a difference in how well people are able to work together. Decision time refers to the length of time one has to gather information, give consideration to all aspects, and make a selection among available options. In today's nursing practice, as in many other fields of endeavor, the decision time is becoming shorter. The decisions nurses will be making in the future will involve greater responsibility and accountability than they have ever experienced previously. This can result in a crisis-management approach, and people tend to function well in a crisis for only a brief period.

All of these factors—leader–follower interaction, the proximity of the leader to the followers, the association among leaders and the leader's leaders, the personality of the organization, job demands, decision time, and many other factors—have been found to have a significant influence on how well people are able to work together. Of all of these, however, the one factor that MUST work in order for the task to be accomplished is the leader–follower relationship. If this relationship does not work, none of the other variables can make it work.

This is what Part II is about—the relationship between the leader and followers, between the head nurse and the staff. This relationship is considered in terms of the nursing leader's communicating, motivating, initiating, facilitating and integrating nursing staff in accomplishing the task group goals: delivery of nursing service to clients.

REFERENCES

1. Deutsch, M. Effects of cooperation and competition upon group process. In D. Cartwright & A. Zander (Eds.), *Group dynamics: Research and theory* (3rd ed.). New York: Harper & Row, 1968, p. 461.
2. Schachter, S. Deviation, rejection and communication. *Journal of Abnormal and Social Psychology,*

1951, 46, 190. Reprinted in D. Cartwright & A. Zander (Eds.), *Group dynamics: Research and theory* (3rd ed.). New York: Harper & Row, 1968, pp. 165–180.

3. Festinger, L. *A theory of cognitive dissonance.* Evanston, Ill.: Row, Peterson, 1957.

4. Heider, F. *The psychology of interpersonal relations.* New York: Wiley, 1958.

5. Asch, S.E. *Social psychology.* New York: Prentice-Hall, 1952.

6. Newcomb, T.N. The prediction of interpersonal attraction. *American Psychologist,* 1956, 11, 575–586.

7. Grant, B.W. A study of anger, cohesiveness, and productivity in small groups (Doctoral dissertation, University of Kansas, 1978). *Dissertation Abstracts International,* 1979, 39, 3916A. (University Microfilms International No. 7824799)

8. Hersey, P. Situational leadership: Developing leadership skills. Notes taken from a workshop lecture, New Orleans, Louisiana, 1981.

4

COMMUNICATION

INTRODUCTION

In this chapter, communication will be defined and a model of the communication process will be described, which we believe is as important to understanding nursing leadership as anatomy and physiology are to understanding nursing care. The way communication is viewed in nursing and organizational theories will be compared and contrasted and some of the major variables that influence or are influenced by communication in small groups and in organizations will be looked at. The process of influencing or persuading people through communication will also be considered. Along the way, a special problem of leadership in nursing will be discussed: hostile audiences. Finally, some suggestions about developing a persuasive speech will be offered.

COMMUNICATION DEFINED

Communication—specifically, interpersonal communication—is a dynamic process involving continual adaptation and adjustments between two or more human beings engaged in face-to-face interactions during which each person is continually aware of the other(s); the process is characterized by being existential in nature, and involving an exchange of facts, feelings, and meanings.[1]

Glueck reports that various types of leaders or managers spend 75 to 95 percent of their time communicating. He contends communication is so important for leaders not only because of the amount of time, but also because it is needed for managerial and organizational effectiveness. Communication enables coordination of all activities and efforts. He also contends power is attained and exercised through persuasive communication.[2]

The size of the audience to whom leaders speak varies. In one-to-one conferences, we speak of *interpersonal communication*. *Small groups* usually consist of up to 20 people, such as a nursing unit staff. In *organizational communication,* the audience may be large segments, such as the agency's entire nursing staff or even all employees. Nursing leaders may also be concerned with *mass communication*. This involves speaking to the public at large to represent the agency and its services. A public relations manager is usually available to advise about this. Top-level and middle-management nursing leaders tend to become involved at this level, while most head nurses and supervisors are concerned with interpersonal, small-group, and organizational communication. Glueck's definition of *organizational communication* is: "Organizational communication is the process by which managers systematically give information and transmit meaning to large numbers of people within the organization and to relevant individuals and institutions outside."[3] We support his statements regarding the importance of communication to effective leadership. According to Humanistic Nursing Communication theory, communication also consists of messages including feelings and facts, which together have meaning (significance, implication, or effect). We would add this to Glueck's definition. Communication is indeed an influence in an organization, and there is strong evidence to support this position. For example, Herzberg, in his research on job satisfaction, found that the communication occurring between the employee and immediate supervisor is a significant factor in the degree of job satisfaction reported by the employee.[4]

Using the semantic differential in their research, Osgood et al. were able to isolate the *connotative* meaning of words, that is, the internal decisions each individual makes about the meanings of words in each message received. Semantic differential is a procedure for measuring meaning in which subjects check on seven-interval bipolar Scales of Adjectives to describe a concept. He identified three bipolar dimensions: evaluative (good-bad); activity (active-passive); and potency (strong-weak). He also found the evaluative dimension accounts for *two-thirds* of the variability in the conveyed connotative meaning of a message.[5] Berlo notes that this evaluative dimension is increasingly used by researchers as an operational definition of attitudes.[6] This evaluative dimension seems to include what we identify in our respective theories as "relationship" (Situational Leadership) or "attitudes" (Humanistic Nursing Communication). It is the consideration of this dimension that we propose is necessary to humanistic and (w)holistic leadership. Thus we believe you need to study the information in this chapter with particular care. Communication is important not only because it increases your potential for being an effective leader, but also because it helps you be a special kind of leader—a humanistic leader having a (w)holistic perspective of your followers and clients as well.

MODELS OF COMMUNICATION PROCESS

The basic paradigm of communication that is frequently used to show the communication process is as follows:

Speaker ⟶ Message ⟶ Receiver
⟵ Feedback ⟵

While there are many models of interpersonal communication available, we have chosen one model that is consistent with our theories of leadership and nursing communication and that can also be applied to small-group and organizational communication. This is Giffin and Patton's model, presented in Figure 4–1.[7] While it is doubtful any one model depicts all aspects of human communication, we believe this model is representative in that it presents enough of the process in the one-to-one relationship to show that communication is indeed not simple at this level. The process gains in complexity exponentially when applied to small-group and organizational communication.

Generally, it is assumed that interpersonal communication is a dynamic, ever-changing process, and that all variables are interacting and changing continually. All of the processes occurring within Person I, the *speaker,* have an influence upon the encoding or development of a message, verbal or nonverbal. These internal processes are the basis of the communication *behaviors* or sensory data perceived by the *receiver,* or Person II, as the *message.* Although *meaning* is generated by Person I, the speaker, the attribution of meaning is made by the receiver, or Person II. This person *decodes* or translates the message as best he or she can, considering the influences of the processes within. Person II now becomes the generator of meaning in a second message or *feedback* to Person I.[8]

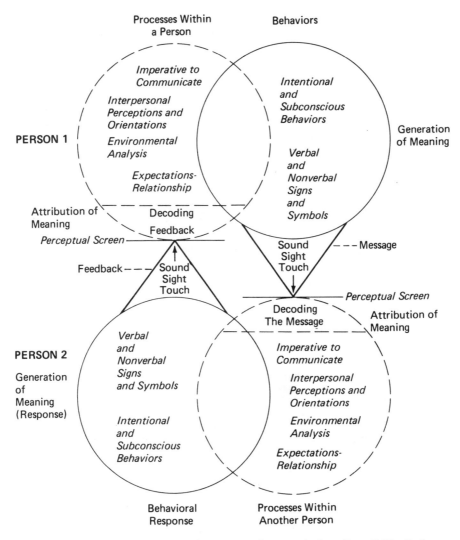

Figure 4–1. The circular process of interpersonal communication. *(From Griffin, K., & Patton, B.R. Fundamentals of interpersonal communication [2nd ed.]. New York: Harper & Row, 1976, p. 20, with permission.)*

In addition to the process within each person, the very language used serves as a perceptual or a "*termi*nistic" screen through which reality is selected. "We hear what we want to hear, either laudatory or critical."[9] Our point is simple. The attribution of meaning lies within *people,* not the message. Specifically, the message and its attribution of meaning lies with the *receiver,* or Person II in the model. Meaning is an individual interpretation: it is connotative. "We attempt to share ideas by means of attributing meaning, *verbal and nonverbal messages.* Based on mutual understandings of the code, we infer the thoughts of the other person and work for rapport. . . ."[10] Consequently, the *feedback* from Person II in the model is the key to assuring Person I the message has been decoded as Person I intended.

There is a rare degree of accuracy in the expression, "getting the message." Intuitively, we seem to have realized that there is more to communication than just comprehending the words. If you "get" what I say, you have the raw information. But if you "get" what I *intend,* if you get what I *mean,* then you are "getting the message."[11]

If you, as a nursing leader, are to be successful as a communicator, you need to listen for feedback in order to know the meaning your followers have attributed to your message. "Words do not have meaning, people do, and people do not mean the same by all words."[12] Research has shown that 75 percent of the time mistakes in judgment tend to be due to miscommunication.[13]

Two of the major leadership and management functions are planning and control; both of these involve communicating to others, primarily about task-related facts or information.[14] This means as a nurse-leader, you need to "tell 'em," and then you need to *listen* and *watch* for feedback to verify your message. When things go wrong, one of the most common complaints of head nurses or supervisors is: "I just don't know what's wrong with these people. . . . I *told* them!"[15] This is similar to your experiences in clinical nursing. You *tell* the diabetics to always carry candy in order to "cover" their insulin. You tell the congestive heart failure patients on low-salt diets that they are not to eat things like salted peanuts. When your patients or clients do not "get the message," they usually suffer some preventable bodily distress or illness. We can state this as a general principle for your consideration:

In the degree you, the speaker, verify by requesting feedback that the receivers, your nursing staff, have heard, processed, and understood your message to mean what you intended, your communication as a leader will tend to be effective.

When your followers do not "get the message," the preventable distress has broader implications because patients or clients, staff, and all the health agency's departments providing services to your unit can be adversely affected. Furthermore, poor performance decreases professional credibility and image. "Only messages are transmitted; and meanings are not in the message, they are in people."[16] So, too, frequent use of "I *told* them . . ." becomes a sign of an ineffective leader.

COMMUNICATION IN NURSING AND ORGANIZATIONAL THEORIES

While it is generally acknowledged by most nursing theorists to be an important concept, communication is not included in the basic conceptual paradigm of the discipline and practice profession: nurse, client, environment, and health. A few nursing theories, however, such as those by Peplau,[17] Travelbee,[18] or Patterson and Zderad,[19] focus on communication as an influential aspect of the interpersonal climate established by the nurse or as a therapeutic intervention. Most theorists include communication as a necessary function of the nursing process. For example, King[20] defines nursing as a process of human interaction that requires the nurse and client to identify health goals for the client and together coordinate efforts to attain these goals. Roy and Roberts,[21] however, view interpersonal communication as a function of the client's state of adaptation: the nurse assesses the client's ability to communicate as part of the total assessment process. Interventions are designed to change maladaptive behaviors, implicitly including communication, to adaptive modes. Generally, then, the communication process seems to be an integral part of nursing, although it may not be specifically mentioned in the theoretical statements. The humanistic or caring theme is, however, predominant in all of the nursing theory literature, and the communication process, verbal and nonverbal, is characteristically the humanizing dimension of the nurse–client relationship.

In a similar manner, communication is not always a major concept in organizational theories, but it is a necessary factor in all. The theories in which it is a major concept include Likert's management systems theory,[22] Blake and Mouton's Managerial Grid,[23] Maslow's theory of motivation,[24] and Herzberg's motivation-hygiene theory.[25] Sometimes the word "communication" is seldom mentioned, but synonyms are used, such as "social esteem," "recognition by others," "interpersonal relationship," and "good working relations." Research based on Likert's theory includes communication data on the direction of flow (upward, downward, and lateral), degree of distortion, and frequency of interactions. Blake and Mouton present descriptive characteristics of the five styles identified on the Managerial Grid, including communication in each. Maslow's theory of motivation implies the communication process throughout, although he does not identify communicating as a basic need specifically. Herzberg's hygienic and motivator factors also imply the communication process; negative attitudes or feelings about one's supervisor are identified as a hygienic factor; that is, if they are not satisfactory, this is viewed as a contribution to job dissatisfaction. On the other hand, recognition in achievement and positive feelings about one's supervisor are motivators as defined by Herzberg. Even in less humanistic theories, communication is there, but under a different label; it may be called "information processing," input-output, or reporting.

Generally, then, it can be concluded that communication is seen by most scholars as an important concept in the processes of nursing and leading. It can be viewed as an independent or dependent variable, or merely as a relevant and revealing type of data indicative of some other concept. For example, there is considerable evidence that communication is influenced by the size of an organization or group, the degree of power a group holds over its members so that they tend to conform, and the degree to which a group sticks together or is cohesive. Communication, therefore, has an influence upon the degree of power, conformity, and cohesiveness characteristic of a group. The amount of supportive or defensive behaviors displayed in a group is also influenced by, and influences, the communication within a group. We agree that communication is important in all of these ways.

THE PROCESS OF INFLUENCING

In fact, we propose that communication is the *core* of leadership, particularly if viewed from a (w)holistic or humanistic philosophical stance. We believe the communication between leader and follower is so important that, if it becomes ineffective and dissatisfying, the leadership attempt will surely fail.

In Situational Leadership theory, the concept of *leadership* is defined as: "The *process of influencing* the activities of an individual or a group in efforts toward goal achievement in a given situation . . ."[26] This process of influencing is achieved through a special type of communication, persuasion. To *influence* is to persuade another to do something by means of argument, reasoning, or entreaty; to convince, to resolve, change, or form another's feelings or opinions in any effective but reputable manner.[27] Persuasion is essentially a humanistic activity in that it emphasizes skills and knowledge, creativity, values, and unity. It is assumed that people can make responsible decisions when exposed to all sides of an issue. The speaker seeks to control others' perceptions of reality through language and to convince others that one particular option is more desirable than another. This leadership attempt requires the speaker to engage the attention of followers and articulate *their* issues, needs, and values. The audience of followers intuitively inspects the speaker for leadership qualities and credibility. Risk is usually involved in that the leader as a speaker publicly takes a stand regarding an issue and proposes a plan; there is risk for the audience of followers in that a change is required of them. In order to motivate them to action, the leader as speaker needs to arouse their feelings to overcome resistance and inertia, ultimately to achieve unity of purpose among them. The persuasive speaker rides this wave of emotional arousal and challenges the audience of followers to choose and to act.[28] Persuasion is usually studied according to the speaker (leader), the message, the context (situation), and the effect as reflected in the behavior of the audience (followers). For our purposes here, we will consider the speaker, the message, and to some degree, the audience; our context, of course, is nursing leadership. If you are interested in further information about persuasion, there are several references that we believe are particularly helpful.[29–33]

The Persuasive Speaker As Nursing Leader

Of all aspects of a speaker, we believe there are three that are crucial to the successful outcome of a persuasive communicative event; *commitment, imagination,* and *trust.* Commitment of the leader and speaker is necessary to spark arousal of feelings in the audience. One way you reveal committment is through controlled expression of your own feelings as appropriate to the problem and situation. For example, a well-known nursing leader in a certain state was attempting to influence a group of health care administrators to set up a program involving telecommunication for meeting the continuing education needs of nursing personnel located in sparsely populated areas of the state. She talked loudly, pounded the table, and would not allow opportunities for discussion and questions. She was gross in the manner in which she pressured the group. By her inability to control her feelings of commitment, she lost her case. The members of the group eventually just got up, mumbled a few social niceties, and left. Nothing was done.

Another way to reveal your commitment is the degree of risk you are taking. How much is being "put on the line" by suggesting a particular plan of action? For example, at a large university-related medical center a few years ago, serious budget problems developed. It was decided by the administrator that certain nursing faculty positions in the school of nursing would be combined with certain supervisory positions in the adjoining hospital. The dean of the school of nursing attempted to persuade the administrator and others that this would severely diminish the quality of the educational program and threaten the accreditation status of the school. The nursing faculty and community supported her, but to no avail. The dean was fired: her risk was high. The change was implemented by compliance, not commitment. Unfortunately she was correct, judging from subsequent events. Her commitment to quality education was clear. She had strong support from the nursing community. She did not, however, have sufficient credibility in regard to budgetary decisions to persuade the key individuals responsible for making the final decision.

In another situation, a nursing service administrator took the position that all nurse aide positions would be eliminated as an economizing effort. The nursing staff were not impressed: "What does she care? She can sit in her office all day, and *she* doesn't have to carry the trays and dirty linen and run around doing nursing aide duties." The nursing staff did not support the director. They resisted the change because they questioned her commitment to quality nursing care and her apparent lack of consideration for them as well as the welfare of the nurse aides. Change occurred through coercion.

Imagination in persuasive speaking requires creativity and originality. The goal of persuasion is to use language to paint the picture of reality you want others to have—to control others' perception of reality. It involves finding unique meanings and describing these vividly and colorfully so that people will remember. Such descriptions serve as goals and aid in uniting group efforts toward achieving this visualization of a future reality. In addition, the design of your speech can enhance the general strategy of a persuasive or leadership effort. Potential designs include using time, space, categories, motivation, causation, repetition, analogy, contrast, and questions and answers; these are used to present different perspectives of the issue, as appropriate. For example, time might be used by including a historical review and projecting the future. A sense of pressure to act might be achieved in followers by suggesting time has "run out." Using space as a design enables a speaker to suggest "moving up to quality" or "climbing out of the pits." These designs can enhance the vividness of imagery you can convey in a persuasive speech.

Trust of you, the speaker or leader, by the audience is a key factor in establishing a followership. Trust is defined as having confidence in the integrity, ability, character, and truth of a person or thing.[34] The following elements have been found to be essential in the behavior of a trusting person:

1. A person is relying on something.
2. This something relied upon may be an object, an event, or a person.
3. Something is risked by the trusting person.
4. The trusting person hopes to achieve some goal by taking this risk.
5. The desired goal is not perceived as certain.
6. The trusting person has some degree of confidence in the object of his trust.[35]

Our formal definition of trust is: ". . . reliance upon the characteristics of an object, or the occurrence of an event, or the behavior of a person in order to achieve a desired but uncertain objective in a risky situation."[36] In our nursing leader–follower context, it is so helpful when each trusts one another. In considering relationships generally, it has been noted that people are miserable without trust. "Misery in a relationship is to expect trust and get tolerance."[37] As professional persons, our greatest asset is our professional reputation. We depend upon one another for providing feedback and for inclusion in important discussions about how things are going generally. Our very livelihood depends upon trusting one another in an increasingly complex and risky clinical practice. We need to trust one another. This is inherent in humanistic communication.

As you speak to your followers in an attempt to influence their beliefs and opinions, there are three characteristics of the speaker of which you need to be aware. Giffin's research has shown these to be important in the development of trust in others: *expertness, reliability,* and *dynamism.* Using the semantic differential and factor analysis, Giffin found these three characteristics seem to define three dimensions of the attitude space of personal trust.[38]

Expertness has to do with the quality of information, skill, ability, and judgment of the speaker. For example, extensive clinical experience, frequently demonstrated skills, education or certification, and a track record of reasonable, accurate decisions would be the basis of credibility for you as a nursing leader.

Reliability means being dependable, predictable, and consistent. This means doing what you promise to do (as in assigning days off for your staff), continually demonstrating a high level of competence in nursing interventions, and consistently behaving in a positive and understanding manner.

Dynamism involves being *"more active than passive, more open or frank than closed or reserved."*[39] This means you will *do* something rather than just stand back when one of your staff is having difficulties. People can expect you to be clear and frank in your evaluations and communications rather than being deceptive and manipulative.

Still another perspective of trust is the trust the speaker or leader needs to have of those listening. One needs to have some sense of psychological safety in order to disclose potentially risky opinions. One also needs to feel that the other nurses will listen and will try to understand what is being said.[40]

Research has shown that the degree of trust increases as communication is increased.[41] This is particularly true, according to Loomis, when certain basic features are expressed:

1. Expression of one's intentions.
2. Expression of one's expectations.
3. Expression of one's planned reaction to violation of one's expectations.
4. Expression of a means of restoring cooperation after a violation of one's expectations.[42]

Gibb's work on defensive communication provides some additional guildelines for developing trust in presenting a persuasive speech. The following statements of principle are based on Gibb's research:

If ideas are presented in a descriptive, problem-oriented, spontaneous way, if opinions are presented in a provisionally held manner, and if an air of equality and empathy prevails, then defensiveness decreases and cooperativeness increases.

If, however, one presents an evaluative, controlling, manipulative manner with neutral feelings, a superior attitude, and dogmatic orders, then others' defensiveness increases.

Generally, with the first approach, Gibb found higher levels of trust and cooperation will tend to result.[43]

Your goal is to convince your audience of followers of your proposals and gain their acceptance of your ideas. People need time to think about your proposals. You need to help them recognize how your ideas interface, not conflict, with their beliefs and values. You can recognize when they begin to be accepting because they will begin to express favorable attitudes toward your ideas and start behaving in accord with your position.[44]

Kelman states people accept a speaker's proposals for three reasons: First, because she or he respects the person making the proposal; second, because the facts and evidence presented to support the proposal are consistent with other things she or he believes; and, finally, if the proposal is accepted, it will lead to potential fulfillment of personal goals.[45]

In his study of social influence, Kelman identified three different ways in which people accept influence: compliance, identification, and internalization. In compliance, an individual does what she or he thinks the influencing agent, or in our context, the nursing leader, wants her or him to do in order to get a favorable response from the leader. The core of this is "social effect." The follower does not believe the opinions expressed, and will stop compliant behavior as soon as she or he is beyond your control as a leader. This is analogous to the (R1) low readiness level of followers in Situational Leadership theory.

Kelman defines identification as acceptance of influence because of a reciprocal-role relationship or a relationship of identity: the motivation here is socially satisfying or the influencing agent is so attractive that the follower wants to *be* the other person. This follower may want to become a leader like you or to take your place as leader. This identifying follower, unlike the complier, does believe the opinions expressed and behaves accordingly. The core of this is "social satisfaction." This is analogous to the moderately ready follower (R2 and R3) of Situational Leadership.

The follower who internalizes your influence as a leader, however, accepts this influence because it is congruent with her or his own beliefs and values. The credibility (reliability, trustworthiness, knowledgeability) of the influencing agent or nursing leader is the motivating source. The values and beliefs are changed and maximized for this individual. The core of this is "value congruence."[46] Internalization of the beliefs, values, and behaviors of the influencing agent or nursing leader is analogous to the (R4) highest level of Situational Leadership.

Thus we can state another general principle:

The success of your leadership attempts to influence others may vary to some degree according to the way your followers accept your influence.

For Kelman's compliers, you need control of resources, rewards, punishment, and so on, and you need to "tell" the follower what to do, when, and how, as noted in Situational Leadership. You need to be attractive to Kelman's identifier and develop a reciprocal role relationship. You need to "persuade" and "participate" in accord with Situational Leadership. According to Kelman's follower who internalizes, you also need to maintain credibility by carefully being truthful and valid in what you say. You need to know. This seems to be the current understanding of how your influence is received by your followers. We suggest that you continually affirm these relationships. You cannot expect uniformity in acceptance of your influence; rather, it is like the sea in its ebb and flow.

In fact, there will be occasions when you must face a group of people who you know will not listen. You know them to be committed to a particular mind-set, and you can consider them a hostile audience or the opposition. Most groups are people who just have not made up their minds, or supporters who already agree with your proposals. It is a challenge to have to speak to a hostile group and try to win them over so that they will at least listen to you. They may never believe you or agree with you. Your goal is that they just listen and try to understand how you figured things out.

We suggest you humanize your approach in three ways. First, early in your speech, acknowledge this difference of beliefs in order to decrease defensiveness and distrust. Second, provide some information about yourself, who you are, and why you believe the way you do; after all, they are probably wondering how you "figured it." Finally, talk about values that you know to be shared by both you and your hostile audience. You certainly want to avoid any language or jargon that would be rude or irritating to them; nor would you want to be disrespectful of any of their beliefs, values, or behaviors. Your goal here is not to win acceptance, but rather, just to get them to listen, understand, and respect you and your position on the issue. Maybe some of them will even reconsider. If you are confronted with destructive criticism, sabotage, or scapegoating, your approach can be generally the same. There are, however, some unique aspects of these offered by Gessner and Sparks, Thorpe, and Johnson-Soderberg that one may wish to consider.[47–49]

Your persuasive approach needs to vary according to other audience characteristics, too. For the undecided audiences, you need to consider ideas, values, and beliefs you share and to provide a lot of information and motivation. For supporting groups, a brief review of the proposals, progress toward goals, and restatement of values is usually appropriate. Here, however, the conclusion of your speech is more important and needs to be unifying and inspiring.[50]

It is time-consuming to spend a lot of time persuading your followers and others to accept some important decision or plan, but you need to remember that it is well worth the investment in terms of ultimate acceptance of your influence and commitment of your followers. As their leader, you need the opportunity to explore all aspects of the issue with your followers so that they, like the patients and clients, can make an informed choice. This is an important process of dialogue and, as suggested in Humanistic Nursing Communication theory, it may include dissent (assertiveness, confrontation, and conflict) on the part of followers and ability to listen, understand, and debate quietly and carefully on the basis of the issues (not personalities) will ultimately tend to strengthen leadership position. Perhaps the loudest dissenter may become the strongest advocate of your chosen position on an issue. It is our position that without followers, leadership does not exist. It is through persuasive communication and dialogue that you and your followers can become unified on an issue and your position as their leader strengthened.

The Persuasive Speech

There are certain elements we believe necessary to consider when developing a persuasive speech. These elements are substance, adaptation, argument, organization, delivery, and language.[51]

Substance

Substance means having something worthwhile to say. You usually need time to research and study the problem or issue. You certainly need to think about implications and perhaps even memorize certain factual information. In your speech, you need to define and state simply the issue and your position in order to hold your listeners' attention. For example, this might be a brief proabortion policy speech a nurse–leader might give to a group of maternity nurses:

> Morally and ethically, most of us believe abortion is wrong somehow. Generally we believe each adult individual has a right to control her own body, and I think people have and will seek to have this control no matter what the law or religion. As a nurse, I value the right of people to have safe care and to decide. As nurses, I believe we need to support the present agency policy of allowing abortions. Don't push the pregnant woman who chooses abortion into "coat-hanger surgery," into dying alone and unattended of infections, shock, or a ruptured uterus. We can prevent that. We know how. We need to respect the decisions of *all* people. We need to help them maintain health. These are our values.

Adaptation

Adaptation refers to designing your speech to this particular audience of followers. For example, in seeking their cooperation and good will, you may need to convince the nursing staff and the volunteers that primary nursing care is preferable to team nursing in delivering nursing care. You need to consider the point of view of the nurses and, when speaking to them, think about how the change will afffect their practice. You will probably need to answer some very specific questions and remember a lot of technical information about each approach. As you think about influencing the volunteers, the ideas and information will need to be rearranged to emphasize their interests. You will probably need a consumer-oriented perspective and will find the questions posed by this group to be more general in nature.

Argumentation

Argumentation involves taking a position for or against an issue and stating clearly the logic you use and your analysis of the evidence. This represents the heart of a persuasive presentation that interacts with and augments all other aspects of the persuasive speech. (See Osborn for suggested references for further information.[28])

Organization

Organization of your presentation needs to follow some logical pattern or sequence. First, you need to provide your audience with an introduction and preview of what you intend to say. Second, in developing the body of your speech, you may find some natural divisions, usually about three, and you will probably want to develop these sections to approximately the same degree and length. Transition sentences between each section and a summary or conclusion serve to bind the entire presentation together.

In addition, you will need to decide whether you want to approach the issue directly or indirectly. Do you want to present a one-sided approach or talk about the ideas in opposition to your preferred choice or position? Research by McGuire shows it is better to "inoculate" an audience with the other side of the issue so they will not be so easily influenced when they hear the other side from the opposition.[52,53] It is often quite effective to consider each argument, pro and con, stating clearly why you believe one particular argument is valid or unacceptable, leading to your position near the end of the body of your presentation. The conclusion of the persuasive presentation often includes a brief review of the issue and arguments, and a challenge to the audience to study the issue carefully and decide.

Delivery

Delivery of a persuasive presentation involves the verbal and nonverbal as well. Body movement, posture, gestures, and voice need to add emphasis to the intent and content of your presentation. Of particular importance is eye contact with your audience. Meaning, sincerity, and trust tend to be enhanced by looking into the eyes of first one, then another member of your audience. Monotone tends to put people to sleep, so do try to use a variety of tone and volume to make your speech lively and rousing.

Language

Language or words are the containers in which meaning is transferred between people; meaning resides in people. If you want your meaning to be transmitted with minimal scrambling, then choose words the audience can immediately understand. Concrete words tend to be better than abstract, ambiguous ones; simple sentences are easier to deliver and for the audience to comprehend. Colorful language (and we do not mean swearing and cursing) is more lively and interesting than ordinary words. Metaphors and "buzzwords" can increase the attractiveness of your presentation. On the other hand, too lively a speech or too much emotion can diminish your professional image and credibility. Watching for nonverbal feedback from those to whom you are speaking will help you judge how you are coming across.

SUMMARY

In this chapter communication was presented as the first function of people management for leadership. The importance of communication generally and for leaders specifically was documented. A model of the communication process was presented that we believe is applicable to nursing leadership. The variety of ways in which communication is viewed in nursing and in organizational theories was looked at. We particularly focused on the process of influence or persuasion as a uniquely important communication process in leadership. Special problems, such as dealing with hostile audiences, have been considered also. Finally, some suggestions are offered for the development and presentation of a persuasive speech. Communication, we believe, is the *core* of effective humanistic leadership in nursing.

REFERENCES

1. Duldt, B.W., & Giffin, K. *Interpersonal communication in nursing*. Philadelphia: Davis, 1983, p. 9.
2. Glueck, W.G. *Management*. Hinsdale, Ill.: The Dryden Press, 1980, p. 564–565.
3. Ibid., 563.
4. Herzberg, F. *Work and the nature of man*. Cleveland: World Publishing Company, 1966.
5. Osgood, C.E., Suci, G.J., & Tannenbaum, P. *The measurement of meaning*. Urbana: University of Illinois Press, 1957.
6. Berlo, D. *The process of communication*. New York: Holt, Rinehart and Winston, 1960, p. 298.
7. Giffin, K., & Patton, B.R. *Fundamentals of interpersonal communication* (2nd ed.). New York: Harper & Row, 1976, p. 20.
8. Ibid., 19–21.
9. Ibid., 21.
10. Ibid.
11. Thayer L., *Communication and communication systems in organizations, management, and interpersonal relations*. Homewood, Ill.: Irwin, 1968, p. 37.
12. Berlo, *Process of communication*, p. 76
13. Kirkpatrick, D. *No nonsense communication*. Brookfield, Wis.: K & M Publishers, 1978.
14. Grosz, M. *General theory of management communication*, (Mimeographed report). Providence, R.I.: Institute of Management Sciences, Research Committee on Management Measurements, 1969.
15. Berlo, *Process of communication*, 176–177.
16. Ibid., 175.
17. Peplau, H.E. *Interpersonal relations in nursing*. New York: Putnam, 1952.
18. Travelbee, J. *Interpersonal aspects of nursing*. Philadelphia: Davis, 1966.
19. Patterson, J.G., & Zderad, L.T. *Humanistic nursing*. New York: Wiley, 1976.
20. King, I.E. *Toward a theory for nursing: General concepts of human behavior*. New York: Wiley, 1971.
21. Roy, Sister C., & Roberts, S.L. *Theory construction in nursing: An adaptation model*. Englewood Cliffs, N.J.: Prentice-Hall, 1981, pp. 43–44.
22. Likert. R. *The human organization*. New York: McGraw-Hill, 1967.
23. Blake, R.R., & Mouton, J.S. *The managerial grid*. Houston, Tex.: Gulf Publishing, 1964.

24. Maslow, A. *Motivation and personality.* New York: Harper & Row, 1954.
25. Herzberg, F., Mausner, B., & Snyderman, B. *The motivation to work.* New York: World Publishing Company, 1966.
26. Hersey, P., & Blanchard, K. *Management of organizational behavior: Utlizing human resources* (5th ed.). Englewood Cliffs, N.J.: Prentice-Hall, 1988, pp. 86.
27. Guralnik, D.B. (Ed.). *Webster's new world dictionary* (2nd ed.). New York: Prentice-Hall, 1980, p. 926.
28. Osborn, M. *Speaking in public.* Boston: Houghton Mifflin, 1982, pp. 264–265.
29. Ibid.
30. Duldt, B.W., & Giffin, K. *Theoretical perspectives for nursing.* Boston: Little, Brown, 1985, p. 33.
31. Toulmin, S.E. *The uses of argument.* New York: Cambridge University Press, 1958.
32. Ehninger, D., & Brockriede, W. *Decisions by debate.* New York: Dodd, Mead, 1973.
33. Beisecker, T.D., & Parson, D.W. (Eds.). *The process of social influence: Readings in persuasion.* Englewood Cliffs, N.J.: Prentice-Hall, 1972.
34. Guralnik, *Webster's,* p. 1527.
35. Giffin, K. The contribution of studies of source credibility to a theory of interpersonal trust in the communication process. *Psychological Bulletin, 1967, 68* (2), 104.
36. Ibid., 105.
37. Luft, J. *Of human interaction.* Palo Alto, Calif.: The National Press Books, 1969, p. 138.
38. Giffin, K. Interaction variables of interpersonal trust. *Humanitas: Journal of the Institute of Man,* 1973, *9* (3), 306–308.
39. Ibid., 307.
40. Giffin, K. The Contribution of . . . , p. 106.
41. Loomis, J.L. Communication, the development of trust, and cooperative behavior. *Human Relations,* 1959, *12,* 305–315.
42. Ibid.
43. Gibb, J. Defensive communication. *Journal of Communication,* 1961, *11,* 141–148.
44. Martin, H.H., & Anderson, K.E. *Speech communication: analysis and readings.* Boston: Allyn and Bacon, 1968, p. 137–147.
45. Kelman, H.C. Processes of opinion change. *Public Opinion Quarterly,* 1961, *25,* 55–78.
46. Ibid.
47. Gessner, B., & Sparks, J.A. Criticism: The other side of nursing. *Mobius,* 1981, *1* (1), 36.
48. Thorpe, R. Sabotage in nursing. *The Journal for Nursing Leadership and Management,* June 1981, 24–25.
49. Johnson-Sonderberg, S. Theory and practice of scapegoating. *Perspectives in Psychiatric Care,* 1977, *15* (4), 153–159.
50. Osborn, *Speaking in public,* 266–270.
51. Ibid., 72, 264–320.
52. McGuire, W.J. Inducing resistance to persuasion: Some contemporary approaches. III. The inoculation approach. *Advances in Experimental Social Psychology, 1,* 191–229.
53. Beisecker, T.D., & Parson, D.W. (Eds.). *The process of social influence: Readings in persuasion.* Englewood Cliffs, H.J.: Prentice-Hall, 1972, p. 197.

5

MOTIVATING

INTRODUCTION

Motivation is commonly defined as a leadership function to arouse, excite, or influence another person to behave in some role or perform some action the person would not ordinarily do. To be motivated refers to some inner drive, impulse, or intention that causes one to act or believe a certain way, or to seek a particular goal.[1] It is the *effect* of persuasive communication. Motivation arises, according to Burke, from the persuasive communication occuring between different entities or kinds of entities, such as leader and follower. Burke, a rhetorical critic and symbolic interaction theorist, describes persuasive communication between different kinds of an abstract paradigm of courtship,[2] and, as in courtship or love, there is "mystery." It is "spiritual" in that change is the result of abstract means. It is for the leader seeking an answer to the fundamental question, "What can I do to motivate followers to get things done?" Certainly one does not expect followers to "love" their leader. Machiavelli advises that it is safer for a leader to be feared than loved, since people are more likely to offend those they love than those they fear.[3]

While perspectives of leadership have changed considerably since the 1500s, Machiavelli's time, the essence of the "mysterious" and the "spiritual" remains in the concept of motivation, particularly in relation to the role of leadership. The belief and expectation remains today that the leader can influence the internal motivation of the followers. We believe there are incentives (external) that a leader can provide to stimulate motivation (internal in followers) so that they will demonstrate appropriate task-related behaviors. We propose these incentives are primarily symbolic—primarily in the way the leader communicates to the followers.

In this chapter, four important perspectives will be discussed that we believe have particular relevance to removing this ancient mystique that surrounds the process of leaders motivating followers. These perspectives include Maslow's needs theory, Herzberg's two-factor theory of job satisfaction, McClelland's study of achievement, and Mead's role theory. Each perspective is briefly described and then related to Situational Leadership and to Humanistic Nursing Communication. The relevance of these perspectives to nursing is noted throughout the discussions.

MASLOW'S MOTIVATION THEORY

Abraham Maslow's theory of motivation has been applied to nursing care for some time, and is probably very familiar to most of our readers. Maslow identified a hierarchy of needs that he proposed as being the basis of motivation for mankind. These needs are arranged in order of priorities on a pyramid, which serves as the classic model for the theory (Fig. 5–1). There are five categories of needs in the hierarchy. Physiological needs have first priority and include such elements as sex, food, water, air, shelter, and survival. Second-priority needs are safety: security, protection, and freedom from fear, chaos, and anxiety. The third priority are social

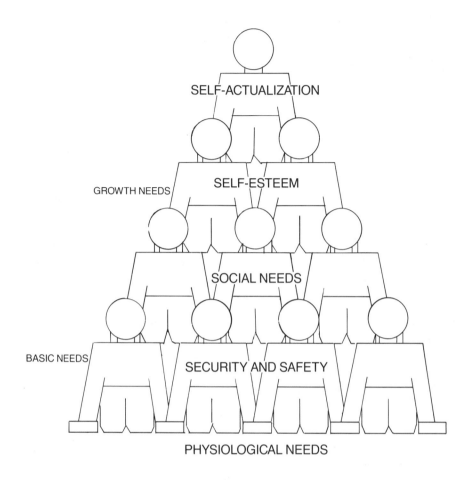

Figure 5–1. Abraham Maslow's hierarchy of needs. *(From Goble, F.G.* The third force: Abraham Maslow. *New York: Pocket Books, 1976, 52.)*

needs, which consist of self-esteem, self-confidence, dignity, and recognition as an individual. Fourth, esteem includes recognition and respect by others, prestige, achievement, status, and attention. Finally, at the top of the pyramid is self-actualization, which is becoming what one can be, the development and utilization of self to one's potential. This hierarchy of needs is grouped into basic or deficiency needs, the first two, and growth needs, or the three remaining.

Generally these needs are interrelated according to a flexible process of emerging. As one need becomes satisfied, human beings become motivated by the next higher need. For example, if physiological needs are met, then safety needs emerge and become salient. Generally, to the same degree that lower needs are satisfied the next higher need tends to emerge and be perceived by the individual; as this occurs, one attempts to meet this next need. Satisfy this need, and still another takes its place; the satisfied need is no longer salient. Humans tend to react, often negatively, when frustrated in meeting a need or when they are unable to satisfy a need. While satisfaction of one perceived need may be related to age, such as physiological needs and safety for infants and small children or self-actualization for older adults, the reemergence of a need is the more common pattern. For example, one may satisfy hunger at breakfast, but by lunchtime, the need to eat is again salient. If the basic needs are not met, a deficiency develops, but if growth needs are not met, there is no deficiency but merely lack of growth to potential.[4,5]

We can use this theory by taking the perspective that the behavior presented by followers may be the result of perceived needs, and we can apply Maslow's work to the readiness of followers as described in Situational Leadership[6] (Fig. 5–2). If a nurse's behavior reflects basic needs (physiological and safety), that nurse tends to fall primarily in the R1 level. A nurse operating at the safety and social need level tends to fall into the R2 level of readiness. Nursing staff who operate at the social and esteem need levels are seen to be at the R3 level of readiness. Finally, nurses who operate out of the need for self-actualization tend to fall into the R4 level of readiness. The process of diagnosing needs that evoke behavior can help you to determine which leadership style will tend to have the highest probability for being most effective in motivating your nursing staff.

For example, nurses generally have been diagnosed as lacking in social needs or self-esteem. Instead of a pyramid, Maslow's model is proposed to be in the shape of an hourglass with a bottleneck at the self-esteem level[7] (Fig. 5–3). If this is true of the nurses who are your followers, then leadership styles S2 and S3 would have the highest probability of providing the external incentives to motivate your nursing staff.

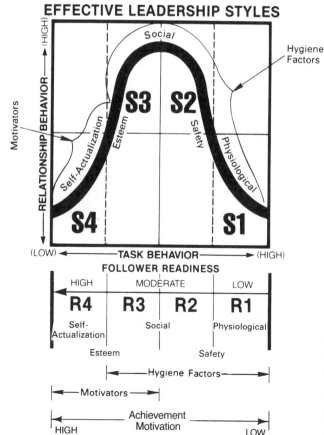

Figure 5–2. Relationship among Maslow's needs theory, Herzberg's two-factor theory, and McClelland's study of achievement. *(Adapted from Hersey, P., & Blanchard, K. Management of organizational behavior: Utilizing human resources [5th ed.]. Englewood Cliffs, N.J.: Prentice-Hall, 1988, 431, 435, with permission.)*

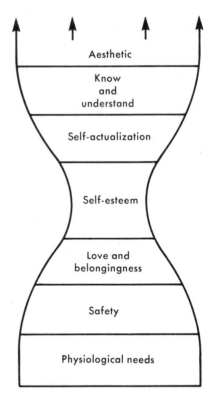

Figure 5–3. Maslow's pyramid model should be an hourglass to demonstrate the bottleneck at self-esteem characteristic of nurses. *(From Chenevert, M. Special techniques in assertiveness training for women in health professions. St. Louis: Mosby, 1976, 34, with permission.)*

The high self-esteem needs would also indicate a need for you as the leader to communicate in a humanistic manner, as defined by the attitudes and patterns of interaction of Humanistic Nursing Communication theory. The degree and character of the humanizing communication, however, vary with the level of needs and the style of communication. While we recommend that one never become extremely dehumanizing, to some degree one needs to engage in monologue and give directives. A leader does relate to followers according to categories or parts. Judgments are made in evaluating performance, and some errors are tolerated. One plays the role of leader. To some degree, the follower will tend to feel isolated, helpless, and powerless. As a general principle:

"As the follower operates out of higher-level needs and demonstrates a higher level of readiness and motivation, then the degree to which humanizing attitudes are used by the leader increases in congruency with the leadership style."

At the R4 level of readiness, the S4 leadership style of delegating is congruent with almost all characteristics of humanizing attitudes. Monological communication, however, particularly in the form of directives, remains in the leader–follower interpersonal relationship.

The patterns of interaction are also important in the leader's communication with followers. Asserting, confronting, and conflicting are appropriate patterns of interaction for a leader to use at all levels of needs. Asserting, for example, is necessary for stating directions and expectations. Confronting is particularly important in intervening in the developmental and regressive cycles. Negotiation of goals and expectations is important in resolving conflicting understandings about the task. Separating is used when promotion or dismissal occurs. Communing is added as communications become dialogical. Separating is also used by the leader in communicating with a follower at the R4 level of readiness because delegating involves some considerable degree of separating between the leader and follower. Interpersonal intimacy, however, would probably not be appropriate in most leader–follower relationships, since this connotes significant personal bonds[8–10] (Fig. 5–4).

Maslow's hierarchy is an excellent method of cross-checking diagnoses of follower readiness and deciding which leadership style of communication is appropriate for motivating nursing staff. Keep in mind, however, that people operate at a variety of need levels simultaneously, and that needs tend to vary with situations. It is also important to note that nurses may find other areas of their lives besides the nursing practice environment in which to satisfy needs.[11]

HERZBERG'S THEORY OF JOB SATISFACTION

It is interesting to note that Frederick Herzberg first conducted research to support his two-factor theory of motivation and job satisfaction in hospitals. This early influence is seen in the labeling of the job dissatisfiers as "hygienic factors," referring to the medical meaning of "prevention" and "environment." Yet many nurses may not be familiar with this theory. Herzberg assumed a humanistic perspective of people and proposed that, if the job dissatisfiers could be identified and eliminated, people would be more satisfied with their jobs and perhaps more productive.[12,13] Because Herzberg and his colleagues used self-reports, interviewing, and content analysis of critical incidents, this theory has been criticized on the basis of researcher bias. Subsequent studies, however, have tended to support the theory.[14]

In the primary supporting study, Herzberg and his colleagues asked over 200 engineers and accountants from 11 industries in the Pittsburgh area what kinds of things about their jobs made them unhappy or happy. The findings showed two distinct categories of needs that were essentially independent of each other, yet exerted different influences upon the job behavior.

The categories that the subjects identified as the cause of unhappiness or job dissatisfaction included: organizational policies and administration, supervision, working conditions, interpersonal relations, money, status, and security. This category was labeled "hygienic factors," later to be relabeled "maintenance factors." These were primarily environmental rather than an intrinsic part of the job. Generally, these hygienic or maintenance factors produced no growth in worker output capacity; they only related with losses in productivity due to work slowdowns. The employees simply worked at the minimal level of their capacity in order to keep their jobs. This means that a nurse could keep her staff nurse position by simply working at 20 to 30 percent of her capacity.

The subjects also identified the sources of happiness or job satisfaction. These items included feelings of achievement, professional growth and development, recognition for accomplishments, challenging work, and increased responsibility. Herzberg labeled this category "motivating factors." These factors were found to have a positive effect on job satisfaction, often resulting in increase of an employee's productivity capacity.

In order to clearly differentiate between the hygienic and motivating factors, we will provide a hypothetical example. Assume that a staff nurse is highly motivated and is working at 90 percent of capacity. She has a good working relationship with her nursing unit manager or head nurse, is satisfied with her pay and other benefits, and with the working conditions

SITUATIONAL LEADERSHIP		HUMANISTIC NURSING COMMUNICATION THEORY		
		Attitudes		Patterns of
Readiness Level	Style	Dehumanizing	Humanizing	Interaction
R1 **LOW**	S1 (HT/LR) "Telling"	Monologue Categories Parts	Equality Positive regard Caring	Assertiveness Confronting Conflicting
Unable, unwilling Unable, insecure			Irreplaceability	Separating
Safety Physiological		Directives Judgment		
Hygiene factors		Tolerance Role-playing		
Low achievement		Isolation Helplessness Powerlessness		
R2 **LOW/** **MODERATE**	S2 (HT/HR) "Selling"	Monologue Categories Parts	Dialogue Individual	Asserting Confronting Conflicting
Unable, willing with supervision Unable, secure or confident		Directive	Equality Positive regard	Separating
Safety, social		Judgment Tolerance		
Hygiene factors		Role-Playing		
Low achievement		Powerlessness	Caring Irreplaceability	
R3 **MODERATE/** **HIGH**	S3 (LT/HR) "Participating"	Monologue Categories Parts Directive	Dialogue Individual Holistic Choice Equality	Communing Asserting Confronting Conflicting Separating
Able, insecure with- out supervision Able, unwilling, & un- committed				
Social esteem		Judgment Tolerance	Positive regard Acceptance	
Hygiene factors, motivators		Role-Playing	Empathy Authenticity	
High achievement		Powerlessness	Caring Irreplaceability Power	
R4 **HIGH**	S4 (LT/LR) "Delegating"	Monologue	Dialogue Individual	Communing Asserting
Able, willing Able, confident, committed		Directive	Holistic Choice	Confronting Conflicting Separating
Esteem, self- actualization			Equality Positive Regard Acceptance	
Motivators			Empathy Authenticity	
High achievement			Caring (Intimacy?) Irreplaceability Coping Power	

Figure 5–4. Relationship between Situational Leadership and Humanistic Nursing Communication. *(Partially derived from similar chart developed by Paul Hersey, with permission.)*

generally. The nursing team with whom she works consists of members who are a congenial group. She even has been assigned her own parking-deck space! Now, suppose her head nurse is suddenly transferred and replaced by a person with whom she is unable to work, or suppose she finds out that someone whose work seems inferior to her own or who has fewer credentials than she has is receiving the same salary or a few dollars more. Since Herzberg's two-factor theory states that performance or productivity depends on both ability and motivation, these unsatisfied hygienic factors (supervision and money) may lead to restricted output: The staff nurse may stay on the job, but quit trying, becoming a "stayer and quitter." The decline in productivity may or may not be intentional, but the quality of nursing care provided by this staff nurse decreases. (See Fig. 5–5 for a graphic illustration of this situation.) According to Herzberg's theory, even if the former head nurse returned and the staff nurse's salary adjusted, productivity would probably only increase to its original level.

Conversely, assume our staff nurse has not experienced this job dissatisfaction and is functioning at 90 percent of her capacity. Suppose she is given an opportunity to mature professionally and satisfy her motivational needs in a situation in which she is free to take some initiative, to be creative, to make decisions without continually needing a supervisor's or physician's approval, to be able to handle problems, and to take responsibility. Suppose she is provided training to prepare her for serving as a nurse on the hospital's new helicopter emergency transport service, or perhaps she is transferred to a nursing unit in which primary nursing is the method used to deliver nursing services. According to Herzberg's two-factor theory, this will have a powerfully motivating effect. If the staff nurse is able to fulfill the new supervisor's expectations in job performance, she may still work at 90 percent capacity. Now, however, she has grown professionally and has increased her nursing skills; she is capable of a greater level of productivity. This is illustrated in Figure 5–6.

Hygienic factors, when satisfied, tend to eliminate job dissatisfaction and work slowdowns, but they do little to motivate an individual to superior performance or increased capacity. Satisfaction of the motivating factors will, however, permit an individual to grow and develop in a mature way, often implementing an increase in ability. Thus hygienic factors affect an individual's willingness or motivation, and motivators have an impact on an individual's ability. As a general principle:

The more a nursing leader pays attention to both the hygienic and motivating factors, the greater the probability of maximizing the nursing performance of her nursing staff in comparison with nursing leaders who ignore these factors.

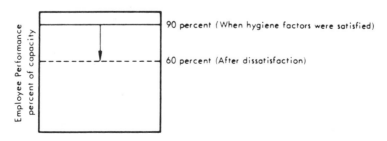

Figure 5–5. The effect of dissatisfying hygienic factors on nursing performance. *(From Hersey, P. & Blanchard, K. Managment of organizational behavior: Utilizing human resources [5th ed.]. Englewood Cliffs, N.J.: Prentice-Hall, 1988, 65, with permission.)*

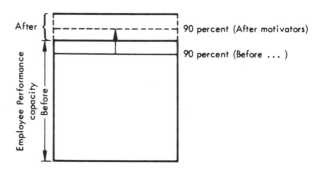

Figure 5–6. The effect of satisfying motivation factors on nursing performance. *(From Hersey, P., & Blanchard, K.* Management of organizational behavior: Utilizing human resources *[5th ed.]. Englewood Cliffs, N.J.: Prentice-Hall, 1988, 66, with permission.)*

The higher the level of job *dis*satisfaction, the greater the percentage of nursing staff capabilities that will be directed toward the hygienic factors rather than toward nursing practice.

Herzberg's two-factor theory can be related to Maslow's motivation theory. The hygienic factors are all related to the physiological, safety, social, and part of the esteem needs. The esteem needs are divided because of definitional differences in status and recognition. Whereas *status* tends to be associated with the position or role one occupies, *recognition* is granted by others because one demonstrates competence and achievement in work. Thus some of the esteem need is satisfied both by the hygienic and motivating factors. The need to self-actualize is related to the motivating factors.

Job satisfaction of nurses has been studied using the two-factor theory. The Herzberg study was replicated by Longest using 195 RNs from 10 Atlanta hospitals to compare nurses' responses with the job satisfaction factors identified by Herzberg. The findings showed some disagreement with Herzberg's list of motivating factors, particularly in interpersonal relations, recognition, and achievement. A very high ranking was given to the interpersonal relationships between the RN and her supervisor as a motivational factor. Recognition and advancement were ranked very low, possibly because, according to Longest, nursing is often described as a profession with limited opportunity for advancement.[15] Jones studied the relationship between expressed anger and job satisfaction, and the data showed an inverse correlation between the number of angry messages received in a given period of time and the degree of job satisfaction. Jones suggests that lowering the number of angry messages received will only decrease dissatisfaction, but in order to increase job satisfaction, supervisors need to increase recognition of nurses' efforts and use similar motivational factors.[16] Duldt conducted a study in which 34 staff nurses, who were given training in coping with anger from alienating co-workers and colleagues were compared with 43 staff nurses who received no such training. A tool based on Herzberg's theory was used, and the subjects were asked how satisfied they were with each factor and how important the factor was to them. In the ranking of factors for all subjects, the item "Communication with the immediate supervisor" accounted for the largest percentage of variance on the satisfaction factor analysis, and "Communication with co-workers" accounted for the largest percentage of variance on the importance factor. The subjects receiving the anger and alienating communication training program showed significantly increased job satisfaction in comparison to the control group.[17]

Herzberg's two-factor theory also can be related to Situational Leadership and Humanistic Nursing Communication theory. Readiness levels R1, R2, and R3 are congruent with the hygienic factors, while R3 and R4 are consistent with the motivating factors. The predominantly dehumanizing communication attitudes and patterns of interaction are consistent with the hygienic factors, and predominantly humanizing ones are appropriate with the motivator factors. (See Fig. 5–4.)

The two-factor theory provides another excellent perspective of nursing staff motivation. Maslow's theory allows you as a nursing leader to think about behaviors displayed by your nursing staff and speculate on diagnosing which need is salient for each individual. In contrast, Herzberg's theory provides an opportunity to obtain information directly from your staff. You can ask the same questions Herzberg used. Ask for a list of the things that give the nurses a great deal of satisfaction in their work, and another list of the things they find dissatisfying. Applying this theory can be as simple as that. You will have an important perspective: You will know how things look from each individual's point of view. You can have their input into what motivates them and build a plan for staff motivation accordingly.

McCLELLAND'S ACHIEVEMENT NEED

When David McClelland, a psychologist, began his 20-year study at Harvard, his objective was to understand some of the forces that produce rapid economic development of some nations. He assumed that these forces lie largely within man and that they come from some fundamental psychological motivation rather than climate, population, division of labor, or politics, as proposed by economic theorists. He ultimately identified four motivational patterns that seem to be learned early in life from within the family and community cultural influences. These four patterns were labeled "affiliation," or a drive to relate to people; "competence," or a drive to do quality work; "power," or a drive to influence people and situations; and "achievement" or a drive to overcome challenges, advance, and grow.[18,19] What McClelland learned about achievement motivation provides some helpful information for us in thinking about how, as leaders, we can create an environment of incentives for motivating nursing staff.

One thing McClelland learned about the achievement need is that it can be isolated and assessed in any group. One classic experiment that revealed the achievement need involved having the participants throw rings over a peg from any distance they chose—the Ring Toss Game. This experiment has since been replicated numerous times, and the results are relatively consistent.[20]

McClelland gave each subject a number of rings and explained simply that the goal was to throw the rings over a stake. He assured the participants that they were not competing against anyone else, and that they were free to stand wherever they liked. Some participants would walk directly to the stake, lean over, and drop the rings in place. The salient need for these participants was probably safety (Maslow), since they seemed unwilling to take even the slightest risk. A fear of failure can often be equated with the need for security above all other considerations. Other participants would stand far from the stake where the chances of success were very slight. These participants might be viewed as having high needs for esteem or self-actualization (Maslow), since they appeared to be motivated by the desire to achieve something beyond reasonable standards of performance. Actually, though, these participants were very much like those who stood directly over the stake to make their toss. They also had a salient need for security and a fear of failure. However, they believed that it is socially unacceptable to drop the rings over the stake at close range. So they moved far away: if they should score a hit, then they would receive praise; if they missed (and they expected to), the miss would be understandable because of the distance involved. These individuals have low needs for achievement.

However, individuals with a high need for achievement seemed to carefully measure the place to stand when tossing the ring so they were most likely to be successful—not too close to make the task ridiculously easy or too far away to make it impossible. *They set moderately difficult but potentially achievable goals.* If their first toss missed, they moved closer to the stake; if they were easily successful on the first toss, they moved back to increase the challenge. Achievement motivation is simply the extent to which people set goals for themselves—not just any goals, but goals that are both challenging and realistic.

McClelland identified certain characteristics of a person having high need achievement. First, *"the high achiever likes situations in which he takes personal responsibility for finding solutions to problems."*[21] Achievement-motivated individuals typically are not gamblers; they prefer to work on a problem if they can influence the outcome rather than depend upon chance. High self-confidence is also involved. High achievers think a lot about what needs to be done and how to do it, so they often can perform better than most.

A second characteristic is *". . . his tendency to set moderate achievement goals and to take 'calculated risks.' "*[22] High achievers will choose to work and play in situations in which they have a chance to affect the outcome. They prefer not to gamble at all. They set their own goals and readily assume total responsibility for achieving the goals.

A third characteristic is that one with *". . . a strong concern for achievement also wants concrete feedback as to how well he is doing."*[23] Children with high achievement needs typically like to work with their hands in a shop or to work with mechanical or electrical gadgets. They are able to get immediate feedback, for example, after wiring up an electric circuit; a throw of the switch and the gadget works or not. Salespeople also receive this instant feedback; they can count the number of sales made each day. Teachers and nurses, however, receive relatively imprecise feedback from the effects of their efforts to impact upon students' intellectual development or clients' improved health status.

McClelland noted that the need to achieve is one of the keys to economic growth:

> . . . men who are concerned with doing things better become active entrepreneurs and create the growing business firms that are the foundation stones of a developing economy. Although some of these heroic entrepreneurs might be regarded as leaders in the restricted sense that their activities established the economic base for the rise of a new type of civilization, they were seldom leaders of men. The reason for this is simple: [high] Achievement n[eed] is a one-man game that need never involve other people. . . . So, in the pure sense, high achievement is not dependent on the judgment of others: he is only concerned with improving his own performance.[24]

Generally, people whose motive is to do things better, often do better work, receive promotions faster, and move up in organizations ahead of those whose achievement need is less salient.

One caution is in order. McClelland indicates that one of the major difficulties in drawing conclusions from most studies that deal with male-female behaviors is that most researchers are inclined to view male behavior as the norm and female behavior as a deviation from the norm.[25] Consequently, the statements about high achievement needs may not apply as appropriately to women as to men. This may not be as applicable to women or men of the 1980s and 90s as it was in the 1960s and 70s when the research was conducted.

The concept of achievement motivation is found to be directly related to the readiness level of followers as described in Situational Leadership. Low achievers tend to cluster in the

R1 and R2 levels of readiness, requiring "telling" or "selling" leadership styles. The high-achievement-needs people tend to cluster in the R3 and R4 levels of readiness, for which the "participating" and "delegating" leadership styles would be most appropriate. In relation to Maslow's theory and the theory of Humanistic Nursing Communication, these are consistent with the classifications described earlier and presented on the chart summarizing the theoretical synthesis. (See Fig. 5–2.)

Clearly, the leadership communication style that has the highest probability of success is S3 and S4, "participating" and "delegating." McClelland notes that interpersonal relationships are more important to women than they are to men. Consequently, disapproval in interpersonal relationships may be more anxiety-provoking for females.[26] Women are also more concerned than men with both sides of an interdependent relationship.[27] Since many roles in nursing practice are composed of interdependent relationships with other professional health care representatives, the high achievement-need-motivated nurse will probably be particularly responsive to the S3 and S4 leadership styles. Concrete feedback to the individual about task performance will be particularly important to include in the incentive plan for the high-need-achievement nurse.

MEAD'S ROLE THEORY

George H. Mead was a professor of social psychology at the University of Chicago who, through his lectures, laid the foundations for what we in nursing know as role theory.[28,29] His ideas were humanistic and focused on interpersonal communication as the basis of socialization of individuals into socially desirable roles. In Mead's role theory, communication functions in humans for the development of the mind, the emergence of self as personality, the creation of social order, and the regulation of behavior toward greater cooperation. Roles are learned through the process of interpersonal communication between the "I" or an independent individual and "Me" or social control. The "generalized other" is the commonly experienced organized community, and the "significant other" is the primary person (the mother or family group) who establishes what it means to be human or socializes the infant into society generally. According to Mead, one "role takes" in the early months of life through conditioning. Later, roles are taken on through play and games. Finally, through communication, one conceptualizes the "generalized other" and takes on a role in society with the attitudes and beliefs appropriate to that role. The "I" sees "Me" seeing "I." In other words, "I see you, seeing me, seeing you." It is a reciprocal process of postive and negative feedback that the "I" learns how to behave, think, and function in society.

Some interesting research by Rosenthal and Jacobson on the concept of labeling offers strong support of Mead's theory.[30,31] *Labeling* consists of describing a person with a particular symbol or word. The way symbols are used tends to influence the way people perceive and evaluate themselves and others. Labeling serves to identify the behavior expected. Thus when you are labeled a "dingbat," "nerd," or "turkey" by your peers, the expected behavior is soon clear. You just act as if you don't have it all together: forgetful, absent-minded, illogical, and unwise.

Rosenthal and his colleagues, in one of many similar experiments, reported some test results to a group of elementary school teachers at a spring faculty meeting. The children were tested, but instead of using the test scores, the investigators randomly selected the control and experimental groups by pulling the children's names out of a hat. Some of the children were reported or labeled as having very good intellectual potential, and others were labeled as having minimal potential. The following spring, the children's grades were reviewed and compared. Those who had been labeled by the investigators as having intellectual potential had shown considerable improvement, while those labeled having little potential made considerably lower grades.

According to Rosenthal, the factors involved in producing this effect involved verbal and nonverbal interpersonal communication. Teachers of the children labeled as having intellectual potential gave more relaxed nonverbal cues such as increased eye contact, relaxed body, frequent smiling, and being nearby frequently. Verbal cues included agreeing with attitudes, beliefs, and opinions expressed by the child and providing realistic feedback about expected performance or behavior. The teachers identified desirable labels with the children, and the children were symbolically motivated to "live up to" the labels. This research design has been replicated on doctors with patients, psychology students with "bright" versus "dull" laboratory rats, camp swimming instructors and their students, and supervisors with employees.

Mead's theory and the research of investigators such as Rosenthal can be applied to the reciprocal role relationship between the leader and follower. The principle seems clear:

> *If the nursing staff is labeled positively, they will tend to live up to the labels; label them negatively and they will probably live up to that label, too.*

Instead of using "stupid," "careless," "bossy," or worse (focus on the school from which the nurse graduated or on the nurse as an associate-degree, diploma, or baccalaureate graduate), it seems logical to use such labels as "wise," "caring," or "assertive," and give more consideration to current behavior and potential than to their educational background.

Further support for Mead's role theory is provided by Peters and Waterman. These two management consultants studied successful versus unsuccessful companies in the United States, seeking to learn what the best-run, successful companies were doing that is different and unique in comparison with less successful companies. One of many characteristics involved the perspective of human beings held by managers. It is assumed that people think of themselves in an illogical manner.

> All of us are self centered, suckers for a bit of praise, and generally like to think of ourselves as winners. But the fact of the matter is that our talents are distributed normally—none of us is really as good as he or she would like to think, but rubbing our noses daily in that reality doesn't do us a bit of good. . . . the lesson that the excellent companies have to teach is that there is no reason why we can't design systems that continually reinforce this notion; most of their people are made to feel that they are winners. . . . In not-so-excellent companies, the reverse is true.[32]

In the role of a nurse leader, therefore, you in a sense become a significant other to your nursing staff. What you say, how you say it, when you say it, and with what interpersonal attitude and communication pattern is proposed as being an essential incentive in motivating your nursing staff. Your staff will tend to live up to the goals, expectations, or labels you set. You provide essential feedback to keep your staff on course, moving toward these goals. You intervene as needed according to Situational Leadership's developmental or regressive cycles with an attitude and interaction pattern that supports your staff's perception of themselves—their self esteem. You provide the primary source for supporting their social esteem needs.

You apply the organizational reward system and personnel policies as additional incentives to support the self- and social esteem, the professional growth and development of your staff.

Ganong and Ganong advise that all nursing leaders need to understand their own motivations and behavior as well as the motivation and behavior of others. Favoring Maslow's theory, they state:

> Motivation is a very personal matter. It stems from the needs of the individual. This is as true at work as it is in other areas of life. In a very real sense, then, you cannot motivate others; they motivate themselves. . . . They do act on the basis of what they feel as a desire, want, yearning, wish, or lack. The problem, of course, is that too often their actions (insubordination, lack of interest, aggressive and unruly behavior, carelessness, quitting the job, joining the union), in response to what they feel as their needs, seem inimical to administrative goals and not in the best interests of patient care. What is the manager to do?[33]

They suggest using survey instruments based on theories. As a nursing leader, you can assess your nursing staff's perception regarding what is currently serving as an incentive and contributing to their job satisfaction or motivation. This needs to be done on a regular basis. The information you receive in this manner can be the basis of an "employee care plan," which is not unlike a client or patient care plan.

> Needs/problems/goals/strengths are identified and action plans/progress notes identified. The conceptual framework for this employee care plan can be based on Maslow's five needs categories, Herzberg's set of hygienic, motivational factors and/or other theoretical/conceptual perspectives.[34]

Thus a program of incentives using interpersonal communication and based on theories and research can be designed to meet the specific motivational needs of your nursing staff.

We suggest the following statements of principle for your consideration and discussion about motivation.

> *If you, when you are the head nurse, use one or more of the motivational theories as a guide to analyze and study the behavior of your nursing staff, then you will have a higher probability of understanding their motivational needs and behaviors and of effectively motivating your staff than you will if you work without a theory.*

> *Since communication with the immediate supervisor has been noted to be a primary source of job satisfaction for nurses, you will want to discipline your communication behaviors and attitudes in a manner that will promote your staff's job satisfaction.*

> *To the same degree that you develop and implement an incentive plan for each staff member, your staff will tend to be highly motivated and productive.*

These statements of principle can serve as initial guidelines for considering how you, as a nursing leader, can have a positive influence upon the motivation of your nursing followers.

SUMMARY

In this chapter, motivation was presented as the second function of people management for leadership. Maslow's needs theory and Herzberg's two-factor theory are identified as two important theories of motivation that are useful perspectives of motivation. McClelland's description was presented of high-achievement-needs people as a type of personality that nurses might present, requiring special consideration from nursing leaders. Mead's role theory was discussed to emphasize the importance of interpersonal communication from a significant other, the nurse-leader, as a source of positive labeling for the staff nurse. Developing a systematic plan of incentives for individuals and groups of nursing staff is also suggested. The primary characteristic of any incentive is support of the positive self-image the nurse-follower may already have.

REFERENCES

1. Guralnik, D.B. *Webster's new world dictionary* (2nd ed.). New York: Prentice-Hall, 1980, p. 929.
2. Burke, K. *A rhetoric of motives.* Berkeley: University of California Press, 1969, pp. 176–177.
3. Machiavelli, N. *The prince.* New York: New American Library, 1980.
4. Maslow, A.H. *Motivation and personality.* New York: Harper & Row, 1964 .
5. Gobel. F.G. *The third force: The psychology of Abraham Maslow.* New York: Pocket Books, 1976.
6. Hersey, P., & Blanchard, K.H. *Management of organizational behavior: Utilizing human resources* (5th ed.). Englewood Cliffs, N. J.: Prentice-Hall, 1988, pp. 430–436.
7. Chenevert, M. *Special techniques in assertiveness training for women in the health professions.* St. Louis: Mosby, 1976, p. 34.
8. Hersey & Blanchard, *Management,* p. 444
9. Leadership Studies, Inc., *Essentials of Situational Leadership: Participant's manual* Escondido, Calif.: Leadership Studies Productions, Inc., 1980 , p. 100.
10. Duldt, B.W., & Giffin, K. *Theoretical perspectives of nursing.* Boston: Little, Brown, 1985, pp. 214–217.
11. Leadership Studies, Inc., *Essentials of Situational Leadership,* p. 111.
12. Herzberg, F., Mausner, B., & Snyderman, B. *The motivation to work* (2nd ed.). New York: Wiley, 1959.
13. Herzberg, F. *Work and the nature of man.* New York: World Publishing Co., 1966.
14. King, N. Clarification and evaluation of the two factor theory of job satisfaction. *Psychological Bulletin,* 1970, *74* (1), 18–31.
15. Longest, B.B., Jr. Job satisfaction for registered nurses in the hospital setting. *Journal of Nursing Administration* May–June, 1974, 46–52. *4* (3)
16. Jones, S. Job satisfaction and expressed anger. (Unpublished master's research project, East Carolina University School of Nursing, Greenville, N.C., 1985.)
17. Duldt, B.W. Coping with alienating co-workers and colleagues: The effects of training on dealing with others' anger. (Unpublished research report available from author, East Carolina University, Greenville, N. C., 1986.)
18. McClelland, D.C. *The achieving society.* Princeton, N. J.: Van Nostrand, 1961, p. 3.
19. McClelland, D.C. *Power: The inner experience.* New York: Irvingston Publishers, 1975.
20. McClelland, *The achieving society,* p. 212.
21. McClelland, D.C. Characteristics of achievers. In K. Davis & J. W. Newstrom (Eds.), *Organizational behavior: Readings and exercises,* Series in Management (6th ed.). New York: McGraw-Hill, 1981, p. 44.
22. Ibid., 45.
23. Ibid., 46.
24. McClelland, D.C. *Power: The inner experience,* p. 252–253.
25. Ibid., 74.
26. Ibid., 86.

27. Ibid., 85.
28. Mead, G.H. *Mind, self and society.* Chicago: University of Chicago Press, 1934.
29. Hardy, M. E., & Conway, M. E. *Role theory: Perspectives for health professionals.* New York: Appleton-Century-Crofts, 1978.
30. Rosenthal, R., & Jacobson, L. F. Teacher expectations for the disadvantaged. *Scientific American,* 1968, *218,* 19–31.
31. Rosenthal, R. The Pygmalion effect lives. *Psychology Today,* September 1973, p. 56.
32. Peters, T.J., & Waterman, R.H., Jr. *In search of excellence: Lessons from America's best-run companies.* New York: Warner Books, 1982, pp. 55, 57.
33. Ganong, J.M., & Ganong, W.L. *Nursing management* (2nd ed.). Rockville, Md.: Aspen, 1980, p. 267.
34. Ibid., 266–270.

6

INITIATING

INTRODUCTION

Initiating means to bring something into practice or use.[1] It is taking the first step, and it is another people-oriented function of the leader. It is taking the responsibility for introducing some new task, ideal, goal, method, or perspective to followers. Leaders are characterized as being able to originate new ideas and to think and act without necessarily being directed to do so. It involves certain personal characteristics such as courage, risk, and wisdom. Leaders need courage to speak up and risk rejection of their attempt to influence or lead others, and they need wisdom to know when to stop trying and accept rejection. Courage, risk, and wisdom primarily come with experience. While we cannot possibly do justice to these issues in this chapter, we do believe the concept of initiating needs to be carefully considered in relation to leadership roles generally and in nursing specifically.

In the Ohio State University studies to identify dimensions of leadership, researchers ultimately identified two distinct dimensions, that of "initiating structure" and of "consideration." Initiating structure refers to:

> . . . the leader's behavior in delineating the relationship between himself and members of the work group and in endeavoring to establish well defined patterns of organization, channels of communication and methods of procedure.[2]

In contrast, *consideration* refers to ". . . behavior indicative of friendship, mutual trust, respect, and warmth in the relationship between the leader and the members of his staff."[3] Initiating structure and consideration are essentially equivalent to the concepts of directive behavior and supportive behavior of Situational Leadership Theory. In this theory, *directive behavior* is the extent to which a leader engages in one-way communication by explaining what each follower is to do as well as when, where, and how tasks are to be accomplished. *Supportive behavior* is the extent to which a leader engages in two-way communication by providing socioemotional support, psychological strokes, and facilitating behaviors. The dimension of consideration and supportive behavior are discussed in the next chapter, "Facilitating."

In this chapter, four aspects are presented of the initiating dimension of leadership, or what the leader is to initiate. These four aspects are structure, communication networks, change, and impact. The ideas of scholars, researchers, and consultants from diverse fields in which leadership is studied are brought together. Where relevant, reference will be made to Situational Leadership and to Humanisitic Nursing Communication theory, with applications to nursing leadership.

STRUCTURE

To enable followers to be productive and achieve task goals, it is the responsibility of leaders to establish and maintain structure within the task or work assignment.

The work assigment refers to the manner in which the tasks are distributed to the follow-ers. Generally, there are three systems used. These are often called "control systems" because the system selected often depends on how much control upper management wants to maintain. These three types are shown in Figure 6–1.[4]

Type I is the simplest and most structured system. In business and industry, the boss controls the activities of three separate functions. The product being worked on moves in assembly-line fashion from one worker to another. This is commonly called the *functional method* of patient care assignment in nursing.[5] One nurse is assigned to medications and procedures for all patients on the unit, a second is assigned to make rounds with the doctors and process all new orders, and a third (along with assisting staff) is assigned to provide routine direct nursing care to the patients. The head nurse typically coordinates all the staff's activities and checks duties off a list as these are reported completed. The head nurse also retains responsibility for communicating with the laboratory, x-ray, dietary, and other depart-ments regarding individual patients' needs. With this approach, some patient care needs often go unnoticed, and occasionally nursing staff have been known to inform patients that "that's not my assignment today." A sense of responsibility is limited, and accountability for quality of care provided is primarily expected of the head nurse.

Type II shows *job enlargement* in that the leader still controls the worker's activities, but the workers see the end product on the assembly line. In nursing, this is commonly called the team method of patient care assignment.[6] Each nurse is assigned to give medications and treatments to certain patients, to be available when these patients' physicians make rounds and process new orders, and provide direct nursing care to these patients. The RNs may also be assigned to give medications and treatments to patients who receive direct nursing care from assisting staff (Licensed Practical Nurses, aides, orderlies, or students). The head nurse, however, continues to coordinate all activities, make all major decisions, and communicate with other hospital departments or community agencies about each patient's needs. The sense of responsibility for quality of nursing care is greater for the nursing staff, but often nurses have been frustrated because of the limited freedom to make suggestions or have input into decisions. Nursing staff often have information about the patient's condition that is not commu-

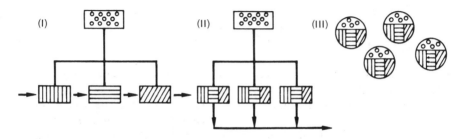

Figure 6–1. Three fundamental types of work assignment or control systems. *(From Hersey, P. & Blanchard, K. Management of organizational behavior: Utilizing human re-sources, [5th ed.]. Englewood Cliffs, N. J.: Prentice-Hall, 1988, 157, with permission.)*

nicated to the head nurse or to the physician because the staff member was not "there," but down the hall with another patient and unaware of the little "summit" meeting between the head nurse and physician. The patient assignments typically would be changed every few days so that one nurse would not have any individual patient very long.

Type III is the least structured, with each follower being assigned all functions, including responsibility for making decisions. In nursing, this is the model for primary nursing care.[7] Each nurse is assigned a case load of patients, usually no more than six or eight, depending on the complexity of care involved. This assignment would begin upon the client's admission and end upon the client's dismissal from the health agency's care, whether hospital or community agency such as home health care. The nurse provides all nursing care: giving medications and procedures, communicating with the physician and processing new orders, and providing direct nursing care. Assisting staff may be available as needed. The nurse coordinates all activities and communicates with other hospital departments or community agencies. The nurse is responsible for developing a plan of nursing care and consulting with other nurses, physicians, health care professionals, or all three, as the necessity for this is determined. The nurses who participate in primary nursing care do sense a greater degree of responsibility, and tend to take a great deal of pride in their practice. The degree of job satisfaction is enhanced, and the accountability to the client (not the patient!) is more salient. The individuality of nursing care is much more evident than with the other two types of job structure, and the quality of nursing care tends to be more humanistic in nature as perceived by the client. The mounting evidence indicates that an all-RN nursing staff providing nursing care within a primary nursing organizational structure is cost-effective in terms of significantly fewer days of hospitalization, less nursing staff required, and reduced nursing staff turnover.[8,9] Thus the structure of the work assignment can have considerable impact on the productivity of a group of people.[10]

In view of the above discussion of structure, we propose the following as a statement of principle:

> *The humanistic leader seeks to maintain minimal task structure and to delegate control of task decisions to the followers; to the degree this is accomplished, the followers will tend to assume responsibility and accountability for the quality and quantity of task performance, to take pride in their work, to experience job satisfaction, and to have a greater sense of individual worth.*

In this way, we believe structure of the task assignment can have a positive influence on productivity.

COMMUNICATION NETWORKS

Communication networks within the task group is a second aspect that is established and maintained by the task group leader, such as a head nurse, supervisor, or nursing manager. Bavelas conducted experiments to determine the kinds of communication networks that commonly emerge and to identify the networks that function most effectively for small task groups.[11] A number of networks were found to emerge and are shown in Figure 6–2.

The most common communication networks are the star (A) and the circle (F). In the star, the person in the center of the star is able to communicate with the other members of the task group, and they can communicate with the leader, but not with one another. In this

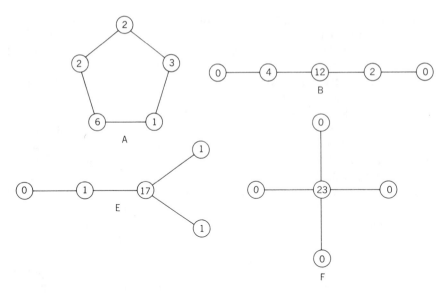

Figure 6–2. Emergence of recognized leaders in different communication networks. The number at each member's position indicates the total number of other group members who identified the person in that position as leader of the group. *(From Bavelas, A. Communication patterns in task-oriented groups. In D. Cartwright & A. Zander (Eds.) Group dynamics: Research and theory [3rd ed.]. New York: Harper & Row, 1968, 508.)*

autocratic structure, the person in the center is the boss and controls all communications. In the circle network pattern, all members are free to communicate all around the circle. Nothing in the pattern favors the leadership role for one group member over another, exemplifying a democratic structure.

Generally, research has shown that the person in the position of highest centrality tends to become the recognized leader, as in the star pattern. The organization within the group develops quickly and tends to be relatively stable. There tend to be fewer errors in task performance. The members tend to maintain the communication network in the star pattern, and the leader usually is happy and satisfied with his or her independence and power. Over time, however, the morale of group members decreases because they have so little opportunity to participate, and ultimately productivity is decreased.

On the other hand, the circle pattern tends to be slow to develop an organization for working on problems, and a leader may not emerge. These groups are slow and often inaccurate in task performance, but morale tends to be high. The members are more independent and enjoy the responsibility, the involvement in checking with other members, and the participation generally. All the group members tend to be happy and satisfied. In emergency situations, the members' relationships are generally good, so they are able to pull together and utilize all resources available to solve problems with a high degree of commitment. In contrast, the star pattern members have little commitment, and in an emergency situation tend to turn to the leader to solve the problem. While the circle pattern members are able to develop numerous checkpoints and correct most of their errors, the star pattern groups need more time to complete the tasks and make up to three and four times more errors.

We propose the following statement of principle for consideration:

In order to maintain a high level of productivity over time, an open, circular communication network within a small task group tends to be most effective because members develop a sense of responsibility, independence, and commitment in comparison with more centralized communication networks.

This statement reflects the research that demonstrates the extent that communication structure can make a difference in a group's ability to function. It can influence the group's capacity to complete a task in terms of speed, accuracy, and adaptability.

CHANGE

As a leader, you are expected to be a change master. For example, you may be asked to plan the change from functional to team nursing as an assignment control system. (See chapters 11 and 13.) This means that you need to know how to initiate change in a manner that will have a high probablity of success. In examining change, Lewin identified three phrases of the change process: unfreezing, changing, and refreezing.[12]

Unfreezing

The aim of unfreezing is to motivate and make the individual or the group ready to change. It is a thawing-out process in which the forces acting on individuals are rearranged so that now they see the need for change. According to Edgar H. Schein, when drastic unfreezing is necessary, the following common elements seem to be present: (1) the physical removal of the individuals being changed from their accustomed routines, sources of information, and social relationships; (2) the undermining and destruction of all social supports; (3) demeaning and humiliating experience to help individuals being changed to see their old attitudes or behavior as unworthy and thus to be motivated to change; (4) the consistent linking of reward with willingness to change and of punishment with unwillingness to change.[13]

In brief, unfreezing is the breaking down of the mores, customs, and traditions of individuals—the old ways of doing things—so that they are ready to accept new alternatives. In terms of force field analysis, unfreezing may occur when either the driving forces are increased or the restraining forces that are resisting change are reduced.

Changing

Once individuals have become motivated to change, they are ready to be provided with new patterns of behavior. This process is most likely to occur by one of two mechanisms: identification and internalization.[14] *Identification* occurs when one or more models are provided in the environment, models from whom individuals can learn new behavior patterns by identifying with them and trying to become like them. *Internalization* occurs when individuals are placed in a situation in which new behaviors are demanded of them if they are to operate successfully in that situation. They learn these new behavior patterns not only because the patterns are necessary to survive but because of new high-strength needs induced by coping behavior. Identification and internalization are not either/or courses of action; effective change is often the result of combining the two into a strategy for change.

Force or compliance is sometimes discussed as another mechanism for inducing change.[15]

It occurs when an individual is forced to change by the direct manipulation of rewards and punishment by someone in a power position. In this case, behavior appears to have changed when the change master (not agent!) is present, but it is often dropped when supervision is removed. Thus rather than discuss force as a mechanism of changing, it should be thought of as a tool for unfreezing.

Refreezing

The process by which the newly acquired behavior comes to be integrated as patterned behavior into the individual's personality, ongoing significant emotional relationships, or both is referred to as *refreezing*. As Schein contends, if the new behavior has been internalized while being learned,

> this has automatically facilitated refreezing because it has been fitted naturally into the individual's personality. If it has been learned through identification, it will persist only so long as the target's relationship with the original influence model persists unless new surrogate models are found or social support and reinforcement is obtained for expressions of the new attitudes.[16]

This highlights how important it is for an individual engaged in a change process to be in an environment that is continually reinforcing the change initiated. The effect of many a training program has been short-lived when the person returns to an environment that does not reinforce the new patterns or, even worse, is hostile toward them.

A major concern in refreezing is assuring that the new behavior does not get extinguished over time. To keep this from happening, reinforcement must be scheduled in an effective way. There seem to be two main reinforcement schedules: continuous and intermittent.[17] With continuous reinforcement, the individuals learn the new behavior quickly, but if their environment changes to one of nonreinforcement, extinction can be expected to take place relatively soon. With intermittent reinforcement, extinction is much slower because the individuals have been conditioned to go for periods of time without any reinforcement. Thus for fast learning, a continuous reinforcement schedule should be used. Once the individual has learned the new pattern, a switch to intermittent reinforcement should insure a long-lasting change.

Implications of this are that to send one or two head nurses or supervisors to "management charm schools" and expect them to plan and to initiate and maintain the desired changes is usually expecting too much. For the most effective initiation and implementation, plans for change need to be sanctioned by the highest administrator appropriate, perhaps even the governing board. Over a period of time nursing leaders need to provide continuous reinforcement throughout the health agency or the nursing service department. As a statement of principle, we suggest the following:

> *To the same degree the individual's environment continually reinforces the desired change, the change process will be enhanced for that individual.*

Situational Leadership assumes that people who work together need a common language. We propose that the communication styles, patterns, and attitudes identified in Situational Leadership and Humanistic Nursing Communication theories can provide a basis of common language for nurses in a health agency. We believe the common language provided by these two theories would enable nurses to work more effectively among themselves and with peers and colleagues.

IMPACT

In the initiation of structure, communication networks, or change, the leader needs to consider the impact of what is being initiated. As a leader, you need to focus on four levels of change as it impacts on people: knowledge, attitudes, behavior, and group or organizational performance.[18] The time relationship and the relative difficulty involved in making each of these levels of change when force or compliance is not a factor is illustrated in Figure 6–3. Of the four levels, the initiation of plans and change in a group or organizational performance is perhaps the most difficult and time-consuming. The future of nursing may in fact be dependent upon how well knowledge of the behavioral sciences is used in understanding and gaining acceptance of plans as well as initiating these plans and change.[19]

Changes in knowledge tend to be the easiest to make; they can occur as a result of reading a book or an article or hearing something new from a respected person. Attitude structures differ from knowledge structures in that they are emotionally charged in a positive or negative way. The addition of emotion often makes attitudes more difficult to change than knowledge.

Changes in individual behavior seem to be significantly more difficult and time consuming than either of the two previous levels. For example, a head nurse may have knowledge about the advantages of increased nursing staff involvement and participation in decision making and may even feel that such participation would improve staff performance, and yet, be unable to delegate or share decision-making reponsibilities significantly with staff. This discrepancy between knowledge, attitude, and behavior may be a result of the nurse's authoritarian management–subordinate upbringing or mentoring. Past experience has led to a habit pattern that feels comfortable. This tends to be true for many people.

While individual behavior is difficult enough to change, it becomes even more complicated when you try to initiate change within groups or organizations. The leadership styles of one or two head nurses might be effectively altered, but drastically changing the level of staff participation throughout an entire health agency might be a very time-consuming process. At this level one is trying to alter customs, mores, and traditions that have developed over many years. As a statement of principle, we propose the following:

As the level of change moves from knowledge, to attitudes, to individual behavior, to group behavior, the amount of time and effort required of the leader in order to effect the changes increases proportionately.

The impact of initiating change affects not only levels of change, as described, but also has impact on the manner in which change is initiated. Now one needs to consider the three interacting dimensions of changing together: levels, cycles, and process of change.

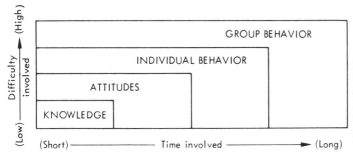

Figure 6–3. Time and difficulty in initiating various changes. *(From Hersey, P., & Blanchard, K. Management of organizational behavior: Utilizing human resources [5th ed.]. Englewood Cliffs, N. J.: Prentice-Hall, 1988, 14, with permission.)*

Cycles of Change

The impact of initiating change affects not only levels of change, as described, but also it impacts on the manner in which change is initiated. There are two ways identified, participative and directive change cycles, which leaders can choose.[20]

Participative Change Cycle

A *participative change cycle* is implemented when new knowledge is made available to the individual or group. It is hoped that the group will accept the data and will develop a positive attitude and commitment in the direction of the desired change. At this level an effective strategy may be to involve the individual nurse or entire group of nurses directly in helping to select or formalize the new methods for obtaining the desired goals. This is group participation in problem solving.

The next step will be to attempt to translate this commitment into actual behavior. This step is significantly more difficult to achieve. For example, it is one thing to be concerned about increasing nurse-follower participation in decision making (attitude), but another thing to be willing actually to get involved in doing something (behavior) about the issue. An effective strategy may be to identify the informal and formal nursing leaders among the staff group(s) and concentrate on gaining their behavioral support for the desired change. Once this is accomplished, organizational change may be effected by getting other people to pattern their behavior after those nurses whom they respect and perceive in leadership roles. This participative change cycle is illustrated in Figure 6–4.

Directive Change Cycle

We have all probably been faced with a situation similar to the one in which there is an announcement on Monday morning that "As of today all nursing staff members of this medical center will begin to operate in accordance with Form 10125 for requisitioning all diagnostic services." This is an example of a *directive change cycle*. It is through this change cycle that many nursing leaders in the past have attempted to implement such innovative ideas as management by objectives, problem-oriented charting, quality assurance, and the like.

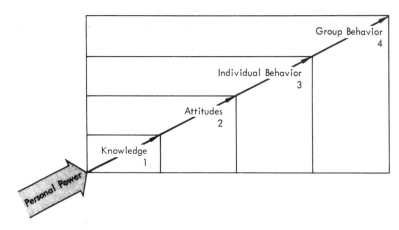

Figure 6–4. Participative change cycle. *(From Hersey, P., & Blanchard, K. Management of organizational behavior: Utilizing human resources [5th ed.]. Englewood Cliffs, N.J.: Prentice-Hall, 1988, 340, with permission).*

This change cycle begins by change being imposed on the total organization by some external force, such as higher management, health laws, or accreditation standards. This will tend to affect the interaction network system at the individual level. The new contacts and modes of behavior create new knowledge, which tends to develop predispositions toward or against the change. The directive change cycle is illustrated in Figure 6–5.

In some cases where change is forced, the new behavior engaged in creates the kind of knowledge that develops commitment to change, and, therefore, begins to approximate a participative change as it reinforces the individual and group behavior. The hope is that "if people will only have a chance to see how the new system works, they will support it."

Is There a "Best" Strategy for Change?

Given a choice between polarities of directive and participative change, most people would tend to give the nod in our society to the participative change cycle. Just as we have argued in discussing Situational Leadership, however, there is no "best" leadership style; there also is no best strategy for planning and implementing change. Effective change "masters" (not agents!) are identified as those who can adapt their strategies to the demands of their unique environment. Thus the participative change cycle is not a better change strategy than the directive change cycle, and vice versa. The appropriate strategy depends on the situation, and there are advantages and disadvantages to each.

Advantages and Disadvantages of Change Cycles

The participative change cycle tends to be more appropriate for working with individuals and groups who are achievement motivated, seek responsibility, and have a degree of knowledge and experience that may be useful in developing new ways of operating—in other words, people with task-relevant maturity, such as nurses and other health care professionals. Once the change starts, these people are much more capable of assuming responsibilities for implementation of the desired change. Although these people may welcome change and the need to improve, they may become very rigid and opposed to change if it is implemented in a directive (the high directive, low supportive style of Situational Leadership theory) manner. A directive

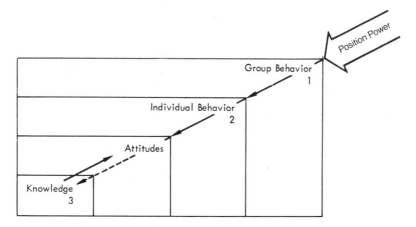

Figure 6–5. Directive change cycle. *(From Hersey, P., & Blanchard, K. Management of organizational behavior: Utilizing human resources [5th ed.]. Englewood Cliffs, N.J.: Prentice-Hall, 1988, 341, with permission.)*

change style is inconsistent with their perceptions of themselves as mature, responsible, self-motivated people who should be consulted throughout the change process. When they are not consulted, and change is implemented in an authoritarian manner, conflict often results. Examples of this occur frequently in hospitals in which a nursing administrator recruits or inherits a competent, creative staff that is willing to work hard to implement new programs, and then proceeds to bypass the staff completely in the change process. This style results in resistance and is inappropriate to the situation.

A coercive, directive change style might be very appropriate and more productive with individuals and groups who are less ambitious, are often dependent, and who are not willing to take new responsibilities unless forced to do so. In fact, these people *might prefer* direction and structure from their leader to being faced with decisions they are not mature or experienced enough to make. Once again, diagnosis is all-important. It is just as inappropriate for a nursing administrator to attempt to implement change in a participative manner with a staff that has never been given the opportunity to take responsibility and has become dependent on its manager for direction as it is to implement change in a coercive manner with a staff that is ready to change and willing to take responsibility for implementing it.

There are other significant differences between these two change cycles. The participative change cycle tends to be effective when induced by nursing leaders who have *personal power;* that is, they have referent information and expert power. On the other hand, the directive cycle necessitates that a nursing leader have significant *position power,* that is, coercive, connection, reward, and legitimate power.

If nursing leaders decide to implement change in an authoritarian, coercive manner, they would be wise to have the support of their superiors and other sources of power or they may be effectively blocked by their staff.

With the participative change cycle, a significant advantage is that once the change is accepted, it tends to be long-lasting. Since everyone has been involved in the development of the change, each person tends to be more highly committed to its implementation. The disadvantage of participative change is that it tends to be slow and evolutionary—it may take years to implement a significant change. An advantage of directive change, on the other hand, is speed. Using position power, leaders can often impose change immediately. This is very appropriate in an emergency or crisis situation in clinical nursing practice. A disadvantage of this change strategy is that it tends to be volatile. It can be maintained only as long as the leader has position power to make it stick. It often results in animosity, hostility, and, in some cases, overt and covert behavior to undermine and overthrow.

In terms of force field analysis, discussed later (see Chapter 9), the directive change cycle could be utilized if the power of the driving forces pushing for change far outweighed the restraining forces resisting change. On the other hand, a directive change cycle would be doomed to failure if the power of the restraining forces working against the change was more frequent and powerful than the power of the driving forces pushing for the change.

A participative change cycle that depends on personal power could be appropriate in either of the cases described. With frequent and powerful driving forces pushing for change in the situation, a nurse-leader might not have to use a high-task, directive-change cycle since the driving forces are ready to run with the change already and do not have to be forced to engage in the new desired behavior. At the same time, when the restraining forces could easily overpower the driving forces, nursing administrators would be advised to begin with participative change techniques designed gradually to turn some of the restraining forces into driving forces or at least immobilize their influence in the situation. In other words, when things are stacked against one, it would seen to be more effective trying to reeducate the forces against the change than trying to force change in a situation when little power is on the side of the change effort.

These two change cycles have been described as if they were either/or positions. The use of only one of these change cycles exclusively, however, could lead to problems. For example, if nursing supervisors introduce change only in a high directive-low supportive style or manner without any movement toward participative change, their head nurses and nursing staff, if they decide to remain, may react in one of two ways. Some may fight the supervisors tooth and nail and organize efforts to undermine them. Others may buckle under to their authority and become very passive, dependent nurses, always needing the superivsors to tell them what to do and when to do it before doing anything. These people say yes to anything the supervisors want, and then moan and groan and drag their feet later. Neither of these responses makes for a very healthy situation within the nursing units, the entire nursing service department, or the health agency. At the other extreme, supervisors who will not make a move without checking with their nursing staff and getting full approval also can immobilize themselves. They may establish such a complicated network of "participative" committees that significant change becomes almost impossible.

Thus in reality, it is more a question of the proper blend of the directive and participative change cycles, depending on the situation, than a forced choice between one or another.[21]

SUMMARY

This chapter presented the initiating process, which is innately characteristic of leadership. Several particular areas are suggested in which a nursing leader is expected to be a self-starter and get things moving. One area is the structure of the task or work to be done; the way a task is arranged and the degree of control required by the nursing leader can influence the productivity and morale of the nursing staff. This has also been found to be true in relation to initiating communication networks among task groups or nursing staff. The manner in which a nursing leader initiates change, the cycles of change, makes a difference in how lasting that change can be. Four levels in people are described, groups of followers or nursing staff; whatever is initiated will move like a wave through these four levels. A reasonable amount of time needs to be allocated for this wave to make its impact. Patience is needed in order to repeatedly restate directives. Wisdom is needed in knowing whether or not to continue initiating.

REFERENCES

1. Guralnik, D.B. *Webster's new world dictionary* (2nd ed.). New York: Prentice-Hall, 1980, p. 725.
2. Halpin, A.W. *The leadership behavior of school superintendents.* Chicago: Midwest Administration Center, The University of Chicago, 1959, p. 4.
3. Ibid.
4. Hersey, P., & Blanchard, K. *Management of organizational behavior: Utilizing human resources,* (5th ed.). Englewood Cliffs, N.J.: Prentice-Hall, 1988, pp. 156–157.
5. Kron, T. *The management of patient care.* Philadelphia: Saunders, 1981, pp. 228–232.

6. Ibid.

7. Ibid.

8. Fagin, C.M. The economic value of nursing research. *American Journal of Nursing,* 1982, *12,* 1844–1849.

9. Felton, G. Increasing the quality of nursing care by introducing the concept of primary nursing: A model project. *Nursing Research,* 1975, *24* (1), 27–32.

10. Hersey & Blanchard, *Managment.* p. 155–157.

11. Bavelas, A. Communication patterns in task-oriented groups. In D. Cartwright & A. Zander (Eds.). *Group dynamics: Research and theory* (3rd ed.). New York: Harper & Row, 1968, pp. 503–511.

12. Lewin, K. Frontiers in group dynamics: Concept, method, and reality in social science; social equilibria and social change. *Human Relations,* 1947, (*I* (1), 5.

13. Schein, E.H. Management development as a process of influence. In Hamptom, D.R. (Ed.). *Behavioral concepts in management.* Belmont, Calif.: Dickinson Publishing Co., 1968, p. 110.

14. Kelman, H.C. Compliance, identification and internalization: Three processes of attitude change. *Conflict Resolution,* 1958, *II,* 51–60.

15. Ibid.

16. Schein, Management development, p. 112.

17. Ferster, C.B., Skinner, B.G., *Schedules of reinforcement.* New York: Appleton-Century-Crofts, 1957.

18. House, R.J. *Management development: Design, implementation and evaluation.* Ann Arbor: Bureau of Industrial Relations, University of Michigan, 1967.

19. Hersey & Blanchard, *Management,* 2, 340–341.

20. Hersey, P, & Blanchard, K. Change and the use of power. *Training and Development Journal,* 1972, *26* (1), 6.

21. Hersey & Blanchard, *Management,* 339–344.

7

FACILITATING

INTRODUCTION

Facilitating is generally defined as making the task easily accomplished in consideration of the needs of the group and their goals. In the human relations movement, the facilitator function was developed to assist participants of sensitivity groups in achieving personal growth and sensitivity to interpersonal relationships. The facilitator served as the role model of being warm and accepting, dialogical, considerate of individual goals and needs, and a "social engineer" in that knowledge and expertise in group dynamics was made available to the group. The functions of the facilitator are recognized as "consideration," a dimension of leadership identified by the Ohio State University Leadership Studies. *Consideration* is defined as the ". . . behavior indicative of friendship, mutual trust, respect, and warmth in the relationship between the leader and members of his staff."[1]

One tenet of the human relations movement is that the real central force of an organization lies in the interpersonal relationships within the work or task group. The implication of this belief is that an organization needs to be developed around the people who make things happen rather than attempting to force people into a preconceived organizational mold, a basic tenet of Taylorism and scientific management of the early 1900s. This earlier management approach allowed the tail to wag the dog, as it were. While extremist facets of the human relations movement have since waned, its influence is still felt today. Most modern management or leadership theories, research, and practice support the idea that recognition of human feelings and attitudes is an important aspect of leadership. Facilitating cooperative behavior among task group members and providing opportunities for the followers' personal and professional growth and development tends to result in a more effective organization.[2]

Facilitating by the leader is analogous to the "supportive behavior" of Situational Leadership theory. Here, supportive behavior is defined as: "the extent to which a leader maintains personal relationships with followers by engaging in two-way communication by providing socio-emotional support, psychological strokes, and facilitating behaviors."[3] Facilitating also involves the humanizing attitudes and patterns of interaction of Humanistic Nursing Communication theory.

The purpose of this chapter is to explore in depth the facilitating process of the people-oriented functions of nurse-leaders in maintaining personal relationships with their followers or nursing staff. The facets of the facilitating process that are discussed in this chapter emphasize the relationship of interpersonal trust, self-disclosure, and feedback in the leader–follower relationship. Using the traditional client–therapist relationship model, similarities and differences shall be distinguished between the roles of therapist and leader.

The concept of trust is a key factor in the development of confidence, and Mead's role theory regarding the development of confidence will be discussed and how this is applied to the organizational context will be described. Likert's contributions to Theory X and Theory Y will be considered, as are contributions of selected scholars. Ways that a nursing leader can develop the facilitating role and establish an interpersonal climate conducive to open communication will be considered. Underlying all, trust remains a particularly delicate issue in contemporary health care organizations in which human values daily vie with pragmatic bureaucracy.

TRUST

The ambiguity of *trust* as a concept is unique, since it is an important element of interpersonal relationships, and thus presents challenges to theorists and researchers.[4] There are several definitions of trust; however, the one by Patton and Giffin,[5] which is a composite of several scholars' views, seems to be most appropriate to the study of nursing leadership:

> Trust is defined here as an attitude in that it involves perceptions, feelings, and behavior tendencies. It involves congnition of a situation,[6] degree of positive or negative feelings,[7] and a potential for action under certain conditions.[8]

Trusting behavior, according to Patton and Giffin, involves the following dimensions, which are, incidentally, used as the definition of trust in Humanistic Nursing Communication Theory.

1. One is relying on another person or persons.
2. There is risk of some potential loss.
3. One is attempting to achieve some goal or gain.
4. This desired goal is uncertain.
5. One's potential loss if this trust is violated is greater than the potential gain if one's trust is fulfilled.[9]

We can apply these dimensions of trusting behavior to nursing. Just as "one relies on another," so clients or patients rely on nurses. Their risk involves some potential injury to their bodies. They are seeking relief from pain or discomfort, and their goal is an improved health status. Whether or not they can achieve this goal is often uncertain. Their potential loss, a diminished health status, is often greater than the potential gain if nurses violate their trust. In a similar fashion, your nursing staff relies on you as their leader. Their risk involves some potential injury to their professional careers and personal livelihood. They are seeking professional and personal gratification and fulfillment through helping others, as well as meeting basic needs and needs for social esteem and self-esteem. Their potential loss, if you violate their trust in you to protect and support them, is loss of professional reputation, isolation and rejection, legal problems, and even possible loss of licensure and the right to practice. Most nurses can even think of specific incidences to further validate the application of these dimensions of trust to nursing in a more personal way.

Patton and Giffin also present a theoretical paradigm in which both interpersonal and intrapersonal trust is involved.

1. Trust of a speaker by a listener, called "ethos" by Aristotle and "source credibility" by C. Hovland, I. L. Janis, and H. H. Kelley;[10]
2. Trust of a listener by a speaker, called "sense of psychological safety" by Rogers,[11] "perceived supportive climate" by Gibb,[12] and "speech confidence" (rather than "anxiety") as described by Giffin, Bradley and Patton;[13]

3. Trust of oneself as a speaker—a person's perception of himself/herself as a communicator capable of achieving a desired goal in a situation perceived as risky or threatening (the opposite of speech anxiety);
4. Trust of oneself as a listener—a person's perception of himself/herself as a listener capable of achieving a desired goal in a situation perceived as risky or threatening.[14]

In applying this theoretical paradigm of trust to the relationship between a nursing leader and her followers, we have the following:

1. The nursing followers must trust the nursing leader.
2. The nursing leader must trust the nursing followers.
3. Both must trust themselves as speakers.
4. Both must trust themselves as listeners.

In other words, the nursing staff need to trust the nursing leader to support them and to tell them the truth. The nursing leader needs to trust the nursing staff to try to understand directives and so on, and to carefully carry out their assignments to the best of their abilities. The nurse-leader and the nursing staff need to trust themselves as speakers in that facts and feelings will be related in as clear and correct a manner as possible. So the leader and the nursing staff also need to trust themselves so that, as they listen to one another, they will honestly try to interpret and understand what is being said in the way the speaker intends.

The trust nurses have in one another influences two factors: communication behavior (patterns of interaction) and the results of interaction. The relationship between these two factors is *reflexive,* according to Patton and Giffin. This means that, as you trust another person, you see this trust reflected back to you in the other person's behavior. It is like looking at yourself in a mirror: You smile and your reflected image smiles back. As the degree of trust between you and another increases in this reflexive manner, your patterns of interaction change, and this change tends to further increase the degree of trust you have for one another.[15] As some of us have experienced, the opposite also tends to occur. Just as trust tends to reflect more trust, so distrust reflects more distrust. It is like the old saying: "What goes around, comes around!" Since leaders establish the interpersonal climate for all group members, you, as the nursing leader, must set the direction of this reflexive interaction by trusting your staff nurses.

What are these communication behaviors that a nursing leader needs to display in order to initiate this reciprocal trusting interpersonal climate? In an extensive review of the speech credibility literature, Giffin concludes that trust of a speaker by a listener tends to be influenced by three characteristics of the speaker:

1. *Expertness relevant to the topic under discussion;* this expertise may be in the form of quantity of pertinent information, degree of ability or skill, or validity of judgment.
2. *Reliability;* this may be perceived as dependability, predictability, consistency, or intentions of the trusted person regarding the goals or objectives of the person doing the trusting.
3. *Dynamism;* that is, behavior perceived as more active than passive and more open or frank than closed or reserved.[16]

We can derive the following general principle from the above:

If you as a nurse-leader, display communication behavior that is noteworthy because of the qualities of expertness, reliability, and dynamism conveyed, then you will tend to be trusted by your followers or nursing staff.

It is important to establish and maintain your nursing staff's trust in you because you need their cooperation and good will in order to accomplish the tasks required of all members of the group. It would not be necessary to have their help if you could singlehandedly provide the nursing care required of all the patients or clients assigned to your clinical unit. What you cannot achieve alone can be accomplished by the total group, you and the nursing staff. In order to accomplish this with the high degree of accuracy required in nursing practice, you need to know your people will tell you the things you need to know. You want them to self-disclose to you.

SELF-DISCLOSURE

In Humanistic Nursing Communication theory, self-disclosure in interpersonal communication is defined as risking rejection in telling how one feels, thinks, reacts, and perceives regarding here-and-now events. When one decides to tell another something about oneself that cannot be discovered through other channels, one is self-disclosing. It is allowing another to know one as one is now. Examples of self-disclosing include: the wife telling her husband she no longer loves him; the nursing student telling the instructor the real reason he or she was late for clinical; or the staff nurse telling the head nurse about having discharged a child without telling the mother how to care for the dressings. It involves interpersonal authenticity, openness, and integrity.[17] It also involves risk because it requires that the self-discloser trust the listener. Thus, a second general principle can be derived from the statement that the speaker must trust the listener before self-disclosing:

> *The nursing staff must trust the nursing leader before they will be able to report (self-disclose) important information about professional (and perhaps personal) matters.*

This is, to some degree, similar to the therapeutic relationship as studied in psychiatric nursing.
    The traditional model of the therapist–client relationship involves self-disclosure on the part of the client. This requires the client to trust the therapist. Before the client can trust the therapist, however, he or she must perceive the therapist as being accepting; the client must feel psychologically safe; the therapist is seen as supporting the client; and the therapist is communicating unconditional postive regard:[18]

> . . . essential for therapeutic movement and change is the experiencing by the therapist of an unconditional postive regard for the client. This means that the therapist communicates to his client a deep and genuine caring for him as a person with human potentialities, a caring uncontaminated by evaluations of his thoughts, feelings or behaviors . . . and places no conditions on his acceptance and warmth. . . . It means not making judgments.[19]

Rogers and Truax also state that this unconditional positive regard is an essential element in developing an effective therapeutic relationship.[22] This attitude of positive regard that the nursing leader has for the nursing staff is crucial in establishing and maintaining an interpersonal climate of trust. The leadership role differs from the therapist role in that the leader of necessity places conditions on the relationship. Judgment and evaluation of performance are necessary to the leadership role in a task group, and the follower is expected to meet specified performance criteria. See page 337–338 of this text for further discussion of positive regard versus disregard of staff by the nursing leader. Positive regard of each nursing staff member as a person is an important aspect in the development of trust.

Jack Gibb, well known for his descriptions of supportive and defensive climates in groups and in management, also considers the role of trust.[20] He identifies six types of nonaccepting leader behaviors that tend to produce a defensive climate and six others that tend to result in a supportive climate. These are as follows:

Supportive	**Defensive**
Descriptive	Evaluative
Problem-orientated	Control-oriented
Spontaneous	Strategy-oriented
Empathetic	Neutral (detached)
Egalitarian	Superior
Provisionalistic	Certain

We suggest that you, as a nursing leader, need to include these supportive leader behaviors in your communication behaviors in order to establish an interpersonal climate in which your nursing staff will self-disclose. Gibb believes high levels of trust and having confidence in people are essential factors in participative management styles having supportive climates. He stresses the importance of trust, confidence, warmth, and acceptance or positive regard as essential to developing a supportive climate. In this climate, the manager as well as the staff shares (self-discloses) information, feelings, and attitudes, and thereby establishes a free exchange of information in all directions. In contrast, defensive management styles have unsupporting climates that include distrust, distortion of data, strategic persuasion, and high control. In this climate, the manager camouflages true feelings and may not share accurate or complete information; people are manipulated in order to reach goals.[21]

There are advantages in being proactive and attempting to establish an interpersonal climate of trust in the task group. According to Likert and Haney, once the distrustful, defensive climate occurs, a cycle of low trust leading to low performance usually is established.[22,23] Without trust and support of the leader, the follower functions with minimal compliance and resentment. "Since I won't get credit for doing anything extra, I might as well give him what he thinks of me," is the perspective of the follower. The follower cannot be expected to break this cycle; this would require responding with high performance in order to win the respect of the low-trusting leader. The leader, however, *can* break the cycle by responding to low performance with high trust.[24] After a nursing staff member has demonstrated some ineffective performance, you as the head nurse, might say, for example, "Well, that didn't work out very well for you that time; since you usually do things so well, I bet you will be able to handle it next time."

Gibb's supportive and defensive climates in management are analogous to Douglas McGregor's Theory X and Theory Y. The assumptions of Theory X about human nature, which are derived from Maslow's hierarchy of needs, are summarized by Hersey and Blanchard as follows:

1. Work is inherently distasteful to most people.
2. Most people are not ambitious, have little desire for responsibility, and prefer to be directed.
3. Most people have little capacity for creativity in solving organizational problems.

4. Motivation occurs only at the physiological and safety levels.
5. Most people must be closely controlled and often coerced to achieve organizational objectives.[25]

The traditional organization has centralized decision making, a superior–subordinate pyramidlike structure, and high control of work by the superiors. (See also the discussions of organizational structure in Chapter 10.) Theory X assumes that most people are motivated by money, fringe benefits, and threat of punishment. A supervisor closely controls the subordinates' work because they cannot be trusted.

Believing that management practices needed to be based on a more accurate understanding of human nature and motivation, McGregor developed an alternate theory, Theory Y. As summarized by Hersey and Blanchard, this theory makes the following assumptions about human nature:

1. Work is as natural as play, if the conditions are favorable.
2. Self-control is often indispensable in achieving organizational goals.
3. The capacity for creativity in solving organizational problems is widely distributed in the population.
4. Motivation occurs at the social, esteem, and self-actualization levels, as well as physiological and security levels.
5. People can be self-directed and creative at work if properly motivated.[26]

If one makes these assumptions, according to McGregor, then the primary task of management is to unleash this potential in people. Thus, Theory Y managers are supportive and facilitating, decision making is decentralized, and people express their feelings and ideas, experimenting and helping one another. Managers help the employees achieve job maturity by allowing them to assume more and more self-control. The managers and employees trust one another.[27]

As we think about Gibb's ideas, we can derive a third principle for establishing a climate of trust:

A nursing staff member will trust you, the nursing leader, more when you respond to the staff member's self-disclosures with acceptance rather than rejection.[28]

For example, you can decide what communication patterns and attitudes you display in response to a nursing staff member who has made a serious mistake—maybe even to the extent that a patient or client is inadvertently injured. Since no one is infallible, there is a probability that such an event will occur. This just goes with the territory of leadership. There is a high probability that you will continue to be associated with and responsible for this staff person long after the mistake has been analyzed, implications noted, reports signed in triplicate, and the incident forgotten. You can choose to view yourself standing beside the staff member as both of you quietly look at the problem before you. This is displaying high trust, positive regard, acceptance, and a supportive climate, described by Gibb, Likert, Haney, and others. Or you can choose to think of yourself standing before the staff member, looking at her as if *she* were the problem. We hope you choose the former and avoid initiating the low trust–low performance cycle.

Research supports the idea that reciprocal self-disclosure increases trust. Tubbs and Baird report several such studies in their discussion of the development of trust, suggesting that "openness begets openness." "These studies tend to support the thesis that *if one wishes to invite disclosure from another person, an effective means of doing so is to engage in the activity oneself.*"[29] Tubbs and Baird note, however, that while high levels of self-disclosure may be pleasing to the discloser, there is a curvilinear effect. Self-disclosure tends to be reciprocal up to a point. Disclosure of very personal information seems to increase anxiety and determines the point at which reciprocity decreases. Reciprocal self-disclosing seems to be saying, "I like you, and I trust you." Some research suggests that a social norm requires that disclosures tend to be of comparable value.[30] So one needs to develop some sense of social wisdom about disclosing comparable information that is not so personal that one experiences regret. As a nursing leader, however, you are rewarding your nursing staff member by self-disclosing something relevant, and in the process you are obligating the staff member to reciprocate further.

We can derive the following principle from this discussion of self-disclosing:

A staff member will trust you, the nursing leader, more when you respond to the staff member's self-disclosure by reciprocally self-disclosing than when you do not.[31]

In the study of superior-subordinate relationships in an organization, the degree of trust existing between leaders and their followers has been found to be an important factor in the followers' decision to communicate openly with the leader.[32] So, in developing your nursing staff's trust, in you as their leader, you need to show acceptance by responding with such comments as, "I can understand how you feel," or "I can see how important that is to you." You need to reciprocate by self-disclosing some comparable information about how you perceive or feel about the subject being discussed. In the process, you can still maintain performance standards when providing feedback.

FEEDBACK

After self-disclosing, the listener provides feedback. In Humanistic Nursing Communication theory, *feedback* is defined as describing another's behavior, beliefs, and so on, plus giving one's evaluation or feelings. The important aspect of feedback is that it provides reality-oriented information about one's self and about relationships. By self-disclosing, one receives the benefits of interpersonal feedback necessary to self-concept.

Self-disclosure and feedback is considered essential to the development of self according to Mead's role theory.[33,34] Mead proposes that roles are learned in the process of social interaction. In the interaction process, people see themselves and the other person(s) as occupants of particular statuses and respond accordingly with appropriate behaviors. Because of the intense contact and influence during childhood, family members and the mother in particular are proposed to be the "significant others" who establish for each person what it means to be human. Communication functions to develop the mind, the self-concept, and social order, for the purpose of regulating behavior and moving each person toward greater cooperation. By interacting with members of a family, and later with co-workers and associates, each person learns role behaviors that are appropriate within the group and develops an understanding of the social world as an organized community, the generalized other.

Thus, it is through this "I see you, seeing me, seeing you" interaction that we develop our self-concept. We assume that the feedback we receive from people whom we trust is honest and authentic. If it is not, we can develop low self-esteem. For example, sexual harassment can be particularly destructive to one's self-concept. It is a dehumanizing interpersonal interaction that not only alienates the harassee, but also provides untrustworthy feedback about one's self, one's capabilities, and one's status in a group or in society generally. It can leave the harassee shaken and distressed if it is not perceived for what it is—the acting out of the harasser's interpersonal inadequacies. Now for that example: Assuming the harasser is a man, the process is described by Duldt in the following manner.

> The typical pattern used by the harasser is to initially praise a woman's work and evaluate job performance very highly. Upon refusal of his sexual advances, however, the harasser's evaluation of the victim's job performance becomes very negative. This is particularly destructive. What can the woman believe—the very positive or very negative evaluation? Even discounting the poor evaluation after rejection, the question remains: Was the positive evaluation true or was it too a sham? How well am I really doing my job? What is reality? Since the harasser is often the supervisor, these questions usually go unanswered. The harassee feels there is no one to trust, and, perhaps worse, begins to doubt her own judgment.[35]

According to Rosabeth Moss Kanter, even in the most impersonal of institutions, the personal and social problem of trust remains. This personal discretion is not a technical but a very human question.[36] Whose feedback can be trusted? These were fundamental concerns of the administrations of Presidents Richard Nixon and Ronald Reagan.

Tubbs and Baird identify four types of feedback: clarifying, personal reaction, judgmental reaction, and interpretation.[37] *Clarifying* is helpful feedback that involves restating the self-discloser's comments to validate your understanding of them in the manner intended. You might preface your feedback with "Did you mean to say . . ." or "If I understand you correctly, you feel that. . . ." The self-discloser then has opportunity to clarify intended meaning so that misunderstandings are avoided.

The *personal reaction* is also a helpful type of feedback because the listener is able to tell the self-discloser how he or she is "coming across." Personal reactions might include, "When you talk about being a graduate of Duke, I feel like you are bragging, and it turns me off," or "When you were supportive of Mary's idea, I felt good." These emphasize the personal and special way of responding to the self-discloser. This type of feedback is often preceded by such phrases as "To me, that seemed . . ." or "In my opinion, . . ." or "My reaction to that is . . ." This allows others the option to have different reactions. While Tubbs and Baird state that this kind of feedback is rarely experienced in normal everyday interpersonal communication, it is exceptionally helpful and constructive.

Judgmental reaction is a type of feedback that adds an evaluation or judgment. It tends to produce defensiveness in the other person and generally is not appreciated. Examples include such comments as, "I don't like it when you talk so much; why don't you just be quiet?" and "I feel uncomfortable when you try to direct the group; why don't you just leave us alone and stop being so bossy?" The first part of each phrase is appropriate, but the evaluation and directive in the second part are unnecessary. It is best to avoid giving unsolicited advice such as this.

Interpretive feedback involves making an observation about the person's behavior and making assumptions about the meaning. For example: "You have been looking really depressed and sad all morning; are you trying to get me to feel sorry for you?" and "You did not

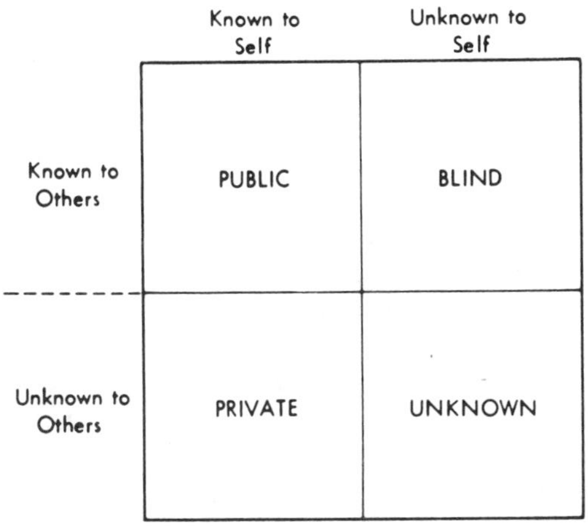

	Known to Self	Unknown to Self
Known to Others	PUBLIC	BLIND
Unknown to Others	PRIVATE	UNKNOWN

Figure 7–1. The Johari window. *(From Hersey, P., & Blanchard, K. Management of organizational behavior: Utilizing human resources. [5th ed.] Englewood Cliffs, N.J.: Prentice-Hall, 1988, p. 276, with permission.)*

meet me at 4 P.M. as we agreed, and I did not wait for you; I think you were making a power play and manipulating me." Such interpretations rarely are accurate, and even if they are true, the person receiving this feedback tends to deny it. Tubbs and Baird state that even highly trained behavioral experts are cautious about making inferences.

The framework developed by Luft and Ingham, called the *Johari window,* provides another perspective of self-disclosure and feedback.[38]* Most nurses are probably familiar with the Johari window from courses in psychiatric nursing, where it is typically applied to general personality. Hersey and Blanchard, however, have used this framework to describe *leadership personality.*[39] This differs from leadership style in that it consists only of an individual's leader behavior as perceived by others. Leadership personality refers to self-perception and the perception of others.

According to this framework, there are communication behaviors (patterns) and/or attitudes displayed by your leader personality that you know about yourself, the *known to self* area. You know the way you are coming across and the impact you are having with people you are attempting to influence. In addition, part of your leader personality is *unknown to self;* you are unaware of how you appear to others. This means you have not been given feedback by others or that you just have not noticed some of the verbal or nonverbal feedback that actually exists in your organizational environment. A third and fourth area of the leader personality includes both communication behaviors (patterns) and attitudes that are *known to others* and *unknown to others.* These four areas complete the window as shown in Figure 7–1.

In the organizational setting, the area that is known to self and to others is labeled the *public* area. That which is unknown to self, you as the leader, is referred to as the *blind area.* As the leader, you are unaware because you have not received feedback from your associates and followers, or you have covertly communicated that you are not able to know or do not want to know this area. An area known only to yourself is the *private* area. You choose not to disclose this to people in the organization, or your associates and followers have not picked up

---

*See also: Luft, J., & Ingham, H. The johari window, a graphic model of interpersonal awareness, *Proceedings of the Western Training Laboratory in Group Development,* Los Angeles: UCLA Extension Office, 1955.

behavioral responses available to them. The area unknown to you and to others is labeled *unknown*. This is analogous to an iceberg; only the tip is seen and the huge part below the water is beyond view.

Feedback in this framework is defined as the extent to which others in the organizational setting are willing to share with leaders how they are coming across. Some managers cut off and eventually stifle feedback by arguing with their followers about their feelings and perceptions. For example, a staff nurse may tell the head nurse that the nursing unit meetings are too long and "generally a waste of my time." The head nurse, rather than listening to the staff nurse's feelings and trying to find out why he or she feels that way about the meetings, responds quickly and harshly, "What do you mean, those meetings are a waste of time? I'm sick and tired of your attitude around here. I think those meetings are the most productive sessions we have had around here for a long time. And I'm sick and tired of this kind of ridiculous comment." If you were the staff nurse, would you try to provide more feedback to this head nurse? Probably not. This staff nurse learned that feelings are not allowed unless they are in line with nursing administration. Without feedback from nursing staff, a nursing leader will develop significant blind areas that will eventually damage effectiveness.

Feelings need to be heard and accepted; it is only behavior that needs to be limited. Everyone is an expert on his or her own feelings and perceptions. Leaders should never say to their staff, "You don't really feel that way," or "That's not true." Obviously, people do know how they feel about things. Leaders need to treat their staff with respect and hope to establish and maintain a relationship in which they feel free to share and talk about their feelings and ideas. As can be seen in Figure 7–2, the more relevant the feedback that takes place within an organization, the more the public area of a leader begins to extend into and displace the blind area and thus the smaller blind area that leader has.

Clearly, the use of feedback is essential to personal growth and development in terms of how people behave in relationships with others. Giffin and Patton describe the behavior of a person who is mature in interpersonal relationships. This person:

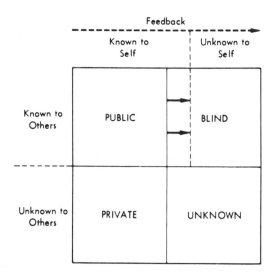

Figure 7–2. The effect of feedback on the Johari window. *(From Hersey, P., & Blanchard, K. Management of organizational behavior: Utilizing human resources. [5th ed.] Englewood, Cliffs, N.J.: Prentice-Hall, 1988, p. 278, with permission.)*

1. Shows confidence in his ability to relate to others—shows trust of self and trust of others.
2. Readily tries new ways of relating to and working with others when old ways are inadequate.
3. Requests and listens to feedback from others regarding (a) how he is perceived and (b) how others feel about these perceptions; he uses this approach particularly when trying out new ways of relating to these others.
4. Evaluates this feedback, carefully discriminating between valid criticism and diatribe, prejudicial attack, or capricious comment.
5. Changes his behaviors with a minimum of tension or confusion *when he chooses to change.*
6. Demonstrates accurate empathy and nonpossessive warmth toward others.
7. Behaves in overt ways that are congruent with his inner feelings.[40]

While Giffin and Patton are concerned with personal relationships in this description of maturity, we suggest this description is equally applicable to self-disclosure and feedback in organizational settings. There are differences, however. First, the most relevant disclosure is not what is said, but how one behaves. Second, disclosures need to be relevant to the organization. With all due respect to the importance of personal disclosures, there is a limited amount of time and energy available in goal-oriented organizations, particularly health care organizations. The focus needs to be, we believe, primarily on organizationally relevant disclosures.

Another principle that we can derive from the discussions of trust, self-disclosure and feedback is as follows:

In order to be an effective nursing leader with a productive nursing staff, look to the verbal and nonverbal behavior of those associates and staff whom you trust to give you authentic, honest feedback.

Developing trusting relationships leads to the open communication associated with self-disclosure and feedback.

As nursing staff members "see you seeing them" as trustworthy, they become more trusting of you as their leader, and they become more self-confident in themselves and their nursing performance. This tripod of Humanistic Nursing Communication theory—trust, self-disclosure, and feedback—serves as the foundation for other leadership concepts. Research has shown that job satisfaction goes up when the leader shows confidence in the member's ability.[41] Confidence is listed as one of the marks of a real professional by Ganong and Ganong.[42] In the health care organizational context, as a nursing leader, you become a significant other to your nursing staff in facilitating their nursing practice by establishing a supportive interpersonal climate. In maintaining high levels of trust, self-disclosure, and feedback, you put the facilitator function of leadership into action.

SUMMARY

We have based our perspective of the facilitating function of leadership on the perspective of Humanistic Nursing Communication theory. The set of elements, trust, self-disclosure, and feedback have been drawn from the concept *communing.* Definitions, theories, research, and examples have been incorporated from a wide variety of sources to support this perspective of facilitating. In an effort to identify specific behaviors a nursing leader needs to incorporate into his or her communication style, five principles have been identified. As cautioned by Peters and Waterman in their book, *In Search of Excellence,* avoid being a victim of the management "gimmicks trap."[43] Recently, this has been Management by Objectives (see Chapter 14), Theory Z (see Chapter 10), and Quality Circles (see Chapter 10). Such plans often are rejected or bureaucratized. The heart of the matter remains the caring leader who facilitates followers' efforts to achieve the goals.

REFERENCES

1. Halpin, A. W. *The leadership behavior of school superintendents.* Chicago: Midwest Administration Center, The University of Chicago, 1959, p. 4.
2. Hersey, P., & Blanchard, K. *Management of organizational behavior: Utilizing human resources* (5th ed.). (Englewood Cliffs, N. J.: Prentice-Hall, 1988, p. 87.
3. Ibid., 172.
4. Tubbs, S. L., & Baird, J.W. *The open person . . . self-disclosure and personal growth.* Patton, B.R., & Giffin, K. [Eds.]. Interpersonal communication series. Columbus, Ohio: Merrill, 1976, p. 18.
5. Patton, B. R., & Giffin, K. *Interpersonal communication in action: Basic text and readings* (2nd ed.). New York: Harper & Row, 1977, p. 431.
6. Newcomb, T. M. An approach to the study of communicative acts. *Psychological Review,* 1953, *60,* (6), 393–464.
7. Thurstone, L. L. Comment. *American Journal of Sociology,* 1946, *52,* (1), 39–70.
8. Edwards, A. L. *Techniques of attitude scale construction.* New York: Appleton-Century-Crofts, 1957, 5–9.
9. Patton & Giffin, *Interpersonal communication,* p. 431.
10. Hovland, C., Janis, I. L., & Kelley, H. H. *Communication and persuasion.* New Haven: Yale University Press, 1953, p. 21.
11. Rogers, C. R. *Client-centered therapy.* Boston: Houghton Mifflin, 1951, p. 41.
12. Gibb, J. Climate for trust formation. In L. P. Bradford et al., (Eds.). *T-group theory and laboratory method.* New York: Wiley, 1964, p. 298.
13. Giffin, K., & Bradley, K. Group counseling for speech anxiety: An approach and a rationale. *Journal of Communication,* 1969, *19* (1), 22–29.
14. Patton & Giffin, *Interpersonal communication* (3rd ed., 1981), p. 367.
15. Ibid., 432.
16. Giffin, K. The contribution of studies of source credibility to a theory of interpersonal trust in the communication process. *Psychological Bulletin,* 1967, *68* (2), 105.
17. Tubbs & Baird, *The open person,* pp. 6–7.
18. Ibid., 18.
19. Rogers, C., & Truax, C. B. The therapeutic conditions antecedent to change: A theoretical view. In C. R. Rogers (Ed.), *The therapeutic relationship and its impact.* Madison: University of Wisconsin Press, 1967, p. 97–108.
20. Gibb, J. R. Fear and facade: Defensive management. In R. E. Farson (Ed.), *Science and human affairs.* Palo Alto, Calif.: Science and Behavior Books, 1965, p. 197–214.
21. Tubbs & Baird, *The open person,* p. 18–19.
22. Likert, R. *New patterns in management.* New York: McGraw-Hill, 1961, p. 103.
23. Haney, W. V. *Communication and organizational behavior.* Homewood, Ill.: Irwin, 1967, p. 12–15.
24. Ibid., 14.
25. Hersey & Blanchard, *Management of organizational behavior,* p. 55.
26. Ibid.
27. Ibid., 54–55.

28. Johnson, D. W., & Noonan, M. P. Effects of acceptance and reciprocation of self-disclosure on the development of trust. *Journal of Counseling Psychology,* 1972, *19* (5), 411–416.
29. Tubbs & Baird, *The open person,* p. 20.
30. Ibid., 20.
31. Johnson & Noonan. Effects of acceptance, p. 411–416.
32. Mellinger, G. D. Interpersonal trust as a factor in communication. *Journal of Abnormal and Social Psychology,* 1956, *52* (3), 304–309.
33. Mead, G. H. *Mind, self, and society.* Chicago: University of Chicago Press, 1934.
34. Hardy, M. E., & Conway, M. E. *Role theory: Perspectives for health professionals.* New York: Appleton-Century-Crofts, 1978.
35. Duldt, B. W. Sexual harassment in nursing. *Nursing Outlook,* 1982, *30* (6), 338.
36. Kanter, R. M. *Men and women of the corporation.* New York: Basic Books, 1977. p. 48–49.
37. Tubbs & Baird, *The open person,* p. 49–50.
38. Luft, J. *Group processes.* Palo Alto, Calif.: Mayfield, 1970.
39. Hersey & Blanchard, *Management of organizational behavior,* 276.
40. Giffin, K., & Patton, B. R. *Personal communication in human relations.* Columbus, Ohio: Merrill, 1974, p. 138.
41. Miles, R. E. *Theories of management: Implications for organizational behavior and development.* New York: McGraw-Hill, 1975, p. 121.
42. Ganong, J. M., & Ganong, W. L. *Nursing management* (2nd ed.). Rockville, Md.: Aspen, 1980, p. 32.
43. Peters, T. J., & Waterman, R. H., Jr. *In search of excellence: Lessons from America's best-run companies* (Warner Books ed.). New York: Harper & Row, 1982, 240–241.

8

INTEGRATING

INTRODUCTION

In this chapter, the integrating process will be explored as the fifth and last people-oriented function of nurse-leaders in maintaining and developing interpersonal relationships between and among all nurses on the staff. The integrated group and the dimensions of integrating nursing staff members will be described: selecting, developing, and mediating. The selection of staff and development of their professional competencies are an important aspect of integrating. We suspect, however, the reader will be particularly interested in the management of disruptive and difficult staff members who interrupt both the problem-solving process and effective nursing practice. Included in the discussions are conflict, its characteristics and management, as well as approaches to conflict resolution. The developmental and regressive cycles of Situational Leadership will be applied, and the concepts of confronting, conflicting, and separating of Humanistic Nursing Communication theory. The similarities and differences will be noted between collaboration and consultation roles in the open dialogue which, by definition, is to exist in an integrated group.

INTEGRATION DEFINED

Integration means bringing all parts together into a whole, or unifying.[1] Generally, integration means removing barriers so as to permit free and equal association among all parts of a whole, or open dialogue among the parts. Synonyms include, *unify, consolidate,* and *merge* as opposed to the antonyms *dissipate, disperse,* and *scatter.* For example, in psychology, a harmonious personality is characterized by the integration of various traits, feelings, attitudes, and behaviors. Many people may associate the desegregation of racial groups in society with this word or concept.

As a leadership function, integration means unifying the group. The leader serves as an integrator by bringing a number of people to work together in a cooperative manner so that they move, operate, and function as a unit in achieving their group or organizational goals. The integrating process is essentially team building. It begins with the selection of staff members, and continues with the development or mentoring of each individual so that personal and professional goals become merged with organizational or team goals.[2] Since one can expect differing viewpoints among group members, conflict is to be expected. Thus a major portion of the leader's integrating function involves managing disruptive individuals to change their behavior and become more cooperative and mediating conflict within a group.

INTEGRATED GROUPS

The conceptualization of an integrated group arose from research sponsored by the National Training Laboratories Institute of Applied Behavioral Sciences in Washington, D.C.[3] This independent institute has been the United State's heart of leadership studies, serving as a center of research and a resource of theory, knowledge, and practice for the armed services and other governmental agencies as well as private businesses and organizations. In a 1968 report of conflict situations in groups, opposing modes of behavior that result in two types of situations are described: *distributive* and *integrative*. A *distributive* situation is one in which one wins only at the expense of another. One such example is a poker game (the winner takes all); another is business transactions involving negotiating. An integrative situation is one in which group members combine their resources to achieve a common goal. Examples of this are a group of children working together on a crossword puzzle, or the precise teamwork of a cardiovascular surgery team of nurses and doctors. Detailed characterizations of the integrative and distributive situations are presented in Table 8–1.[4] We believe the integrative and distributive modes of group behavior are generally consistent with the concepts of humanizing and dehumanizing communication as described in Duldt's Humanistic Nursing Communication theory.

TABLE 8–1. INTEGRATIVE AND DISTRIBUTIVE INTERGROUP CONFLICT SITUATIONS AS IDENTIFIED BY THE NATIONAL TRAINING LABORATORIES.

Integrative Approach	Distributive Approach
1. Behavior is purposeful in that goals held in common are pursued	1. Behavior is purposeful in that one's own goals are pursued
2. Openness	2. Secrecy
3. Accurate personal understanding of own needs and accurate representation of them	3. Accurate personal understanding of own needs, but these are publicly disguised or misrepresented: Don't let them know what you really want most, so that they won't know how much you are really willing to give up to get it
4. Predictable: while flexible behavior is appropriate, it is not designed to take the other party by surprise	4. Unpredictable, mixed strategies, utilizing the element of surprise
5. Threats or bluffs are not used	5. Threats or bluffs
6. Search behavior is devoted to finding solutions to problems and utilizing logical and innovative processes	6. Search behavior is devoted to finding ways of appearing to become committed to a position: logical, nonrational, and irrational arguments alike may serve this purpose
7. Success demands that stereotypes be dropped, that ideas be given consideration on their merit regardless of sources, and that hostility not be induced deliberately. In fact, positive feelings about others are both a cause and an effect of other aspects of the integrative approach	7. Success is often enhanced (where teams, committees, or organizations are involved on each side) by forming a bad stereotype of the other, by ignoring the other's logic, by increasing the level of hostility. These tend to strengthen in-group loyalty and convince others that you mean business
8. A pathological extreme occurs when one will assume that whatever is good for others and the groups is necessarily good for oneself. Cannot distinguish own identity from group or other person's identity. Will not take responsibility for own self	8. A pathological extreme occurs when one assumes that everything that prevents the other from reaching *his* goal also must facilitate one's own movement toward *his* goal; thus, one would state his own goals as being the negation of other's achievement

From Patton, B.R, & Giffin, K. Problem-solving group interactions. New York: Harper & Row, 1973, p. 94, with permission.

According to Duldt's theory, if the participant(s) in a conflict situation communicate with a humanizing attitude, this is "conflicting with dialogue," and the interpersonal relationship tends to move toward communing, or toward being integrated: to come together, to consolidate, and to unite. If the communication is characterized by a dehumanizing attitude, however, then the interpersonal relationship tends to move toward separation, or toward being "distributed," to scatter, to divide, and to break up. Specifically, Duldt proposes the following relationship statement:

> To the degree that conflict tends not to re-establish trust, self-disclosure, and feedback, and to the degree that dehumanizing communication attitudes continue to be expressed by another, to that degree one tends to terminate the relationship by separation.[5]

In this manner, communicating humanizing attitudes in a conflict situation as defined in Duldt's theory is congruent with the National Training Laboratories' modes of behavior characteristic of integrative and distributive conflict situations. In the development of an integrative group, selection of the group members or nurse-followers who have a track record for behaving in a manner congruent with the integrative approach is of major importance.

SELECTION OF FOLLOWERS

People do not *have* to have similar personalities to be compatible. We suggest the following principle for your consideration:

> *The degree of integration achieved by a group tends to vary with the degree to which the members hold similar perceptions of one another's roles and maintain a commitment to the same goals.*

It is necessary that the people, whom you, as a head nurse or similar nursing leader, select share perceptions of one another's roles and have a commitment to common goals. Marriner states that selecting a nurse who predictably fails to achieve the organization's expectations can be an expensive mistake.[6] Risks are often necessary, however.

It is often more appropriate for you to select key followers who can provide expertise in areas in which you have shortcomings, rather than surround yourself with followers who are all similar to you. Some large companies and agencies have created problems for themselves by using a testing and selection process that eliminates personalities incongruent with the "company norm." This process involves measuring values and styles of the top administrative people and then selecting new people according to these measures. It is assumed that if these administrative leaders got to the top, their values and styles must be what is needed to be successful in this particular organization. This assumption identifies what is believed to be the best style for this particular organization.

One reason this process of hiring the "company norm" became popular is that it leads to a more harmonious organization. It is believed that if the leaders and followers have the same set of values and behave in similar ways, then they will tend to get along with minimal conflict, that is, form an integrative group. Research and practice, however, have shown that this process leads to management "inbreeding," which tends to stifle creativity and innovation. To be effective in the long run, we believe healthy organizations and nursing staffs need an open dialogue so characteristic of the integrative group. There needs to be a certain amount of conflict, confrontation, and differing points of view to encourage new ideas and patterns of behavior so that the nursing practice within the health organization will maintain its ability to adjust to external competition, unique client population needs, and innovative approaches to planning and implementing individual patient or client care. Health agencies that are forced to break a policy of promoting only from within and hire some key nursing staff from outside in effect encourage open dialogue.

What is needed in health agencies is greater emphasis on team building of integrative groups and hiring nursing staff and key nurse-leaders who complement rather than replicate a nursing executive's style. For example, a high-relationship, low-task nursing executive may select a high-task, low-relationship first-level nursing leader who can more easily eliminate dead wood and enforce adherence to required policies and procedures in a nursing staff that has a poor performance history. If each person understands the other's role and is committed to common goals, they can complement each other and be successful as nursing leaders.[7]

If you, as a nursing leader, have determined you have a narrow range of leadership styles according to Situational Leadership theory, then you can expand your flexibility without changing your own behavior by selecting nurse-followers whose best communication style differs from your own. In this manner, you can develop a wider range of potentital styles within your nurse-follower group, styles that can be brought to bear on the variety of situations you and your nursing followers face. Again, it is important that each understand others' roles and have a commitment to the same goals and expectations.[8]

Tappen notes that you may not always be free to choose followers, but at least you can expect to influence the final decisions. She also stresses the importance of having a well-defined purpose or goal for a nursing staff group, team, committee, or the like.[9] Certainly one needs to match nursing expertise with the task to be performed; home health nursing or intensive care nursing expertise needs to be matched to home health and intensive care projects.

One may be severely limited by the number of qualified people available, and consequently the desirable integrative, collaborative behaviors may risk becoming a lower priority for you in the selection process. Rather than compromise your group's success, you may consider other ways of acquiring the needed expertise, such as through consultation services, visiting other agencies to learn from others' experiences, or attending workshops.

Collaborative behaviors are important communication skills in the development of an integrated group. We suggest the following principle:

> *As collaborative communication behaviors increase, the integration of the group tends to increase proportionately.*

Collaboration differs from consultation in certain important ways. Langford defines collaboration as an interaction

> . . . characterized by activities directed toward an agreed upon goal by two or more persons among whom exists a norm of equity and mutual recognition of complementarity of their knowledge and abilities.[10]

The specific collaborative behaviors which, according to Langford, are so desirable include the following:

1. Share a mutual respect for the expertise of their collaborators.
2. Define a common goal through discussion.
3. Accept mutual responsibility in reaching the common goal.
4. Participate in mutual review upon reaching the common goal.
5. Communicate in an honest, open face-to-face mode.
6. Share decision making power as peers, equitably.
7. Share knowledge for the benefit of the group of collaborators.
8. Offer support to collaborators through positive statements regarding their contribution.
9. Understand the common language or terms common to the problem at hand.
10. Have mutually acceptable roles.[11]

In contrast, *consultation* involves asking an expert for professional or technical advice or opinions. Langford notes that the decision-making power does not lie with the consultant, but is retained by the leader. For example, an ill person may consult a physician, but ultimately decides whether or not to follow the physician's advice.[12] Noted nursing authors have pointed to the differing educational process in medical and nursing education. Generally, medical education emphasizes consultation, whereas nursing education emphasizes collaboration.[13-15] This may be a factor in the failure of some interprofessional health teams to become integrated and effective.

The number of members selected can also make a difference in the degree of integration of a group. A general principle can be stated as follows.

As the number of members increases, the amount of communication necessary to achieve agreement on an issue increases.

Small groups, up to six or eight members, can usually achieve consensus rather easily. Gillies notes that as the group size increases from six to twelve, the degree of consensus decreases, particularly if there are time limitations. Smaller groups allow greater opportunity for participation on the part of each member, and thus members tend to have higher morale in comparison to larger groups.[16]

While you may offer a nurse an opportunity to join a particular nursing staff, committee, or team, the nurse you have selected may decline. There are certain properties of a group that may influence such a decision. Cartwright describes, among others, three major reasons people want to join groups: the *group* is attractive because of its reputation for success or importance; the *group members* are particularly attractive; the group *tasks* are attractive because the person is able to successfully perform them.[17] These incentive properties of a group vary according to individual motives: one's need for affiliation, recognition, security, money, or whatever other factors might fulfill an individual's needs. Expectation of outcomes of membership refers to whatever benefits one might derive from the group. Nurses may also have a comparison level, that is, some average value of the total possible outcomes of memberships in all the different groups available to an individual.[18] Gillies suggests some reasons nurses might have for declining membership in a group. The nursing audit committee may be considered more powerful and prestigious than the nursing procedure committee. A friend may already be a member of the group. The membership may be perceived as necessary to career advancement.[19] The nurse may be experiencing burnout or job dissatisfaction, or may be in stressful situations that negate new commitments. While disappointing, such decisions need to be respected. You want the nurse who does join your group or unit staff to be interested and willing; if you have to work too hard at convincing someone to join, you may have a follower whose loyalty and commitment is less than desirable.

In selecting nursing staff, comparable information needs to be obtained from all applicants.[20,21] All the usual policies and procedures of the health agency, plus state and federal regulations as well, need to be followed carefully. Further discussion of the selection of nursing staff is presented in Chapter 11 of this text.

DEVELOPING INTEGRATIVE BEHAVIORS

The development of individual nursing staff members into an integrated group is analogous to team building. The following principle can be stated:

The integration of a group is dependent to a considerable degree upon the leader's ability to analyze performance and identify problems limiting individual and group performance and to intervene with correctives.

It involves analyzing group performance and identifying intragroup problems that impede individual and group functioning. According to Dyer, teams are: ". . . groups of people who must rely on group collaboration if each member is to experience the optimum of success and goal achievement."[22] Dyer compares this integrative leadership function to coaching. Football coaches must be able to analyze team efforts, identify what is preventing the members' achievement, and develop a strategy for removing the obstacle so that the team members are freed to perform well, increasing the probabilities of winning. The key factor here is problem recognition. Just as a good football coach can spot in an instant when someone fails to block, when a team member fails to cover his man, or a quarterback executes a play inaccurately, so the nurse-leader can quickly note when an ICU nurse fails to keep current nursing notes, when an oncological nurse is slow to respond to a patient's request for pain injections, or any nurse demonstrates inadequate knowledge of commonly used drugs or equipment.

The above examples are typical nursing practice behaviors, however. The behavior problems which you need to spot quickly are those of a disruptive group member, the member whose behavior is indicative of a *distributive* rather than integrative approach. Look again at these approaches (Table 8–1). We believe other behaviors can be added, behaviors such as those listed by Porter-O'Grady:

Speechmaking	Chronic Complaining
Repetition	Withdrawing
Interrupting	Separating
Sidetracking	Subverting
Emotionalizing Issues	Personalizing Issues
Aggressive Behavior	Accusations
Sarcastic Language	Threats[23]

In addition, Bramson has a unique list of difficult people that we believe is consistent with distributive behaviors:

Sherman Tanks, Snipers and Exploders
The Silent, Unresponsive Person
The Super-Agreeables
The Wet Blanket
Bulldozers and Know-It-All Experts
Indecisive Stallers[24]

Porter-O'Grady and Bramson provide some good suggestions for interacting with people who exhibit these disruptive behaviors and defusing the effects. The reader may want to refer to their books for further information.

Confrontation

You need to know what to do once you have identified such distributive behavior. In deciding how to intervene, you need to describe to yourself how you would like this individual to behave. How do you want her to change? Then, the simplest way to intervene is often the most effective; just tell 'em. Use confrontation. Be as tactful and positive as possible; be private; be humanistic; be confrontive with caring. Use persuasive capabilities to convince the nurse that a change in behavior is important. After all, as the leader, you control the nurse's evaluation (and potential promotion and salary increases), and thus you are in a better position than most to influence a follower.

Duldt defines *confronting* as using information a person gives you and pointing out inconsistencies. It is an attempt to become highly involved with the person and a challenge to the confrontee to improve interpersonal skills. Generally, the term is used when the confronter deliberately or inadvertently does or says something that causes the confrontee to think about, examine, question, or change some aspect of behavior. There are four steps in the process of confronting.

First, get the confrontee's *attention:* "I have something important to tell you. I think it may be helpful to you, and I want you to listen to me." When saying this, look the individual in the eye, and speak in a quiet, confidential manner. If you feel comfortable touching the confrontee, you may lightly touch a hand, arm, or shoulder to get attention. If the confrontee is angry or generally unapproachable, touching will probably not be appropriate. Ask her or him to go with you to an office, the coffee shop, or some comfortable, private place where you both can talk without interruption for a few minutes.

Second, give the behavioral *facts:* "This is how you have been behaving . . ." or "This is what you said . . ." are sentence "stems" to initiate the confrontation when in private. For example: "When the other staff members made suggestions for handling the new patient's problem you threw a wet blanket on it by immediately saying it wouldn't work, there's no use trying, or administration will never give us permission to do that. The effect of such comments just pulls everyone down and stifles any further suggestions." Speak in an even, quiet manner, without anger or other strong emotional overtones to your own verbal and nonverbal behavior. It is important to prevent unnecessary defensiveness in the confrontee, although you can anticipate some tension, of course.

Third, in a similar manner, continue by telling how this kind of behavior makes you *feel* as the leader, "I think this kind of behavior is detrimental to getting staff members to share their ideas, and I don't like it. I want everyone to feel comfortable about making suggestions for improving the way we practice nursing on this unit."

Finally, request a specific *change* in the confrontee's behavior. "I want you to stop telling other staff members their ideas won't work. I expect you to identify at least three positive features about any new idea before you even suggest one that is negative. I expect you to be more supportive and more cooperative with the other nursing staff".

In response, you can expect three general reactions: defensiveness, counterattacks, or acceptance. The first two can be confronted, too, in a manner similar to that described above. Often the confrontee will apologize and indicate unawareness of the problem he or she was causing. Sometimes such behavior is merely a bad habit easily broken, and a confrontation does not seem to create much tension. Before the confrontation ends, you need to extract a promise from the confrontee to change by a certain point in time, such as within a week. An appointment can be made at the end of this time to discuss the confrontee's progress and establish future goals.

Care needs to be taken when confronting another. If the individual is known to be coping with too many other problems, there may be nonengagement and the confrontation will fail. If the confrontee clearly states, "I am not ready to listen to you now," do respect this and arrange to discuss it another time.[25-27] To avoid confusion and misunderstandings, it is best to confront the nurse-follower with one issue or behavior at a time. Be timely and specific in your confronting, and be consistent in that you respond in the same way to the same behavior.

Other Interventions

In addition to confrontation, there are several other strategies you can choose to implement as you deem appropriate. You can apply the Situational Leadership developmental cycle to introduce small, successive steps toward the kind of behavior you expect. Certainly recognition or positive feedback, probably in private at first, needs to be given for progress. You can identify an appropriate role model for the nurse-follower to observe. As a leader, you might help your nurse identify a potential mentor for more individualized and personalized guidance than you can appropriately provide as leader.

If the nursing staff member refuses to change or to meet expectations, then separation may be the next step. As the leader, you have to determine how much deviation from the established behavioral norm is too much. You might suggest a transfer to another unit, an extended vacation or leave of absence to think things over, or dismissal. If you can discuss the situation with the disruptive staff member, you may find that the person is unhappy in the group and is already looking elsewhere. Separation can be a mutually agreeable option, and often it is an opportunity for reassessment of capabilities and successful career redirection.

MEDIATING

A third dimension of the integrating function of a leader is settling differences between people by mediating, a positive, diplomatic intervention to handle intragroup conflict.[28] Conflict may range from quietly stating differences of opinion between two or more members of a group to arguing, name-calling, and competitive behavior, to disruptive behaviors such as withdrawing, scapegoating, destroying another's property, or actually fighting. Using the definition of Humanistic Nursing Communication theory, *conflict* indicates a need for a decision about an issue in which there is risk of loss or possible gain, in which there is a choice between two or more alternatives, and in which values are involved.[29] Differences of opinions between nursing staff often need to be resolved rather quickly because of the care and pressures of patients' or clients' needs. The risk of loss or possible gain often has to do with the health (or illness) state of the patient.

For example, a patient in the ICU cardiovascular unit is supposed to be moved "now" to a step-down care unit to avoid being charged for another day in ICU, but the patient's blood pressure or pulse might still be somewhat unstable. The nursing staff may disagree about whether or not to move the patient. The risk of moving a patient with unstable vital signs includes having the patient go into cardiovascular shock or "go bad" while on the elevator or in the hallway without all of the technical equipment, emergency drugs, and telephone typically available in the immediate area of the patient's ICU bed. There are a number of options possible, including transporting with extra equipment as a contingency. These conflict situations typically revolve about the value of human life or humanistic values versus money, insurance, availability of rooms, and similar bureaucratic, business-office requirements. Thus solutions or decisions in nursing and health care are not all black and white, right or wrong, but many shades of gray. It is in this gray area that values and perspectives vary, and conflict is born.

Conflicting

Consequently, we believe conflict cannot be prevented, but, in fact, needs to be expected. It is the leader's role to manage the conflict situation by intervening in a mediating role. Thus, we believe it is helpful to have some knowledge of the characteristics of conflict situations.

Conflict situations can be characterized as being humanizing or dehumanizing. When humanizing, the leader and followers believe and behave in the following manner:

1. Everyone recognizes that it is normal for differences to occur and to expect conflict; they understand that conflict is necessary to effective problem solving; everyone learns to disagree in a productive manner.
2. Everyone needs to hear the different views, give fair consideration and critically evaluate each view, and reach a consensus after a full discussion of the issue.
3. Everyone supports the maintenance of an open climate of communication so that ideas can be expressed without punishment or embarrassment.

We propose the following statement of principle:

When disagreements and conflict are handled in a humanizing manner, the effect upon the group interpersonal climate tends to be constructive.

There will be a tendency for wiser decisions to be made, decisions that are better than any one member could make alone. There is considerable research to support this proposition.[30] The effect of a humanizing approach is to promote personal and professional growth as well as an increase in motivation and commitment because of the high involvement interpersonally in analyzing and selecting the best possible resolution to the issue. The problem-solving discussions of the issues broaden members' understanding of the nature of the issue and its implications. The members have an opportunity to share and clarify their values with one another. This humanistic approach also allows more alternatives to be identified from which the best possible solution can be selected.

In contrast, conflict situations can also be approached in a dehumanizing manner. The group members' beliefs and behavior are as follows:

1. People do not believe disagreements or conflicts can be constructive, but are either win or lose situations.
2. The interpersonal climate is closed, competitive, and unfriendly.
3. The group lacks a sense of direction, unity, and commitment to a common goal.
4. The members frequently and habitually display disruptive behavior.
5. Members tend to become frozen to their own viewpoints and to perceive others as lacking credibility; they do not *listen* to one another.
6. Discussions frequently and quickly move from the issue to personal attacks as viewpoints polarize.
7. Once a solution or decision has been reached, the members have little satisfaction about the outcome, and tend to feel interpersonally cold and distant about one another.*

We propose the following principle for your consideration:

When disagreements and conflicts are approached in a dehumanizing manner, the effect tends to be disruptive to the group's productivity as well as interpersonal climate.

Since the group's energy is consumed by the disruptive and dehumanizing behaviors and attitudes, the total effect is to impede progress toward the task. In addition, individual members tend to feel threatened, narrow their perceptual processes, and increase their defensive behaviors, as described by Gibb.[31,32]

Like Duldt, Blake, Shepard, and Mouton also speak of attitudes in conflict situations. They have identified three attitudinal mind-sets that people can have about conflict within a group. First, the conflict is seen as inevitable and agreement as impossible; second, the conflict is not inevitable, but agreement is impossible; or third, given conflict, agreement is possible. Blake, Shepard, and Mouton propose that these attitudes lead to predictable behavior, varying according to how the stakes are perceived, that is, how much the issue involved is valued. The higher the stakes, the more active the behavior. The attitudes, behaviors, and outcomes are illustrated in Figure 8–1.

If people think that conflict is inevitable and agreement impossible, then, according to Blake, Shepard, and Mouton, their behavior will range from passive to very active. When the stakes are low, they will tend to be passive and willing to let fate (a flip of the coin, perhaps) decide the conflict. When the stakes are moderate, they will permit a third-party judgment to decide the conflict. Finally, when the stakes are high, they will actively engage in a win-lose confrontation or power struggle.

If people think that conflict is not inevitable, but that if it occurs, agreement is impossible, they will be passive and indifferent if the stakes are low. When the stakes are moderate, they will isolate themselves from such a conflict situation. When the stakes are high and they find themselves actively involved, they will eventually withdraw.

If people think that although there is conflict agreement is possible, they will be passive and attempt to smooth over the situation when the stakes are low. When the stakes are

---

*The descriptions of humanizing and dehumanizing beliefs and behaviors about conflicts are drawn from unpublished, copyrighted (1977) materials developed by B. W. Duldt and distributed as handouts in seminars and workshops.

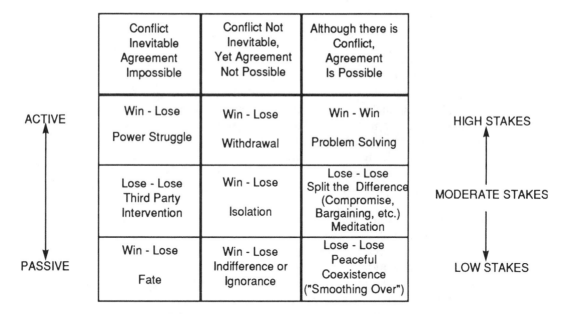

Conflict Inevitable Agreement Impossible	Conflict Not Inevitable, Yet Agreement Not Possible	Although there is Conflict, Agreement Is Possible
Win - Lose Power Struggle	Win - Lose Withdrawal	Win - Win Problem Solving
Lose - Lose Third Party Intervention	Win - Lose Isolation	Lose - Lose Split the Difference (Compromise, Bargaining, etc.) Meditation
Win - Lose Fate	Win - Lose Indifference or Ignorance	Lose - Lose Peaceful Coexistence ("Smoothing Over")

ACTIVE ↑ PASSIVE

HIGH STAKES ↑ MODERATE STAKES ↓ LOW STAKES

Figure 8–1. Three basic attitudes toward conflict and the behavior each evokes as involvement ("stakes") increases and decreases. *(From Hersey, P., & Blanchard, K. Management of organizational behavior: Utilizing human resources [5th ed.]. Englewood Cliffs, N. J.: Prentice-Hall, 1988, p. 355. An adaptation from Blake, R.R., Shepard, H., & Mouton, J.S. Managing intergroup conflict in industry. Houston: Gulf Publishing Co., 1964, p. 13.)*

moderate, they will engage in bargaining or some form of negotiation. If the stakes are high, they will actively engage in problem solving.

Knowledge of these characterstics or types of conflict can be helpful in managing conflict. We propose that if you, as a nurse-leader know about the attitudes your nursing staff members have about conflict and what the "stakes" are for them—what they value—then you may be able to predict their behavior with a reasonable degree of accuracy.

Resolving Conflict

In managing intragroup conflict, Meyer suggests three options.[34] First, there are conflicts that you, as the leader, must appear to resolve, but that may not need to be resolved. For example, two or more staff members may have a long-standing disagreement about an issue that is esoteric and rhetorical rather than immediately relevant to the group's activities, such as purchasing a CAT scan machine, although there are no means of financing it. This is not a staff nurses' decision. It is irrelevant to the main stream of nursing issues, yet these person(s) talk and talk. They fail to make progress, neglect their legitimate concerns, and lose credibility. These machines are extremely expensive, and generally only large medical centers or research centers have one; indeed, there may be only one to a city or region. You might have the vice-president of nursing set up a committee and appoint these staff members to serve on the committee. Without financing and broad support, little progress can be expected. Your staff then have a forum in which to act out their disagreement, and others on the committee may be able to help them resolve their differences. It looks like you did something, when the conflict was merely moved out of your territory to allow the chairman of the committee to deal with it. (Harry Truman would label this "buck passing.") With careful neglect by the vice-president (limited secretarial services, no budget allocation, no goals, and no specified time to report), the disagreement will probably fade away in a little while.

Second, there are conflicts that need to be resolved and can be resolved only by you, the leader. Typically, these include disagreements about resources, space, or scheduling. These are legitimately leader or manager conncerns and sources of power; decisions about these things are not to be delegated. You will need to listen to all viewpoints, spend a respectable period of time taking all suggestions under advisement, and then tell your staff of your decisions. Overlapping assignments, duplication of efforts, and inadequate staffing are also management errors that need to be corrected quickly to eliminate confusion and conflict among staff.

Third, there are conflicts that need to be solved, but it must appear as if *you* have not resolved them. For example, it is seldom wise to publicize and openly deal with disagreements over personal issues (verbal attacks or boisterous laughter on night duty) or disagreements that involve those disruptive individuals described earlier in this chapter. You may be able to manage the disagreement quietly and informally in a series of private confrontations and dialogues with each individual separately.

We would suggest a fourth possibility. There are some disagreements that serve you well by remaining unresolved. For example, your staff may complain bitterly about lack of certain resources or space, and argue about it in front of your supervisor. As the head nurse, you may have in fact managed to satisfy your staff's needs to a considerable degree. It is to you and your budget's advantage for your supervisor to witness your staff's quarreling over who gets to use the (whatever), when, and how long. With a little more justification, your unit budget may eventually be increased because of the intragroup conflict.

As mediator, you have certain responsibilities, as suggested by Gillies. First, you need to determine whether one or both groups are willing and want to find a mutually satisfactory solution; if none do, then there is no point in attempting to mediate and negotiate. Second, as mediator, you are to choose the time and place for the opposing parties to meet, and you are to serve as the discussion leader (or referee). Third, because certain people (low-status, minorities, or women) tend to speak less frequently and defer to others (high-status, ethnic groups, or men) you need to provide opportunities for the former to speak. Fourth, during the discussions, you need to redirect the conversation as necessary to keep the comments focused on the topic or theme being discussed at the time; you need to keep them moving forward, toward their goal. Fourth, you can be helpful by restating the arguments or positions of each party to one another. This requires that each listen to the other. It is sometimes helpful to require that each person must restate what the opposition has just said before stating his or her own thoughts. Each side needs to be encouraged to give feedback to the other. Overall, as mediator, you need to respect the dignity of each participant and require the same of all involved.[35]

In mediating disagreements and conflicts among your nursing staff, it is usually appropriate for you to bring the clashing groups together. Dyer proposes that there are certain things everyone needs to agree about before coming together. All need to agree:

1. To get together to work on problems;
2. That there are problems that can be solved;
3. That all individuals have some responsibility for working toward solving the problems;

4. That they are not expected to like one another at the conclusion, but to understand one another better and be able to work together;

5. That they are not expected to place blame on someone for the problem, but are expected to consider differences and come to a consensus about solutions.[36]

Dyer also suggests a "start, stop, continue" format for the meeting. Each individual or group is to list what they believe the other side needs to start, stop, or continue doing in order to solve the problem or issue. This format is based on expectation or the "perceptions of appropriate behavior for one's own role or position or one's perceptions of the roles of others within the organization."[37]

In a conflict situation, the opposing factions have differing expectations. If your nursing staff is able to openly discuss their own expectations, and carefully listen and understand the others' expectations, then the staff may be able to enlarge their *shared* expectations, and in turn, become committed to common goals in the process of negotiating positive outcomes.

Conflict Resolution Outcomes

There are several outcomes possible in conflict resolution. In a study conducted by Lawrence and Lorsch in six organizations, the findings show the two highest performing organizations used confrontation (win-win) to a greater degree than the other organizations; forcing (resorting to authority) and soothing were other options considered in the study.[38] Burke reports on another study comparing five outcomes of conflict resolution. It was found that the more effective supervisors used the following resolution outcomes in the following order: confrontation, soothing, compromise, forcing, and withdrawal. Less effective supervisors used confrontation, forcing, withdrawal, soothing, and compromise, in that order.[39] To force or use authority will result in a staff's feeling dominated or put down. To use compromise requires both sides to lose something of value, and no one is really satisfied. To use the soothing approach is merely avoiding the whole situation; everyone is frustrated; no one wins. This, like withdrawing, merely avoids the conflict temporarily; unresolved disagreements and conflicts may be avoided temporarily, but will come out again and again to produce disruption. Thus as a general principle, the following can be stated:

> *The effective leader tends to use confrontation as an initial approach to conflict situations rather than force, withdrawal, soothing or compromise.*

The Aftermath

Filley notes that the aftermath of a conflict has implications for future relationships among the people involved.[40] (See Fig. 8–2.) If the outcome is a defeat for one group or a concession of some sort, the resulting attitudes are about the same. One group will perceive themselves as winners, the other as losers. If people feel they are losers, then they will probably feel cool and alienated interpersonally toward the winners and expect to win next time. You can expect them to be less cooperative, less trustful, and quick to negatively distort what is said to them.[40] In the future, you can expect to have more conflicts. The approach you, as leader and mediator, select to use has been found to be related to the degree of assertive and cooperative behavior your nursing staff will display in the period after the conflict has been resolved.[41] Thus, the following principle can be stated:

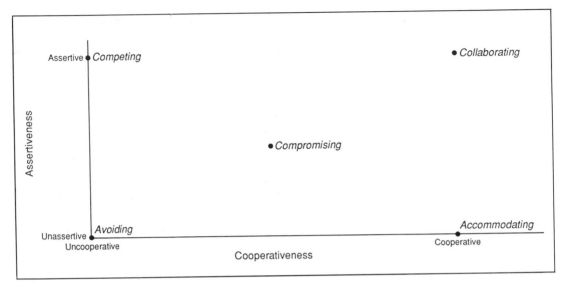

Figure 8–2. The residual effects of various approaches to conflict resolution in regard to degree of assertiveness (active or passive) and degree of cooperativeness of nursing staff after the conflict has been resolved. *(Reprinted by permission of the publisher from Schmidt, W.H. Conflict: A powerful process for (good or bad) change.* Management Review, *December 1974, p. 9. © 1974 AMACOM, a division of American Management Association, New York. All rights reserved.)*

To the degree in which collaboration and a problem-solving approach are used by the leader and members of the group, the resolution of conflict situations tends to involve shared agreements and cooperation.

Both parties need to believe that they are winners and have been dealt with fairly. The solution needs to be an integration of the needs, expectations, values, and perceptions of both parties. Integrated solutions are necessary to maintain an integrative group of nurses.

An Example of a Conflict Situation
An example of dehumanizing and humanizing approaches to conflict resolution is provided by Filley to demonstrate the superiority of a win-win outcome.

Nine of the state's top prison officials met to design an ideal correctional institution. In the course of the discussion, one group member proposed that uniforms traditionally worn by prison guards be eliminated. The group then began a lengthy argument about whether or not uniforms should be worn. One group member suggested that the issue be resolved democratically by vote. As a result, six people voted against the uniforms and three voted in favor of them. The winning members looked pleased while the losing members either got angry or withdrew from further discussion.

A group consultant present at the time suggested that the members take another look at the situation. Then he asked those in favor of uniforms what they hoped to accomplish. Those officials stated that part of the rehabilitative process in correctional institutions is that of teaching people to deal constructively with authority, and saw uniforms as a means for achieving that goal. When asked why they opposed uniforms, the other group members said that uniforms created such a stigma that guards had an additional difficulty laying to rest the stereotypes held by inmates before they could deal with them on a one-to-one basis. The group consultant then asked the group what ways might be appropriate to meet the combined goals, namely, teaching people to deal with authority and avoiding the difficulty of stereotypes held about traditional uniforms. While working on the problem, the group generated ten possible solutions, including indentification of prison personnel by name tags, by color-coded casual dress, or by uniforms for guard supervisors but not for guards in constant contact with prisoners. After discussing the various alternatives, the group decided upon the third solution.[42]

In the first discussion, the disagreement was resolved by vote, but the participants had produced a win-lose solution with the expected negative feelings on the part of the losers. In the second discussion led by the consultant, an integrated group developed as a problem-solving approach was used. The win-win solution was acceptable to all members. The long-term effect of such an outcome is predictable.

While each disagreement or conflict will vary, there are some common themes that tend to occur as a conflict is resolved. As a mediator in the resolution process, it is helpful to be sensitive to the direction in which the opposing individuals or groups need to move. Douglas has developed a model for conflict resolution which is helpful in review[43] (see Figure 8–3).

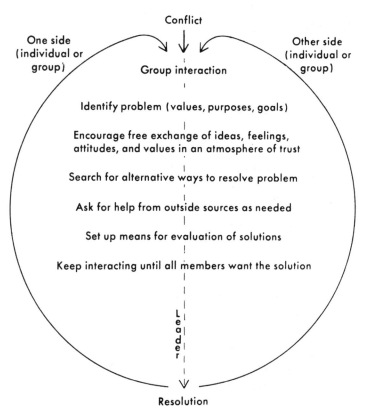

Figure 8–3. A model for conflict resolution. *(Reproduced by permission from Douglass, L.M. The effective nurse: Leader and manager (2nd ed.). St. Louis: The C.V. Mosby Co., 1984, p. 177.*

After getting the individuals to agree to try to resolve their differences, it is necessary that values, purposes, and goals be clarified and understood in addition to defining the issue or problem. Development of an open climate and free exchange of feelings and facts will tend to move the group toward collaborative communication behaviors and problem solving. When appropriate, others may be drawn into the discussions as resource people or as consultants. The group must describe what their hopes or goals are as these descriptions become the criteria for evaluating the alternative solutions. Only when everyone in the group is satisfied with the decision or solution and feels good about it will the conflict be resolved. This is a process that needs to be activated again and again with each issue that arises. We believe consistent humanistic behaviors and attitudes on the part of the leader tend to have a positive and releasing effect on the followers, and can increase the integrative processes within the group.

SUMMARY

In conclusion, the people-oriented leadership function of integrating has been defined as a process of team building through selection of nursing staff, management of disruptive nursing staff, and mediation of disagreements and conflicts. Applying selected aspects of Situational Leadership and Humanistic Nursing Communication theory, we have advocated confrontation, the developmental cycle, collaborative communication, and problem solving as particularly applicable. The nurse-leader establishes the interpersonal climate in which a nursing staff or followers can become an integrated group and achieve "win-win" outcomes. We believe an integrated nursing staff is a successful staff.

REFERENCES

1. Guralnik, D. B. *Webster's new world dictionary* (2nd ed.). New York: Prentice-Hall, 1980, p. 732.
2. Argyris, C. *Integrating the individual and the organization*. New York: Wiley, 1964, p. 7.
3. *1968 reading book*. Washington, D.C.: National Training Laboratories Institute of Applied Behavioral Sciences, 1968.
4. Patton, B. R., & Giffin, K. *Problem-solving group interaction*. New York: Harper & Row, 1973, p. 93.
5. Duldt, B.W., & Giffin, K. *Theoretical perspectives for nursing*. Boston: Little, Brown, 1985, pp. 222–225, 250.
6. Marriner, A. *Guide to nursing management*. St. Louis: Mosby, 1980, p. 80.
7. Hersey, P., & Blanchard, K. *Management of organizational behavior: Utilizing human resources* (5th ed.). Englewood Cliffs, N. J.: Prentice-Hall, 1988, p. 161.
8. Ibid., 297.
9. Tappen, R. M. *Nursing leadership: Concepts and practice*. Philadelphia: Davis, 1983, p. 241.
10. Langford, T. *Managing and being managed: Preparation for professional nursing practice*. Englewood Cliffs, N. J.: Prentice-Hall, 1981, p. 94.
11. Ibid., 97.
12. Ibid., 99.
13. Ibid.
14. Nolan, M. G. Wanted: Colleagueship in nursing. *Journal of Nursing Administration,* 1976, *7* (3), 41
15. DeTornyay, R. Doctor and nurse—restraining forces in teamwork. *Hospital Forum,* 1974, *17,* 4–6.
16. Gillies, D. A. *Nursing management: A systems approach*. Philadelphia: Saunders, 1982, p. 152.

17. Cartwright, D. The nature of group cohesiveness. In D. Cartwright & A. Zander (Eds.). *Group dynamics: Research and theory* (3rd ed.). New York: Harper & Row, 1968, p. 98–103.
18. Grant, B. W. *Anger, cohesiveness, and productivity in small task groups.* (Unpublished doctoral dissertation, University of Kansas, 1978). *Dissertation Abstracts,* 1979, *39,* 3916 A. (University Microfilms International No. 7824799, 63.)
19. Gillies, *Nursing management,* p. 152–153.
20. Ibid., p. 200.
21. Stone, S., Firsich, S. C., Jordan, S. B., Berger, M. S., & Elhart, D. *Management for nurses: A multidisciplinary approach* (3rd ed.). St Louis: Mosby, 1984, p. 210–216.
22. Dyer, W. G. *Team building: Issues and alternatives.* Reading, Mass.: Addison-Wesley, 1977, p. 4.
23. Porter-O'Grady, T. *Creative nursing administration: Participative management into the 21st century.* Rockville, Md.: Aspen, 1986, p. 164.
24. Bramson, R.M. *Coping with difficult people . . . in business and in life.* New York: Random House, 1981.
25. Duldt, B. W., and the Community Education Staff of Metropolitan Medical Center: *Participant's manual for anger workshops; Facilitator's manual for anger workshops;* and *Anger, a training film.* Minneapolis: Metropolitan Medical Center, 1983.
26. Egan, G. Confrontation in laboratory training. In *Encounter: Group processes for interpersonal growth.* Belmont, Calif.: Brooks/Cole, 1970, pp. 287–335.
27. Egan, G. Confrontation. In Berger, M. S., et al. (Eds.). *Management for nurses: A multidisciplinary approach,* p. 165–180.
28. Guralnik, *Webster's dictionary,* p. 881.
29. Duldt & Giffin, *Theoretical perspectives for nursing,* p. 216, 222–223, 252.
30. Harnack, R. V., & Fest, T. B. *Group discussion: Theory and technique.* New York: Appleton-Century-Crofts, 1964, p. 21–31.
31. Ibid.
32. Gibb, J. Defensive communication. *Journal of Communication,* 1961, *11,* 141–148.
33. Blake, R. R., Shepard, H., & Mouton, J. S. *Managing intergroup conflict in industry.* Houston: Gulf Publishing Co., 1964, p. 13.
34. Meyer, J. W. Organizations as ideological systems. In Sergiovanni, T., & Corbally, J. (Eds.). *Leadership and organizational culture.* Chicago: University of Illinois Press, 1984, Chapter 11.
35. Gillies, *Nursing management,* p. 373–375.
36. Dyer, *Team building,* p. 91.
37. Hersey & Blanchard, *Management of organizational behavior,* p. 147.
38. Lawrence, P. R., & Lorsch, J. W. *Organization and environment: Managing differentiation and integration.* Division of Research, Graduate School of Business Administration, Harvard University, 1967.
39. Burke, R. J. Methods of resolving superior-subordinate conflict: The constructive use of subordinate differences and disagreements. *Organizational Behavior and Human Performance,* 1970, *5,* 393–411.
40. Filley, A. C. Types and sources of conflict. In Berger, M. S., et al. (Eds.). *Management for nurses: A multidisciplinary approach,* p. 149.
41. Schmidt, W. H. Conflict: A powerful process for (good or bad) change. *Management Review,* December 1974, p. 9. © 1974 AMACOM, a division of American Management Association, New York.
42. Filley, A. C. *Interpersonal conflict resolution.* Glenview, Ill.: Scott, Foresman, 1975, p. 33.
43. Douglass, L. M. *The effective nurse: Leader and manager* (2nd ed.). St. Louis: Mosby, 1984, p. 177.

III

MANAGEMENT OF THE TASK

Regardless of the type of organization or the level of management, there are certain functions that are the core of task management. Early in the study of organizational behavior, scholars identified a classic set of managerial functions to which we subscribe: planning, organizing, directing, and controlling. Because of the unique characteristics and concerns of nursing, we have added the function of staffing.

In part III, each of these functions is considered in depth. *Planning* refers to determining what needs to be done. *Organizing* involves designing an organizational structure to accomplish the task. *Staffing* includes developing job descriptions, personnel policies, and placement of qualified people in jobs or positions. *Directing* transforms all preceding efforts into action through utilization of material and human resources. *Controlling* is the system of checks and balances that maintains the direction of all efforts toward the original goals and objectives of the organization. Part III, then, focuses on these five functions of a leader in the management of the task.

9

PLANNING

INTRODUCTION

This chapter is devoted to the theory, research, and practice of planning as the first task-oriented function of nurse-leaders. Also considered will be the issues of allocating time to plan, and, briefly, nurses' current and future roles in planning.

THE SIGNIFICANCE OF PLANNING

Alvin Toffler concludes his popular book, *Future Shock,* by noting that the ultimate objective of society is more humane, foresighted, democratic planning and that the present period is ". . . the turning point in history at which man either vanquishes the processes of change or vanishes, at which, from being the unconscious puppet of evolution he becomes either its victim or its master."[1]

Since this statement was published in 1970, some notable events have proved Toffler correct—too correct. A salient example is the starvation of the Ethiopians in Africa. According to news analysts, the lack of effective agricultural planning caused erosion of soil, rapid water runoff, and, finally, devastating drought and crop failures. One distinctly unique capability of human beings is to plan, to generate ideas about many alternative futures, and to choose the most desirable outcome, the preferred future. Application of this unique human capability is particularly relevant in the delivery of health care and nursing services.

Changes within society that have an impact on delivery of health and nursing care include laws, economics, technology, role specialization, ecology, and ethics. Specific issues confronting nurses include aspects that many health care professionals have not had to consider before, at least to the degree presently required. Examples include financial monitoring, marketing, Medicare and other federal programs, megahospital chains, Diagnosis Related Groups, pre-payment plans, and health maintenance organizations.

One significant change will concern *who* decides how the health care dollar is spent. Historically, the physician has usually decided, in approximately 80 percent of the cases, who enters the health care system, the length of hospitalization, what services and resources are used in providing care, and so on. Soon this will no longer be true. The consumer, third-party providers, and nurses as health care managers within health care agencies will soon be making about three-fourths of these decisions. It is estimated that over 50 percent of the decisions presently being made by physicians will be made by nurses as first-line managers in home health agencies, health maintenance organizations, hospices, and similar health care agencies. It has been predicted that these changes will occur within the next one or two decades.[2]

There is no question that change is occurring. The issue is this: how can nurses as leaders adapt to the inevitable barrage of changes occurring daily so that the delivery of nursing and

139

health services is kept viable and current?[2] To be effective nurse-leaders, nurses need to be prepared to be "change masters," not "change agents," as most professional graduates are described by nursing faculties. Agents act for someone else, such as an agent for an insurance company or a trustee in managing an estate. Masters are experts highly skilled in some endeavor and are self-directed. As a general principle, we suggest the following:

> *To the same degree nurses are able to master planning skills and strategies, nurses will be able to direct and control change and to select a preferred future.*

Professional nursing education programs prepare nurse-leaders to plan nursing care or patient care management, and there are ample models for nurses to follow in conducting nursing practice: team nursing, primary nursing, and problem-oriented practice.[3] The focus here, however, is on planning for the delivery of nursing services, for organizing, staffing, directing, and controlling human resources, and other resources as well, within the scope of larger health care organizations.

DEFINING PLANNING

According to the dictionary, *planning* is a detailed scheme, program, or method worked out beforehand for the accomplishment of an object, project, or goal. It can take the form of a drawing, diagram, outline, or narrative describing in detail the process of achieving a goal.[4] Synonyms for *plan* as a noun are blueprint, design, game plan, project, plot, scheme, and strategy. For *plan* as a verb, the synonyms include arrange, layout, map, set out, and arrange.[5] *Plan* is derived from the Latin *planum,* meaning level ground.

The role and function of planning is to effect change. This is the first function of management: the effectiveness of all subsequent functions, organizing, staffing, directing, and controlling, depends upon planning. That planning is a process is generally supported in the literature of many disciplines.[6,7] For example, Koontz and O'Donnell state it is an intellectual process in which there is conscious determination of courses of action.[8] As a part of the nursing process, planning is an integral role in the art and science of nursing: assessing, diagnosing, planning, implementing, and evaluating.[9]

Planning Theory

While theories of planning, that is, organized perspectives of planning, are rare, according to Troub,[10] planning is a process that involves a wide range of activities directed toward initiating change. While there are a number of definitions of planning and statements about planning in the literature, most seem to consist of a shopping list of activities in which one engages when planning. There are two exceptions, however. Googins et al emphasize an interactional theoretical framework that stresses the need to obtain acceptance of a plan by others.[11] Troub's theory of planning evolution provides a historical perspective of how planning becomes more complex as human societies have moved from feudal through agricultural and industrial to postindustrial (high-tech) phases of socioeconomic development.[12]

Troub identifies four evolutional levels of planning. Type I, or *preadaptive planning,* is characterized by prophecy or technological predictions, with the planner having no control over future events. Thus one can only preadapt for such events as drought, flood, and similar problems. This level of planning is consistent with feudal systems and agricultural societies.

Type II, or *innovational adaptation,* is characterized by technological predictions, and some degree of control is possible by creating systems of control. This is typical planning in an industrial society. Intraorganizational planning is prevalent, and cognitive planning occurs within individual organizations.

Type III, or *complex anticipative planning,* is based on obtaining information about interacting systems in future prediction, designing of significant control systems, and directing changes across time toward preferable outcomes. This type of planning is characteristic of postindustrial societies.

Type IV, *creative design of a chosen dynamic future,* is characterized by conscious creation of novel futures and the creation of (not adaptation to) control systems and processes to result in new outcomes or to guide and control outcomes. This is characteristic of high-technology (or whatever comes after postindustrial) societies, and it involves use of professional decision makers (consultants, attorneys, and so on) and collective decision making at all levels of societies. Troub states that this society has been at Type III for several centuries, and he proposes it is moving to Type IV, a holistic planning level.

> Computers carry on conversations of sorts, and artificial intelligence seems to be on its way. More recently humans have created pseudolife, and they are evolving entirely new biological organisms. These organisms are patentable, produced by both public and private enterprise, and contracted for and sold in markets. Serious negotiations are in process about whether to limit endeavors which may lead to humans evolving themselves biologically. In this setting, growing potential for a fourth mode of evolution, self-conscious evolution involving introduction of Type IV planning efforts, does not appear too surprising.[13]

Nurses are already involved in providing high-tech, high-touch care. This is particularly true for those practicing as clinical nurse-specialists or in intensive care areas. It is highly probable that soon, these nurses will become increasingly involved in health care projects at Troub's Type IV level of planning.

White's predictions about health professions personnel by the year 2000 indicate that more than 700,000 physicians will be practicing in the United States, and this is expected to exceed this society's needs by approximately 20,000 to 70,000 around 1990.[14] This surplus of physicians will undoubtedly change the functions and relationships of other health professionals, particularly nurses. Whereas nurses have predominantly been employed in hospitals and similar health agencies, Andreoli and Musser predict the graying of America will create a demand for geriatric nursing care and services in home health, adult day care centers, day hospitals, hospices, and community-based mental health centers.[15] In schools, they forecast that:

> Nurses will continue to carry out stress counseling, health assessment, screening programs, sex education classes, physical fitness programs (beyond competitive sports), and organization of peer support groups around risk factors such as obesity, substance abuse, smoking, and stress.[16]

These services provided by nurses are already established in business and industry. Nine times more nurses than physicians are currently practicing in occupational health settings.[17] Andreoli and Musser also note potential conflict between physicians and nurses as the doctors take back some of the functions historically passed over to nursing. This includes patient education and counseling and moving into underserved rural and inner-city areas where nurses have been the primary health care providers. Administrators of hospitals are expected to replace physicians with highly skilled clinical nurses in some clinical areas to contain costs. Nurses' relationships with physicians and hospital administrators will need considerable attention and planning in order to maintain effective working relationships.[18]

A General Framework for Planning Is Needed

The primary question remains: How can nursing leaders adapt to the inevitable changes through planning? Troub's Type IV planning, creative design of a chosen dynamic future, is probably the holistic planning needed: it is consistent with the holistic philosophical perspectives of nursing and of health care. Andreoli and Musser have identified some changes in nursing and health care delivery for which we need to plan. What is now needed is a general framework for planning.

There is a natural tendency to wonder where nursing fits in Troub's levels of planning. The teaching in generic nursing programs tends of necessity to focus on planning nursing care for individual clients and for small groups. It is proposed that, while the curriculum objectives and content may reflect a higher level, the clinical practice of contemporary generic nursing students probably is at Level II (innovational adaptation). While other health care providers may be prepared for and are participating on higher levels, nurses seem to consider it a stroke of good luck to become involved in a group using Type III or IV planning. Most do not seem to expect even to be involved. Too many nurses and nurse-educators seem to think and behave as if students and practicing nurses are to be *reactive* rather than *proactive*.

There is a world of difference between being reactive and being proactive. According to the dictionary, to *react* means to respond to a stimulus or to return an opposing action, force, or influence. To be *reactionary* means to politically advocate a particular response.[19] To be *proactive* means to go before (pro) and to initiate action or change (active) with exemplary forcefulness of inspiration to others.[20] This definition implies that, in being reactive, one reacts to *others'* plans and consequently lacks self-direction. On the other hand, being proactive implicitly necessitates aggressive planning, which provides direction for one's efforts to which others then must react. Thus greater control is possible so that one's preferred future becomes a probability, not just a possibility.

Where are nurses in relation to being reactive and proactive?

First, Ashley's work documents the reactionary mode that nurses in the United States have used for over a century in seeking the recognition, social sanctions, and protection granted to physicians, dentists, and other health professionals. She attributes this to the fact that nurses have predominantly been women and consequently second-class citizens. Thus, they have felt they had no right to achieve their ambitions.[21] This self-labeling phenomenon is reflected in the reactive tone of the American Nurses' Association (ANA) Code of Ethics for Nurses (1976). (See Appendix A.) By comparison, the statements of the American Medical Association (AMA) Principles of Medical Ethics (1980) seem more proactive, emphasizing exposing incompetence within and without the association's ranks, advancing scientific knowledge, and choosing clients, associates, and contexts. Perhaps the most appropriate observation is that attributed to the comic-strip character, Pogo: "We have met the enemy, and they are US!"

Second, new graduates complain of insufficient preparation for leadership roles. Seeking to identify the management and leadership competencies that neophyte nurses need to function effectively in contemporary job settings, Brown used five categories to define competencies: planning, organizing, staffing, directing, and controlling. Her findings show the neophyte nurses ranked planning items lower than nurse-educators and nurse-administrators; there were no differences among the three group means on the other four competencies. Approximately one-third of the neophytes, nurses who had graduated from a generic BSN program within one year, indicated the nursing educational program had not prepared them adequately in leadership skills, and that the employing institution did not offer adequate assistance in filling the void.[22]

Third, the followership as well as leadership in nursing may be changing. Corona proposes a theory of followership to describe and explain contemporary nursing leadership.[23] Assuming every role has a complementary role, she notes the individual's right to civil disobedience—to openly defy leadership because of one's individual moral convictions. Since the Nuremberg trials, followers are held responsible for their individual actions regardless of a leader's influence. This concept of civil disobedience has been used effectively in the United States by the civil rights movement, environmentalists, and other groups. Perhaps this influence is now flowing through the ranks of nurses. The result may be a followership that no longer just quits and withdraws, but is learning how to engage in dialogue with leaders, making the followership a more divergent, tougher group to lead.

While this is mere speculation, it is interesting to note that in the past 50 years there has been an absence of outstanding, nationally recognized leaders in nursing. In addition, individuals seem to be in nursing leadership positions for very brief periods. For example, the average tenure in recent years of deans or heads of nursing education programs is commonly estimated to be three years. Generally, such positions need to be held by one individual for five to seven years in order to implement and evaluate programs and administrative stances. This phenomenon of rapid leadership turnover may reflect the turbulent interval necessary as the followership and leadership learn how to engage in dialogue without terminating relationships.

Corona stresses the importance of two factors in persuading followers.[24] First, *moral* leadership involves decision making based on the greatest benefit to the majority rather than personal gain and on considering the characteristics and capabilities of the followership and client population. Essentially, this is a humanistic perspective of human values. The second factor is the character of communication necessary to influence the followership to accept a potential leader's proposals and decide to follow. This is the heart of Situational Leadership theory: If the followers decide to follow one person, then this person becomes a leader. The following principle is based on the above discussion:

If our nursing leaders would consider the moral issues, communicate to persuade and influence, and maintain a proactive stance in planning for our preferred futures, then the turbulence and unrest among nurses would tend to decrease.

There is hope in turbulence, however; it often means growth is occurring.

THE PLANNING PROCESS

The general framework for planning that we propose includes four sequential steps of the planning process: diagnosing, deciding, interacting, and changing. Each step has a set of dimensions that interact to shape and mold the development of a plan. The first and most important step is that of diagnosis.

Diagnosing

Broadly defined, *diagnosing* is an art and science involving skillful interviewing and intuitively knowing the right question to ask. Sensing the contextual climate of the health care agency and establishing effective patterns of observation and data collection are also involved. Finally, one needs to develop ways to process and interpret data. As a general principle, we suggest the following:

> *Depending on the degree of accuracy in diagnosing the need for change, the nurse-leader can be effective in initiating planning efforts.*

In diagnosing for planning and change, nursing leaders need to determine (1) what *actually* is happening now; (2) what is *likely* to be happening in the future if no planning effort is made; (3) what nurses and others would *ideally* like to be happening in this situation; and (4) what or who is *blocking* or preventing progression from actual to ideal.[25] There are three interacting dimensions to diagnosing: perceiving, identifying, and analyzing.

Perceiving

Perceiving involves looking at the situation through the eyes of each person or representative group involved: the nurses, clients and their families, other health care providers, third-party payers, and society in general. Ideally, to get the full picture, the nurse-leader needs to look at the situation from as many points of view as possible of the people who will be affected by any changes. Reality, however, sometimes restricts such a broad perspective. It may even be difficult for nurse-leaders to have access to people and information beyond the nursing unit or service.[26] If nursing is to be involved in Troub's Level IV planning, however, this broad perspective seems to be an imperative.

Identifying

The second dimension, identifying, consists of describing the problem, a discrepancy between what is actually happening (the real) and what you or someone who hired you (point of view) would like to be happening (the ideal). Until you can explain precisely what you would like to have occurring and unless that set of conditions is different from the present condition, no problem exists, no change is necessary, and no planning is needed. To the same degree in which a discrepancy exists between the real (actual) and the ideal, you need to plan for changes. The identifying dimension of planning involves change efforts that attempt to reduce the discrepancies between the real and the ideal.

It is in problem identification that the concepts and theoretical frameworks presented in this text begin to come into play. For example, two important potential areas for discrepancy are output-end result variables and intervening variables.

In examining *end-result variables,* the questions are: Is the hospital, nursing staff, or individual nurse doing an effective job in providing the needed type and scope of nursing care to a specified population? Are short-term goals being met? How does the long-term picture look in terms of shifts in client population characteristics, mortality, morbidity, and the like? Are the agency's philosophy, objectives, departmental programs and policies, therapeutic protocols, and nursing care plans being put into operation appropriately and effectively? Are services coordinated to the greatest benefit of the client so that there are seldom lost hospital days when tests or patient education are not being done? If these are working out sufficiently well, but discrepancies between the real and ideal still exist, then *intervening variables* need to be considered.

If performance is a problem, then you can look at the condition of the human resources as an intervening variable. For example, how much turnover, absenteeism, or tardiness is there? What about error rates in administering medications and treatments, and how frequent are the accident rates, such as patients falling out of bed? What about the accident rates among personnel? How often are personnel on workmen's compensation? The theories that you have been reading can generate all kinds of diagnostic questions for planning change in the situation you are examining, such as the following ones:

What leadership, decision-making, and problem-solving skills are available? What is the motivation, communication, commitment to objectives, and climate (morale)? (Use Likert's work.)

What is the readiness level of the people involved? Are they willing and able to take significant responsibility for their own performance? Do the head nurses, supervisors, and others acknowledge the nurses' expert ability and responsibility? (Use Hersey and Blanchard's work.)

What need level seems to be most important for nurses right now? (Use Maslow's motivation theory.)

How are the hygiene factors and motivators? Are nurses getting paid enough? How are the working conditions? Is job security an issue? How are interpersonal relations? Do nurses complain about the head nurse or supervisor? Are nurses able to get recognition for their professional accomplishments? Is there much challenge in patient care assignments? Are there opportunities for professional growth and development? Are nurses given the power to function along with the responsibility? (Use Herzberg's theory of motivation.)

The questions and the theorists they represent point out that the material in this book was meant to be used. *Good theory is just common sense organized.* Use the theories presented to help you to sort out what is happening in your situation and identify what might need to be changed.[27]

Analyzing

Problem identification flows almost immediately into analysis, the third dimension of diagnosing. Once a discrepancy (problem) has been identified, the goal of analysis is to determine why the problem exists. The separation of problem identification and analysis is not always that clear, however, for identifying areas of discrepancy is often a part of analysis.[28]

Once a discrepancy has been identified in the end-result variables or intervening variables, the most natural strategy is to begin to examine *causal variables*—the independent variables that can be altered or changed by the organization and its management, such as leadership or management style, organizational structure, or organizational objectives. In other words, can you identify what in the environment might have caused the discrepancy? Again, different theorists come to mind and stimulate various questions.

What is the dominant leadership style being used? How does it fit with the maturity level of the people involved? (Use Hersey and Blanchard's work.)

What are the prevailing assumptions about human nature adhered to by nursing administration and the agency administrator? How well do those assumptions match the capabilities and potential of the nurses involved? (Use McGregor's work.)

Are nurses able to satisfy a variety of needs in this environment? How do the opportunities for need satisfaction compare with high strength needs of the nursing staff involved? (Use Maslow's motivation theory[29].)

How do the expectations of the various situational variables compare with the leadership style being used by nurse-administrators? (Use Hersey and Blanchard's Situational Leadership.)

Again, these theories and questions are presented to suggest how the concepts studied can help you to analyze problems that exist in your environment and provide guidelines for developing strategies for planning.[30]

Deciding

The second step in the planning process is *deciding*. Most probably think of John Dewey's steps of problem solving in order to logically arrive at a decision.[31] One has to realize, however, that these steps (as well as the steps of planning that are currently being described) are not the way real-life decisions are made. Typically, there is a mixture of task and relationship behavior blended in this process, and the individuals or groups deal with each step in a variety of ways.

Generally, to *decide* means that after all pertinent facts (and feelings) have been considered, a conclusion is reached, a verdict pronounced, or a judgment made.[32] As a general principle, the following can be stated:

> *By reviewing relevant values and data, the leader can confidently decide which areas, issues, or factors need to be given priority for planning.*

There are three interacting dimensions of deciding that we shall consider: valuing, surveying, and selecting.

Valuing

Values are beliefs and opinions that are arranged in a hierarchical order according to importance, as defined by McNally, who provides the following criteria for a true value:

1. It is prized and cherished.
2. It is a part of a pattern, i.e., repeated.
3. A value is freely chosen from among alternatives only after due reflection.
4. A value is positively affirmed and acted upon.[33,34]

The dimension of valuing involves weighing the preferred and potential options in relation to beliefs, attitudes, and moral or ethical codes that significantly influence the behavior of individuals and groups involved in the situation. This may be extended to include cultural mores, laws, religious beliefs, and personal as well as organizational philosophies. In fact, after diagnosing the problem, you may realize that the ideal is unrealistic and may be in conflict with a highly valued aspect of nursing care. While values may be considered a barrier by some,[35] we propose that early consideration of values is an asset in providing wisdom and direction to the planning process.

For example, a common theme today is cost-effective health care, yet you may value an all-RN staff and primary nursing as the best way to organize delivery of nursing services. Eason, Lee, and Spickerman provide their nursing students with the following problem involving calculating the basic annual budget to cover a unit of 36 patients with all RNs. No differential pay, overtime, or fringe benefits are included in the calculations.

To make the calculation as simple as possible, a salary of $10.00 per hour is used. Students find the number of paid hours per year, 2080, by multiplying 40 (the number of hours worked per week) by 52 (the number of weeks in the year). The salary for one nurse is obviously $20,800. Next the students calculate the money necessary to pay 33 RNs at this rate: $686,400 is an astronomical figure! Many students recalculate believing they made an arithmetic error. Students are reminded that this is an overly simple example: that accurately budgeting for personnel is a complex management task. Just to provide customary fringe benefits the institution would have to allocate an additional 15% to 20%.[36]

That's a lot of money—and perhaps too costly for the clientele your agency serves, too.

The relevance and implications of factual information, however, can interact with the value systems of interested individuals to impel support for planning. People will form special groups to *do something (plan)* about the problem.[37] For example, parents in Atlanta and later elsewhere who became concerned about the disappearance of their children formed special groups to do something about the problem. In a short time, children were being fingerprinted, educational programs were implemented to teach children how to recognize potential kidnapers and what to do to protect themselves, and so on. Another example is the group called MADD (Mothers Against Drunk Driving). Members of this group have lost a child in an auto accident caused by a drunk driver. The point is that people will do something to protect what they value highly. These people place high value on their children's safety and welfare, they formed planning groups, and they made significant changes in the way these particular problems were handled in their communities and states.

It is your value system that determines which facts are relevant, and it is imperative that before you plan, you determine the value systems of the various people who will be affected by the planning.[38] Corona stresses the need for leaders to communicate messages that are consistent with nursing values.[39] These values are summarized in the nursing code. Research in the area of interpersonal perception indicates that when value systems of individuals are congruent, the interpersonal interactions tend to be satisfying; when value systems are incongruent, people tend to withdraw and avoid one another.[40]

Even though management based on the assumptions of Theory X is perhaps no longer widely appropriate, in the opinion of McGregor and others, it is still widely practiced. Consequently, a large majority of the people in the United States today are treated as immature human beings in their working environments. In attempting to analyze this situation, Chris Argyris,[41] now of Harvard University, has compared the bureaucratic-pyramidal values (the organizational counterpart to Theory X assumptions about people) that still dominate most organizations, including health care agencies, with a more humanistic-democratic value system (the organizational counterpart to Theory Y assumptions about people) as illustrated in Table 9–1.[42]

According to Argyris, following bureaucratic or pyramidal values leads to poor, shallow, and mistrustful relationships. Because these relationships do not permit the natural and free expression of feelings, they are deceptive or nonauthentic and result in decreased interpersonal competence.

Without interpersonal competence of a "psychologically safe" environment, the organization is a breeding ground for mistrust, intergroup conflict, rigidity, and so on, which in turn lead to a decrease in organizational success in problem solving.[43]

TABLE 9-1. TWO DIFFERENT VALUE SYSTEMS AS SEEN BY CHRIS ARGYRIS.

Bureaucratic/Pyramidal Value System	Humanistic/Democratic Value System
1. Important human relationships—the crucial ones—are those related to achieving the organization's objectives, *i.e.,* getting the job done.	1. The important human relationships are not only those related to achieving the organization's objectives but those related to maintaining the organization's internal system and adapting to the environment as well.
2. Effectiveness in human relationship increases as behavior becomes more rational, logical, and clearly communicated; but effectiveness decreases as behavior becomes more emotional.	2. Human relationships increase in effectiveness as *all* the relevant behavior (rational and interpersonal) becomes conscious, discussible, and controllable.
3. Human relationships are most effectively motivated by carefully defined direction, authority, and control, as well as appropriate rewards and penalties that emphasize rational behavior and achievement of the objective.	3. In addition to direction, controls, and rewards and penalties, human relationships are most effectively influenced through authentic realtionships, internal commitment, psychological success, and the process of confirmation.

From Hersey, P., & Blanchard, K. Management of organizational behavior: Utilizing human resources *(5th ed.). Englewood Cliffs, N.J.: Prentice-Hall, 1988, p. 59, with permission.*

If, on the other hand, humanistic or democratic values are adhered to in an organization, Argyris claims that trusting, authentic relationships will develop among people, will result in increased interpersonal competence, intergroup cooperation, flexibility, and the like, and should result in increases in organizational effectiveness. In this kind of environment, people are treated as human beings, both organizational members and the organization itself are given an opportunity to develop to the fullest potential, and there is an attempt to make work exciting and challenging. Implicit in following these values is

> . . . treating each human being as a person with a complex set of needs, *all* of which are important in his work and in his life . . . and providing opportunities for people in organizations to influence the way in which they relate to work, the organization, and the environment.[44]

We believe the humanistic-democratic value system as described by Argyris is most congruent with the values of nursing as a discipline and profession. Using this as a broadly based value system, you, as a nursing leader need to study facts, opinions, and beliefs to determine specific factors that are uniquely valued by the people to be affected by your planning. Belock identifies three ways in which values are exposed:

1. *Personal value claims* are reflected in such statements as: "I like . . . ," "I prefer . . . ," "It is important to me that . . ."
2. *Market value claims* are manifest in the statements a person makes when trying to convey what a certain object is worth in the market-place.
3. *Real value claims* assert that a certain thing is better (i.e., of greater worth or merit) than other conceivable and available alternatives according to particular criteria, i.e., money, energy, or time. People making such a claim are not referring to the common or even expert opinion of what a particular thing is worth—nor are they merely expressing a personal opinion. They are claiming that a certain idea is better than another idea because, all things considered, it outweighs its alternatives in terms of explicit and important criteria. Moral value claims represent a particular kind of real value claim.[45]

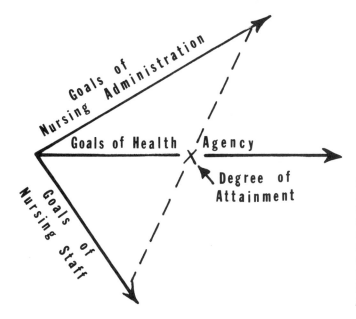

Figure 9–1. Directions of goals of nursing administration, nursing staff, and the health care organization—moderate organizational accomplishment. *(Modified from Hersey, P., & Blanchard, K.* Management of organizational behavior: Utilizing human resources *[5th ed.]. Englewood Cliffs, N.J.: Prentice-Hall, 1988, p. 137.)*

There is a considerable amount of literature available regarding value clarification and the value of human life in clinical care problems. The Karen Quinlan case and Baby Jane Doe episode are recent examples of evaluating difficult clinical situations in relation to individual values, laws, and religion. The concern here is with the values relating to leadership roles in planning and decision making about human resources in particular, but other resources as well.

Another way to get a handle on values is to look at the integration of goals. Generally, the degree to which individuals and groups perceive their own goals as being satisfied by the accomplishment of organizational goals is the degree of integration of goals. When organizational goals are shared by all, this is what McGregor calls a true "integration of goals."[46,47]

To illustrate this concept, divide an organization or a health agency into two groups, nursing administration (leaders) and nursing staff (followers). The respective goals of these two groups and the resultant attainment of goals of the health agency to which they belong are illustrated in Figure 9–1.*

In this instance, the goals of nursing administration are somewhat compatible with the goals of the health agency but are not exactly the same. On the other hand, the goals of the nursing staff are almost at odds with those of the health agency. The result of the interaction between the goals of nursing administration and the goals of nursing staff is a compromise, and actual performance is a combination of both. It is at this approximate point that the degree of attainment of the goals of the health agency can be pictured. This situation can be much worse when there is little accomplishment of health agency goals, as illustrated in Figure 9–2.

In this situation, there seems to be a general disregard for the welfare of the health agency. Nursing administration and staff see their own goals conflicting with those of the health agency. Consequently, morale and performance will tend to be low, and health agency

---

*In reality, the schematics presented in the following pages are simplifications of vector analyses and therefore would be more accurately portrayed as parallelograms.

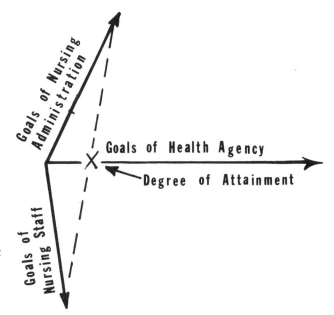

Figure 9–2. Little organizational accomplishment. *(Adapted from Hersey, P., & Blanchard, K. Management of organizational behavior: Utilizing human resources [5th ed.]. Englewood Cliffs, N.J.: Prentice-Hall, 1988, p. 138.)*

accomplishment will be negligible. In some cases, the health agency goals can be so opposed that no positive progress is obtained. For any organization, the result often is substantial losses, or draining off of assets and resources. (See Fig. 9–3.) In fact, in the business world, organizations are going out of business every day for these very reasons; this may also be true for hospitals and other health agencies.

The hope in an organization of any type is to create a climate in which one of two things occurs. The individuals in the organization (both leaders and followers) either perceive their goals as being the same as the goals of the organization or, although different, see their own

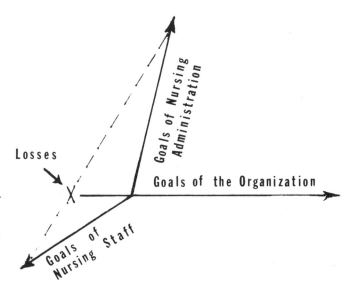

Figure 9–3. No positive organizational accomplishment. *(Adapted from Hersey, P., & Blanchard, K. Management of organizational behavior: Utilizing human resources [5th ed.]. Englewood Cliffs, N.J.: Prentice-Hall, 1988, p. 138.)*

goals being satisfied as a direct result of working for the goals of the organization. Consequently, the greater the integration of an individual's goals and objectives to the organization's goals, the greater will be the organizational performance, as illustrated in Figure 9–4. Integration of goals is often approached effectively by using the process of management by objectives (MBO). (See Chapter 14 for a description of this process.)

Generally, you need to determine what value system you want to guide your planning. What leadership theory is most congruent with your chosen value system? In what situations do you expect to engage in planning as a leader? We propose as most congruent with nursing the humanistic-democratic value system, Situational Leadership as the leadership theory, and the Humanistic Nursing Communication theory to develop and maintain interpersonal relationships. We believe exploration of value systems and appropriate dialogue will tend to result in the development of congruency of values to guide planning and to facilitate the acceptance of these plans. Having considered congruent values, decisions in the planning process can be discussed.

Surveying

Surveying is the second interacting dimension of deciding. This consists of looking over all of the data and potential solutions associated with the situation. You need to carefully inspect the information that has particular relevance to the value system established. It is in scrutinizing the data that the value system can serve as a guide in picking out the important facts.

The kind of information or facts to be surveyed will vary with the situation. Budgets can be expected to be included. In this period of conversion to Diagnosis Related Groups (DRGs) and soaring health care costs, cost containment has become a highly valued factor. Another kind of information is the length of hospitalization and acuity (degree of illness). As the DRG conversion occurs, nurses have noted the patients are sent home earlier and sicker. This increased patient care load caused by higher acuity is often further complicated by decreasing the number of nonprofessional personnel on the nursing staff. The nurses, then, are pressed into doing more non-nursing duties, such as busing trays and carrying linen. Staffing by primary care, team nursing, and other approaches are being studied carefully from a budgetary perspective. Maternity nurses are concerned because they do not have opportunities to teach infant care to new mothers, who now go home in 24 to 48 hours after delivery, rather than three or four days as was formerly the case. Public health nurses express concern about whether or not someone will be at the home to help patients who are still ill, uninformed about self-care, or both.[48] Home health nursing agencies seem to be a reasonable direction for planning to meet this evolving gap in health care. Computerized staffing patterns and personnel surveys of absenteeism, turnover, tardiness, and job satisfaction of nurses also are relevant data.[49] Patients' evaluations of care received while hospitalized are

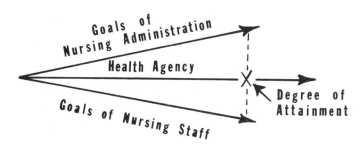

Figure 9–4. An integration of the goals of nursing administration, nursing staff, and the health agency organization—*high* organizational accomplishment. *(Modified from Hersey, P., & Blanchard, K. Management of organizational behavior: Utilizing human resources, [5th ed.]. Englewood Cliffs, N.J.: Prentice-Hall, 1988, p. 139.)*

also important. The kind of service clients and patients would like to have is probably highly relevant data, too.

Another aspect of surveying is generating potential solutions. This calls for creativity and new perspectives. One technique is called *brainstorming*. The four rules are:

1. *Criticism is ruled out.* Adverse judgment of ideas must be withheld until later.
2. *"Free-Wheeling"* is welcomed. The wilder the idea the better; it is easier to tame down than to think up.
3. *Quantity is wanted.* The greater the number of ideas, the more likelihood of winners.
4. *Combination and improvement are sought.* In addition to contributing ideas of their own, participants should suggest how ideas of others can be turned into *better* ideas; or how two or more ideas can be joined into still another idea.[50]

This is an ideal technique for a small group of planners. It allows the members freedom from inhibition of self-criticism or squashing by others. The goal is to generate more "alternative approaches to a specific problem."[51] Someone is to record all the ideas for later consideration.

A second, more complex approach is called the Delphi Method, developed in the Rand Corporation.[52] This technique is particularly helpful for groups that are larger and composed of individuals of varying social status, occupations, and professions. Opinions are given in writing, and ownership of the statements may be withheld for a while in order to focus on *what* the suggestion is rather than on *who* made it. The relative degree of attractiveness or status of group members seems to have a strong influence upon the communication within a small task group. For example, the amount of communication from low-status members to high-status members tends to increase, and there tends to be pressure among the group members to conform to the attractive or high-status member's opinions.[53,54] Temporarily withholding the source of an idea allows due consideration of *all* potential approaches and tends to increase the quantity of ideas generated.

Selecting
The third interacting dimension of deciding is *selecting*—choosing the most preferred approach, solution, or future. Patton and Giffin suggest three criteria for evaluating any proposed plan:

1. Will this proposal produce the desired changes in the current situation? Will it meet the need for change as we have identified it?
2. Can this proposal be implemented by us? Is it a workable suggestion?
3. Does this proposal inherently contain serious disadvantages?[55]

These seem to be very practical questions to ask as you consider your options.

Another useful technique, force field analysis, was developed by Kurt Lewin for diagnosing situations, and this may be useful in looking at the variables involved in determining the potential impact of initiating a change, its possible influence on effectiveness, and your options in selecting on a course of action.[56]

Lewin assumes that in any situation there are both driving and restraining forces that influence any change that may occur. *Driving forces* are those forces affecting a situation that are pushing in a particular direction; they tend to initiate a change and keep it going. In terms of improving productivity in a work group, pressure from a supervisor, incentive earnings, and competition may be examples of driving forces. "Career ladders" is another example that has been developed in many health agencies to systematically recognize nurses who demonstrate advanced clinical knowledge and competencies. This system enables nurses to advance and be promoted while remaining at the bedside. In the past, staff nurses could only achieve higher pay and rank by going into nursing educational or administrative positions.[57] The career ladder system generally provides three options: clinical, educational, and administrative. Agencies having this system report lowered turnover rates. (See Appendix F.)

Restraining forces act to restrain or decrease the driving forces. Apathy, hostility, and poor maintenance of equipment may be examples of restraining forces against increased production. *Equilibrium* is reached when the *sum of the driving forces equals the sum of the restraining forces.* In this example, equilibrium represents the present level of productivity, as shown in Figure 9–5. In nursing, increases in patient or client load, staff shortage or vacancies, and staff burnout are common factors in limiting quality and quantity of nursing care services.

According to Lewin's technique, this equilibrium, or present level of productivity, can be raised or lowered by changes in the relationship between the driving and the restraining forces. For illustration, look at the dilemma of a new head nurse who takes over a nursing unit in which the quality and quantity of nursing care (productivity) is high but whose predecessor drained the human resources (intervening variables). The former head nurse had upset the equilibrium by increasing the driving forces (that is, being autocratic and keeping continual pressure on the nursing staff) and thus achieving increases in output in the short run. Because the head nurse did this, new restraining forces developed, such as increased hostility, antagonism, and burnout. At the time of the former head nurse's departure the restraining forces were beginning to increase, and the results manifested themselves in turnover, absenteeism, and other restraining forces, which lowered the quality and quantity of nursing care (productivity) shortly after the new head nurse arrived. Now a new equilibrium at a significantly lower level of nursing care (productivity) is faced by the new head nurse.

Now, just assume that the new head nurse decides not to increase the driving forces but to reduce the restraining forces. The head nurse may do this by taking time away from the usual nursing care assignments and engaging in problem solving, in-service training, and development of interpersonal relationships. In the short run, output will tend to be lowered still

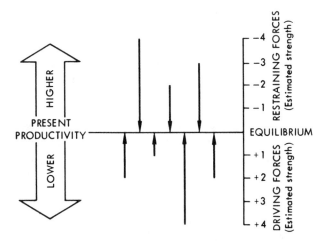

Figure 9–5. Driving and restraining forces in equilibrium. *(From Hersey, P., & Blanchard, K. Management of organizational behavior: Utilizing human resources. [5th ed.]. Englewood Cliffs, N.J.: Prentice-Hall, 1988, p. 136.)*

further. If commitment to objectives and technical know-how of the group are increased in the long run, these may become new driving forces. Along with the elimination of hostility and apathy, the new driving forces will now tend to move the balance to a higher level of output. Certainly the support of the health agency administrator, the medical staff, and others would be necessary. The patient or client census would also need to be lowered during this period of lowered productivity expectations, so that the safety of these people would not be jeopardized while the restraining forces were being reduced.

Nurse-leaders are often in a position in which they must consider not only output but also intervening variables, not only short-term but also long-term goals. A framework that is useful in diagnosing these relationships is available through force field analysis.[58]

Interacting

The third element in planning is *interacting*. As a general principle:

> *The quality and quantity of persuasive communication tends to directly influence the degree of acceptance and support received by a proposed plan for change.*

Interacting involves talking with people to convince them of the necessity, appropriateness, and value of a plan. Effective interpersonal relationships and communication skills are an imperative to enable the ultimate implementation of plans. Implementation of a plan is achieved only by working through others. Interacting involves three interrelated dimensions: negotiating, bargaining, and consolidating.

Negotiating

This is the process of communing and conferring with others in order to reach an understanding. Diplomacy and tact is necessary in order to deal with people, and listening is as much a part of negotiating as talking. Dialogue is necessary to identify values, goals, preferences, and needs for you as a nursing leader and for your followers and colleagues. As a leader, you need to be sensitive to the desires and expectations of the people whose support you need in order for your plan to be implemented.

Bargaining

This is finally developing an agreement, contract, or deal that is acceptable to most of the people involved. In seeking support for your plan, you may not want to have a contract in the legal sense, but rather an informal alliance with individuals or groups who will be affected by the plan's implementation. This alliance or coalition is based upon agreements or consensus about the details of the plan and how the plan can be of the greatest benefit to all concerned.

Consolidating

Finally, *consolidating* means to unify and to firmly establish support for one's plan. Acceptance needs to be openly supported and even celebrated, perhaps, in order to strengthen the individuals' commitment to the plan and each one's role in its development and implementation.

It is this process of interacting (negotiating, bargaining, and consolidating) that is particularly important in effective planning. Corona emphasizes the leader's message as needing ". . . to be consistent with the actions of the group of followers and in the best interests of the organization or profession."[59] She also emphasizes that the nursing leader's communication needs to include all of the facts so that an informed followership can make a decision to follow.

Googins states: "Plans are *conceived* through cognitive skills and *realized* through planner's interactive skills."[60] According to Situational Leadership, the very heart of leadership is activated at this interacting stage: ". . . leadership is *the process of* influencing *the activities of an individual or a group in efforts toward goal achievement in a given situation.*"[61] To influence is to gain acceptance of plans, and this brings us to the last element of planning.

Changing

One cannot plan without considering the changes that will occur upon implementation of a plan. Change is briefly introduced and defined in Situational Leadership (see page 17). It is also considered earlier in this text in relation to the people-oriented concept of initiating. The levels, cycles, and process of change are equally appropriate to consider again in relation to the task-oriented concept of planning. Thus it is suggested that readers at this point may want to review the material about change in Chapter 6, Initiating.

ALLOCATING TIME FOR PLANNING

The buzz words *time management* have been a popular topic of seminars and workshops recently. This is based on the premise that those with responsibilities need to control the way they spend time (as if it were money!). Time management suggests that specified periods are to be allocated according to priorities and goals. It would seem particularly necessary to allocate time for planning because, human nature being what it is, planning is easily neglected, yet it is so important. As a class assignment, one of the graduate students in nursing conducted a survey about planning habits of middle-management nurses in a local medical center (a nonrandom sample of convenience). Much to her chagrin, only a few of the approximately 20 head nurses and supervisors could clearly identify how, what, when, and where they engaged in planning. They "just sort of did it along with everything else." It was concluded that most of the nurses apparently were in a reactive rather than proactive mode in regard to planning. This is truly a shame because of lost potential and possibilities for quality nursing care and development of professional capabilities. If this is also true for our readers, then the following discussion may be of particular interest and personal relevance.

Googins emphasizes the need for *reflection* and suggests nurse leaders ". . . deliberately set aside time to consider prior episodes, activities, linkages, individuals, and actual and potential resources."[62] Although we have not found documentation about how much time nursing leaders spend in planning, Steiner provides information about "ideal" allocations of time for planning in an average business.[63] (See Fig. 9–6.) We can generally superimpose typical health agency administrative levels by substituting head nurse for Steiner's "group supervisor," supervisors for "section supervisor," and so on in order to estimate the time nursing leaders at the various levels might reasonably allocate to planning. In addition, Glueck provides information about the type of planning generally expected at the various management levels.[64]

At upper management levels, planning usually involves strategies, policies, projects, programs, and budgets. Middle management planning usually involves policies, procedures, rules, projects, programs, and budgets. For the supervising level, Glueck states planning typically includes rules, projects, programs, budgets, and schedules. Planning strategies are unique to upper management, according to Glueck, procedures unique to middle management, and schedules to supervisors. Until specific information about time allocations and types of planning at the various levels of nursing leadership is available, these charts can serve as a helpful

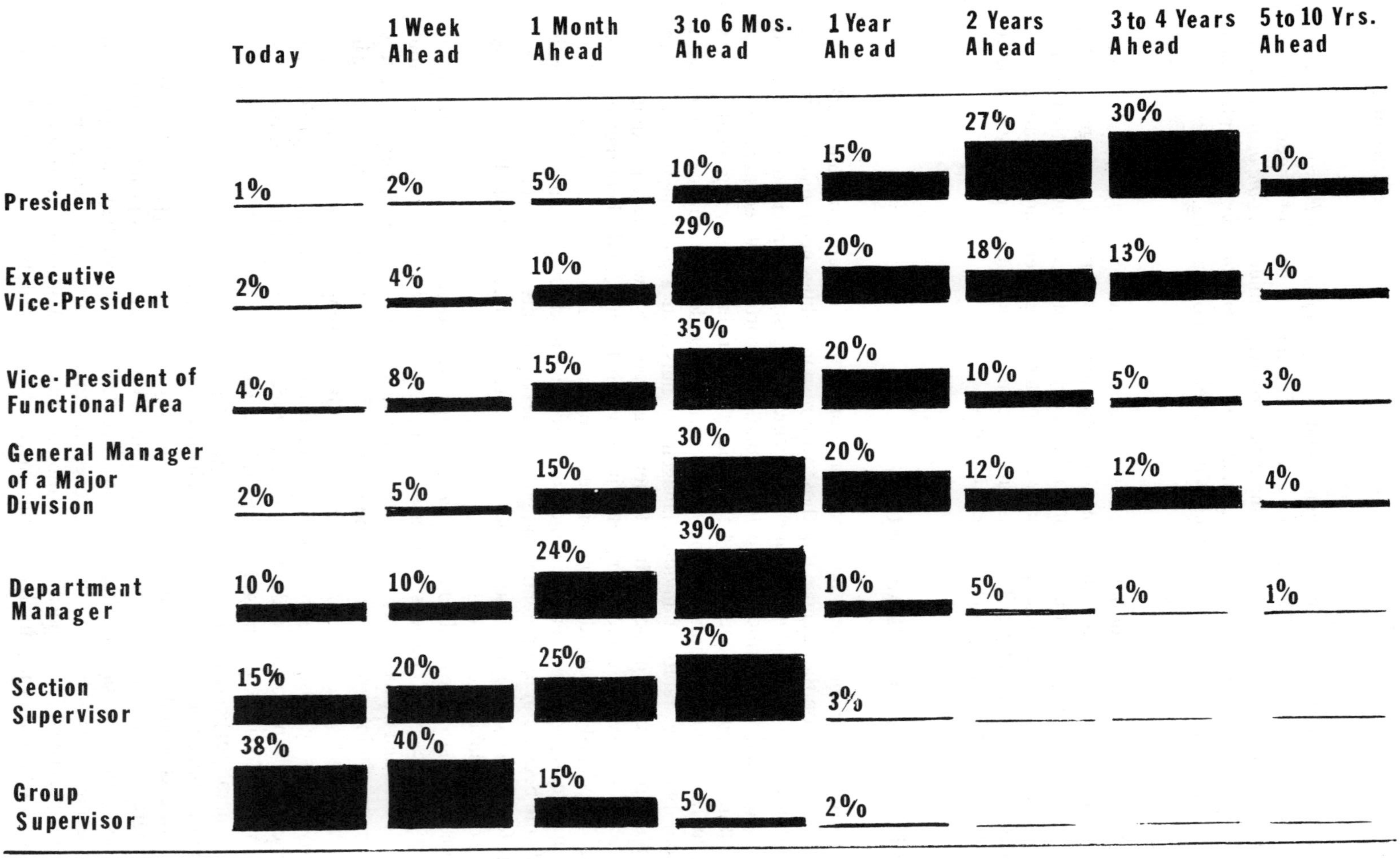

	Today	1 Week Ahead	1 Month Ahead	3 to 6 Mos. Ahead	1 Year Ahead	2 Years Ahead	3 to 4 Years Ahead	5 to 10 Yrs. Ahead
President	1%	2%	5%	10%	15%	27%	30%	10%
Executive Vice-President	2%	4%	10%	29%	20%	18%	13%	4%
Vice-President of Functional Area	4%	8%	15%	35%	20%	10%	5%	3%
General Manager of a Major Division	2%	5%	15%	30%	20%	12%	12%	4%
Department Manager	10%	10%	24%	39%	10%	5%	1%	1%
Section Supervisor	15%	20%	25%	37%	3%			
Group Supervisor	38%	40%	15%	5%	2%			

Figure 9–6. "Ideal" allocations of time for planning in the "average" company. (Reprinted with permission of The Free Press, a division of Macmillan, Inc. from Steiner, G.A. Top management planning. copyright © 1969 by The Trustees of Columbia University of The City of New York. 1969, p. 26.)

estimate of what can be expected of a nursing leader at the various administrative levels within a health agency.

One specific study of managers' use of time is reported. Mintzberg found the managers he studied generally did not set aside specific periods of time for planning and other managerial functions. Instead, their attention was found to be fragmented so that nine minutes was the average amount of time they devoted to any one issue.[65-66]

In allocating time for planning, there are some strategies in time management that may be helpful in avoiding common pitfalls, and we suggest that you may want to look at some of the solutions identified by experts in time management.[67-69] Procrastination is one failing high on the time mismanagement list: "If it doesn't get done today, just put it off until tomorrow," "I work best under pressure," "Long hours just go with the title," and "If I want it done right, I better do it myself," are not necessarily true, but myths one uses as excuses.

A close contender for first place in misuse of time is the "open-door policy." Nursing staff need to know you, as their leader, are available, and if absolutely necessary, they can interrupt you by opening your closed door. The closed door needs to mean you are working. Nursing staff will understand, particularly if you post hours you will be available in your office and if you make rounds frequently and regularly so that you *are* available. Another pitfall is the desk stacked high with work to be done; one has an overwhelming sense of panic just looking at it.

Delegating analysis and planning to a committee without a budget, secretarial support, or a deadline for producing a final report is another. Typically, the committee members miss meetings, and the task falls to one member, often the person who delegated the task in the first place. The result is that the analysis never quite gets done, so planning just cannot happen. Thus time mismanagement is not only a problem for each one as individuals, but it occurs in the development of task groups or committees within the organization, too.

NURSES' ROLE IN PLANNING

As was indicated earlier, most nurses currently are playing an influential role in providing clinical nursing care of patients or clients within a clinical service or health care agency. Increasingly, nursing leaders in middle-management positions, such as head nurses and supervisors, are becoming responsible for planning budgets for their clinical unit. This was not true generally as recently as 1978. Indeed, nurses' role in health care in society is in transition, and the part they play in planning health care is a significant part of that total perspective.

By definition, planning is a first function of leadership; thus nurses realistically can expect to fulfill a major portion of leadership in the future health care in society. In response to McCarty's question, "What will nursing be like in the year 2000," numerous leaders in nursing education and practice responded that nurses would be participating in policy making at the highest levels.[70] The respondents also indicated nurses will be planning, often in collaboration with other health care professionals, to meet health care needs not only locally, but also at state and national levels. A greater portion of nursing practice will be in outpatient clinics, community-based agencies, home health care, and long-term-care facilities, with practice in acute care areas in hospitals accounting for only a small percentage of the total. Having more control of nursing practice, it is anticipated that nurses will be the ones to set limits to patient care costs and cost cutting. These current and future roles of nursing and of the health care system are graphically presented by Porter-O'Grady.[71] (See Figs. 9–8 and 9–9.) In making the transition to the expanded roles and functions, nurses will need to become experts in planning.

158

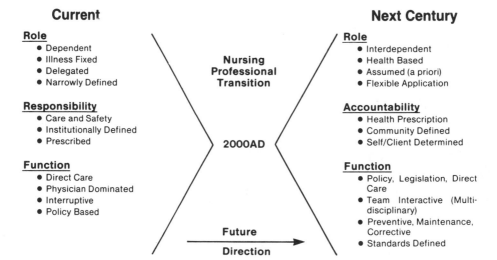

Figure 9–7. Role transition into the 21st century. *(Reprinted with permission of Aspen Publishers, Inc. from Porter-O'Grady, T. Creative nursing administration: Participative management into the 21st century. Salem, Mass.: Aspen, 1986, p. 204.)*

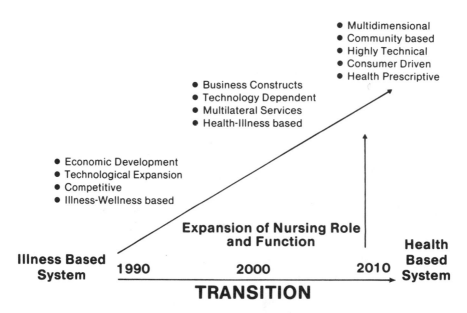

Figure 9–8. Health system focus 2000 A.D. *(Reprinted with permission of Aspen Publishers, Inc. from Porter-O'Grady, T. Creative nursing administration: Participative management into the 21st century. Salem, Mass.: Aspen, 1986, p. 219.)*

SUMMARY

In this chapter, a definition of planning has been presented, the first task-related function of management and leadership. Observations have been presented of the unique and pressing need for nursing leaders to be proactive in approaching planning for the preferred future of nursing in practice and educational settings. The process of planning has been discussed according to four steps: diagnosing, deciding, interacting, and changing. Some suggestions have been presented for the amount of time needed for planning and types of planning generally appropriate at the various levels of management within organizations such as health agencies. The current and future roles of nursing have been considered in regard to planning for nursing and health care.

Finally, a word of caution that little attention has been devoted to another important aspect of planning. Generally, health care agencies are viewed as an open system. The implications of this perspective are that all aspects of an organization are interrelated; planning and implementing a change in any one part of the health care agency or system probably will have an impact on other parts of the system. Thus a plan for one part of the nursing care system needs to be studied carefully in order to determine its potential impact on the total agency, even the total health care system for the community or area.

REFERENCES

1. Toffler, A. *Future Shock*. New York: Random House, 1970, pp. 485–486.
2. Amos, L. K., President of the American Association of Colleges of Nursing. Reassessing nursing education priorities in a cost containment era: How do we see the future and what do we plan to do about it? Speech presented to the Southern Council on Collegiate Education for Nursing, Atlanta, Georgia, November 1, 1984.
3. Rowland, H.S., & Rowland, B. *Nursing administration handbook*. Germantown, Md.: Aspen, Corporation, 1980, pp. 343–357.
4. Guralnik, D. B. (Ed.). *Webster's New World Dictionary* (2nd ed.). New York: Prentice-Hall, 1980, p. 1088.
5. Grove, P. B. (Ed.). *Webster's new dictionary of synonyms*. Springfield, Mass.: Merriam, 1968), pp. 611–612.
6. Dejmozka, E. L., & Kapel, D. E. (Eds.). *American educators' encyclopedia*. Westport, Conn.: Greenwood Press, 1982, p. 401.
7. Harris, C. M. (Ed.). *Dictionary of architecture and construction*. New York: McGraw-Hill, 1975, p. 366.
8. Koontz, H., & O'Donnell, C. *Principles of management: An analysis of managerial functions* (5th ed.). New York: McGraw-Hill, 1972, p. 113.
9. George, J. B. *Nursing theories: The base for professional nursing practice*. Englewood Cliffs, N. J.: Prentice-Hall, 1980, pp. 12–26.
10. Troub, R. M. A general theory of planning: The evolution of planning and the planning of evolution. *Journal of Economic Issues,* 1982, *16* (2), 382.
11. Googins, B., Capoccia, V. A., & Kaufman, N. The interactional dimension of planning: A framework for practice. *Social Work,* July–August 1983, 273–277.
12. Troub, A general theory of planning, p. 384–386.
13. Ibid., 389.
14. White, D. HRSA predicts health professions balance by 2000. *Washington Actions on Health,* July 23, 1983.

15. Andreoli, K. G., & Musser, L. A. Trends that may affect nursing's future. *Nursing and Health Care,* 1985, *6* (1), 47–51.
16. Ibid., 49.
17. U.S. Department of Health, Education and Welfare. *Healthy people—The Surgeon General's report on health promotion and disease prevention, 1979.* Washington, D.C.: U.S. Government Printing Office, 1979.
18. Andreoli & Musser. Trends, p. 48–50.
19. Guralnik, *Webster's Dictionary,* p. 1181.
20. Ibid., 14, 1132.
21. Ashley, J. *Hospitals, paternalism and the role of the nurse.* New York: Teachers College Press, 1979, p. 116.
22. Brown, S. T. Leadership and management competencies needed by neophyte nurses (Doctoral dissertation, North Carolina State University). *Resources in Education,* February 1985 *20*(2). (Educational Microfilms #248-795)
23. Corona, D. F. Followership: The indispensable corollary to leadership. In Hein, E. C., & Nicholson, M. J. (Eds.). *Contemporary leadership behavior: Selected readings.* Boston: Little, Brown, 1982 , pp. 85–89.
24. Ibid.
25. Hersey, P., & Blanchard, K.H. *Management of organizational behavior: Utilizing human resources* (5th ed.). Englewood Cliffs, N. J.: Prentice-Hall, 1988, pp. 334–336.
26. Ibid.
27. Ibid., 335.
28. Ibid.
29. Ibid.
30. Ibid.
31. Dewey, J. *How we think.* Boston: Heath, 1910.
32. Guralnik, *Webster's Dictionary,* p. 366.
33. McNally, J.M. Values: Part I. In Hein, E. C., & Nicholson, M.J. (Eds.). *Contemporary leadership behavior: Selected readings.* Boston: Little, Brown, 1982, p. 103.
34. *Supervisor Nurse: The Journal for Nursing Leadership and Management,* May and June 1980.
35. Tappen, R.M. *Nursing leadership: Concepts and practice.* Philadelphia: Davis, 1983, pp. 425–426.
36. Eason, F.R., Lee, B.T., & Spickerman, S. Analyzing costs, a learning module. *Nursing Educator,* in press; tentatively scheduled for July–August, 1988.
37. Patton, B.R., & Giffin, K. *Decision-making group interaction* (2nd ed.). New York: Harper & Row, 1978, pp. 135–136.
38. Ibid.
39. Corona, Followership, p. 85–89.
40. Jones, E., & Thibaut, J. Interaction goals as bases of inference in interpersonal perception. In R. Taguri & L. Petrullo (Eds.) *Person perception and interpersonal behavior.* Stanford, Calif.: Stanford University Press, 1958, pp. 157–178.
41. Argyris, C. *Interpersonal competence and organizational effectiveness.* Homewood, Ill.: Irwin Dorsey Press, 1962.
42. Bennis, W. G. *Organizational development: Its nature, origins and prospects.* Reading, Mass.: Addison-Wesley, 1969, p. 13.
43. Ibid.
44. Ibid.
45. Belock, M., et al. *Approaches to values in education.* Dubuque, Iowa: Brown, 1966.
46. McGregor, D. *The human side of enterprise.* New York: McGraw-Hill, 1960.
47. McGregor, D. *Leadership and motivation.* Boston: MIT Press, 1966.
48. Unit leaders tell where cost cutting hurts. *The American Nurse,* 1985, *17* (1), 1, 15.
49. Ibid.

50. Patton & Giffin, *Decision-making group,* p. 149.
51. Ibid.
52. Ibid., 163–164.
53. Festinger, L. Informal social communication. *Psychological Review,* 1950, *57,* 271–282.
54. Cartwright, D., & Zander, A. *Group dynamics: Research and theory.* New York: Harper & Row, 1968, p. 494.
55. Patton & Giffin, *Decision-making group,* p. 153.
56. Lewin, K. Frontiers in group dynamics: Concept, method, and reality in social science: Social equilibria and social change. *Human Relations,* 1947, *I* (1), 5–41.
57. Potter, D. O. (Ed.). *Practices.* Spring House, Pa.: Springhouse Corporation, 1984, p. 421–425.
58. Hersey & Blanchard, *Management of organizational behavior,* p. 135–137.
59. Corona, Followership, p. 87.
60. Googins, Interactional dimension, 273.
61. Hersey & Blanchard, *Management of organizational behavior,* p. 86.
62. Googins, Interactional dimension, 276.
63. Steiner, G.A. *Top management planning.* New York: Macmillan, 1969, p. 26.
64. Glueck, W.E. *Management.* Hinsdale, Ill.: Dryden, 1977, p. 246.
65. Peters, T.J., & Waterman, R.H. *In search of excellence.* New York: Harper & Row, 1982, p. 7.
66. Mintzberg, H. *The nature of managerial work.* New York: Harper & Row, 1973, pp. 31–35.
67. Mintzberg, M. The manager's job: Folklore and fact. *Harvard Business Review,* July–August 1975, 49–61.
68. Rowan, R. Keeping the clock from running out. *Fortune,* November 6, 1978, 76–83.
69. LeBoeuf, M. *Working smart: How to accomplish more in half the time.* New York: McGraw-Hill, 1979.
70. McCarty, P. How can nurses prepare for year 2000? *The American Nurse,* 1987, *19* (3) 3,6,10,18.
71. Porter-O'Grady, T. *Creative nursing administration: Participative management into the 21st century.* Salem, Mass.: Aspen, 1986, pp. 201–220.

10

ORGANIZING

INTRODUCTION

The second task-oriented function of management generally and of nurse-leaders specifically is *organizing,* the focus of this chapter. After defining the concept and noting its significance, the source of power and the delegation process used to establish power centers or leadership positions throughout the organization will be discussed. Included also are some important organizational principles. The relationship will be established between selected models of organizational structure and leadership theories. While it is recognized that pure forms do not actually exist, models will be presented of organizational charts and each evaluated in relation to theories and contemporary trends. Discussion of variables that are influenced by structure are noted as appropriate throughout; these include power, communication, and task. Some historical and contemporary issues that are unique to organizational structures of hospitals and health agencies and have implications for the autonomy of nursing practice within organizations are discussed. These include the placement of the medical staff in the hospital hierarchy, formal and informal (grapevine) communication patterns, and placement of the nursing unit. The organization within the nursing unit is also considered, particularly in reference to the structure of committees.

DEFINITION AND SIGNIFICANCE OF ORGANIZING

As a second function of management, *organizing* is generally defined as establishing a formal structure within which plans are implemented. According to the dictionary, *organizing* means to bring into being; to establish or to institute something such as a corporation or an organization; and to make into a whole with unified and coherent relationships. It is derived from the Latin word, *organizare,* meaning to provide an organic structure.[1] Marriner states: "Organizing involves establishing a formal structure to provide for the coordination of resources to accomplish the objectives and determining position qualifications and descriptions."[2] Specifically, Talcott defines an organization as a social unit "deliberately constructed and reconstructed to seek specific goals."[3] Etzioni supports this definition and notes that organizations as human groupings are characterized by:

1. being deliberately planned divisions of labor, power, and communication responsibilities;
2. having a power center(s) which directs all resources toward goals, continuously monitoring performance and, if indicated, revising the structure to increase efficiency;
3. shifting personnel through hiring, firing, transfer and promotion.[4]

Etzioni suggests, as a matter of clarification, there are two synonyms for organization that one needs to avoid: *bureaucracy* and *institution. Bureaucracy* tends to have a negative connotation because most people immediately think of the bureaucratic red tape of large agencies, particularly government agencies such as the Internal Revenue Service. Typically, there is one decision-making unit in a bureaucracy; thus hospitals do not fit this definition. A *bureaucrat* is one who blindly follows routines, petty regulations, and properly filled-out forms, making no exceptions for individuals or circumstances (that is, no common sense). *Institution* can mean a large organization such as Du Pont, or institutions such as marriage, or persons such as disreputable relatives (former President Carter's brother Billy was an institution unto himself). *Formal* organization refers to structure, the first characteristic mentioned above, and *social* organization can mean a Thursday night bowling team or a local chapter of organized crime. Consequently, Etzioni suggests use of the terms *organization* or *organizing* to avoid misunderstandings.

The significance of organizations and organizing has two interlocking facets: *power* and *cooperation*. First, it is through carefully designed placement throughout the organization of centers of power (leadership or management positions) that the goals and objectives of an organization are achieved. Power in the organization refers to authority, responsibility, and accountability. Second, the systematic distribution and interdependence of each unit's tasks and functions requires and consequently promotes cooperation among all employees—followers and leaders or managers. Each individual is interdependent with others in order to achieve goals. Acceptance of organizational goals is in itself a source of motivation to cooperate. In addition, employees' acceptance of the influence of those in power center positions tends to promote cooperation among all involved. Organization of tasks and people provides the elements of power and cooperation to achieve goals.

DELEGATION OF POWER

An official source of power is from the legal arm of society. After establishing a need, a group may petition a state attorney general, requesting to be licensed or commissioned as a single corporate body in the eyes of the law in order to conduct a business. When granted, this license authorizes the group to organize a business, such as a health agency. Thus the ultimate source of organizational power lies within this legal authorization.

The petitioning group usually becomes the governing board, which then delegates power to administrators to develop and manage the organization. *Delegation* is the process of assigning part or all of one's power to others. Just as a delegate to a convention is empowered to speak and act for others,[5] so the organizational administrators and managers are empowered to speak and act for the governing board. This implicitly means the delegate must be trustworthy as well as capable and willing.

The process of delegation is exemplified in the organization of a hospital. The governing board usually appoints the hospital administrator and delegates power to this position. The hospital administrator or president, then, appoints and delegates power to a small group of managers, often labeled vice-presidents. One of these, a vice-president of nursing (VPN), is empowered to plan and establish a unit of nursing services. This process of delegating power is continued until all management positions are filled. Thus, we can state the first organizational principle, often labeled the *unity of command* principle:

Each individual in an organization is to report to one person for final direction.[6]

This leader–follower relationship is to be respected by all others.[7]

Each position within an organization needs to have some relative degree of *authority, responsibility,* and *accountability;* these are three necessary elements of power. Authority can be delegated, but accountability and responsibility cannot. A second organizational principle is labeled *requisite authority:*

> *When a leader delegates a task, the corresponding authority over resources needed must also be delegated.*[8]

One answers or is accountable to the delegator for the accomplishment of an assignment, even if the assignment is completed by a subordinate of the delegatee. Individuals decide whether or not to accept responsibility; if accepted, then the responsibility remains with the individual. A third organizational principle is that of *continuing responsibility:*

> *The leader retains responsibility for a delegated task.*[9]

Thus, the governing board retains accountability to society, legally and ethically, for the quality and quantity of nursing services provided by this hospital. The VPN delegates authority to the nursing administrators or middle managers, but personally accepts and retains responsibility for nursing services and accountability to the hospital administrator and, ultimately, to the board of trustees. Generally, authority is delegated to layers or levels of positions as centers of power throughout the organization. Individuals filling positions on the same level in the organizational hierarchy have relatively equal authority, although their tasks and functions may differ considerably. For example, the vice-presidents would be expected to have equal authority at their level; at a lower level directors of programs or areas would have equal authority, and so on down through the hierarchy.

The centers of power delegated to positions are distributed throughout the hospital organization and form a chain of command for decision making, delegation, and communication. A *line* position is on a direct line of delegated power from the top; for example, the head nurse is in a direct chain of command from the vice-president of nursing position. A fourth organizational principle is:

> *Issues are to be solved at the lowest level possible before moving up the chain of command, without bypassing a line position.*[10]

For example, individuals in head nurse positions typically have delegated authority to make decisions about hiring, disciplining, or firing personnel, budgeting and spending money, and determining nursing personnel's duty hours and days off or staffing, among other things. In contrast, there are staff positions without authority, which are in an *advisory and support* relationship to those in line positions. Those in staff positions usually provide the services or make the products, gather data, develop reports, and provide information for those in line positions to consider in making decisions and developing directives, policies, and procedures. An example of a powerless staff position is that of charge nurse. Typically, this position is filled by one of the unit nurses on the head nurse's days off, and it carries all of the responsibility and accountability of the head nurse position, but not the authority. Any decisions of significance are held until the "real" head nurse returns. Clinical nurses, instructors for in-house educational programs, and some clinical nurse-specialist positions are additional examples of staff positions.

ORGANIZATIONAL STRUCTURE AND LEADERSHIP THEORY

Basically, there are two types of organizational structure, centralized and decentralized power centers, and there are four models for displaying the structure: tall, flat, circular, and matrix. Of course, there are many variations of these in reality, and these distinct categories are used primarily for discussion purposes. According to Lawrence and Lorsch, however, research has shown that there is no one best way to organize. These authors propose that as long as the numerous specialties in an organization are differentiated and a high degree of collaboration provides for integrating services of many departments to achieve a combining of resources to effect quality health care, the organization will tend to be successful.[11] Langford notes that each hospital needs to be structured to accommodate its own unique situation.[12]

The decisions about the kind of structure to be used for an organization are usually made during the initial planning phase of an organizational structure. As a general principle, we propose:

> *The kind of structure selected tends to be consistent with the theoretical and philosophical perspective of the relationship among the governing board, management, and employees.*

For example, if one believes an organization is made most effective by holding as much power as possible in the highest power center, such as the governing board and the top administrators, then one tends to choose a *tall* structure with many levels of power centers throughout the organization, and to choose an *autocratic* administrative perspective or theories for leadership roles. Conversely, decentralized structures are often *flat,* with few power centers, tending to be congruent with *participative* leadership perspectives or theories. Figure 10–1 presents a continuum of organizational structures, extending from centralized to decentralized. Brief descriptive statements of Situational Leadership theory and Humanistic Nursing Communication theory are placed at correspondingly appropriate points along the continuum. The reader may also wish to consider the placement on this continuum of other organizational or leadership theories as a point of discussion.

One must understand that just because an organizational structure is flat, with few levels of power centers, it does not necessarily follow that participative management is practiced throughout the agency. While the planning group or the governing board may have indicated a particular philosophical or theoretical preference, individuals selected to serve in the management role in the power center positions may not play the role accordingly. (See the discussion of participative versus directive change in Chapter 6.)

Organizational Structure			
Centralized			**Decentralized**
Tall	Circular	Matrix	Flat
Autocratic and Hierarchical		Participative and Democratic	
Situational Leadership Theory (Hersey & Blanchard):			
Style 1	Style 2	Style 3	Style 4
"Telling"	"Selling"	"Participating"	"Delegating"
Humanistic Nursing Communication Theory (Duldt & Giffin):			
Dehumanizing			Humanizing
Management communicates monologically with directives, disregarding of employees' needs, abilities, suggestions, and so on.		Management communicates dialogically, noting with positive regard, employees needs, abilities, suggestions, and so on.	

Figure 10–1. Continuum of Organizational Structure and Related Perspectives of Leadership Theory.

For example, a hospital's structure may indicate decentralization, and the hospital administrator may behave in a congruent manner by delegating appropriate authority to several vice-presidents. An individual serving as Vice President of Nursing (VPN), however, may tend to perceive people as untrustworthy and unwilling to accept responsibility. This person, as VPN, tends to retain authority. Thus only with this VPN's personal review and authorization will nursing area managers, supervisors, and head nurses be able to spend money, hire and fire personnel, or change policies. In such a case, every power center in the hospital's nursing service unit is limited to accountability and responsibility without adequate power. Even in such circumstances, some of the head nurses may use a participatory management approach to the extent they are able. The way in which the management role is actually played by people placed in organizational power centers can vary to some degree from that proposed by the structure displayed in the organizational chart. It is only with considerable effort, however, that excessive variances are maintained, and those individuals who cannot support the perspectives advocated by those in high power positions tend to leave. Over time, cognitive balance tends to occur.

ORGANIZATIONAL CHARTS

The organizational structure is typically displayed on an organizational chart, which graphically indicates relationships of the power centers and accountability, that is, formal communication networks, among the power centers or management positions. Line relationships are typically indicated by dark, solid lines on organizational charts; staff relationships are usually shown as broken lines. (See the discussion of structure in Chapter 6.)

Tall Structures

A *tall* or pyramid-model organizational structure typically has several levels of power centers or administrators, emphasizing authority. This structure is considered efficient for very large, formal agencies or institutions (see Fig. 10–2). Rowland and Rowland state this structure is particularly appropriate for units having ritualistic and routine tasks to perform.[13] It was originally described by Max Weber.[14] Langford and Marriner note the classic characteristics of tall organizational structures that have been typical of hospitals' bureaucracy:

a. There are well defined formal relationships between manager and employee.
b. Job descriptions are clearly described, especially routine tasks.
c. Personnel are treated in an impersonal and distant manner.
d. There is a well-developed system of policies and procedures which limit decision-making.
e. Each individual reports to one manager.
f. Authority is to be proportionate with responsibility.[15,16]

In addition, since employees are not trusted, the *span of control* becomes important; this refers to the number of subordinates each administrator manages. In the pyramid, this ranges from 1:3 at the upper levels to 1:6 at the bottom.[17] Although research has shown that productivity is higher when close supervision is impossible,[18] the low span of control promotes close supervision.

Some disadvantages of the tall pyramid model have also been noted by Langford and Marriner. First, the emphasis on control, authority, and productivity tends to prevent rather than promote normal, healthy interpersonal communication and personality. Second, some supervisors who do not have the technical competence of their subordinates seem to become bothered by this; their insecurity is displayed by self-serving and inappropriate behaviors, such

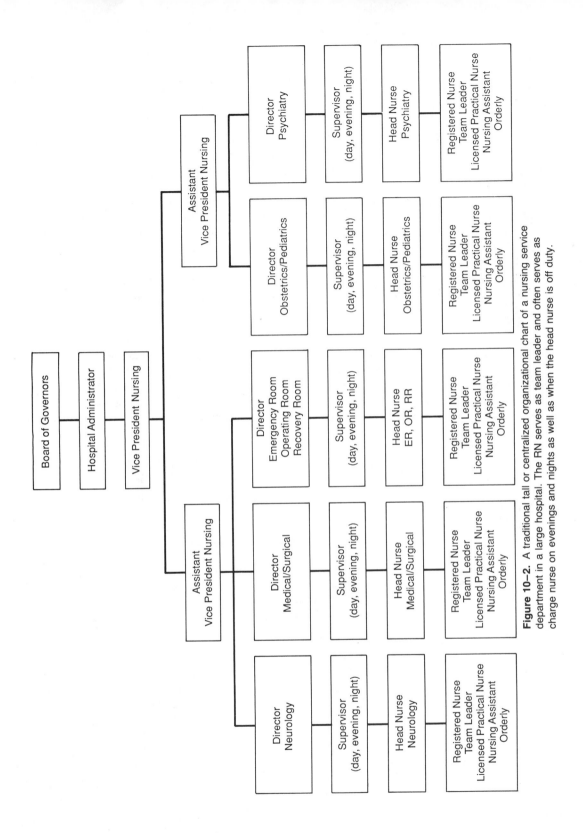

Figure 10–2. A traditional tall or centralized organizational chart of a nursing service department in a large hospital. The RN serves as team leader and often serves as charge nurse on evenings and nights as well as when the head nurse is off duty.

as expecting too much deference. Third, since little kingdoms can develop as managers maintain control of their territory, the managers' protective resistance to change can be a problem. Fourth, as units become more specialized in task, technology, or function, there is a tendency to communicate in an impersonal manner to others.[19,20] Finally, it is possible that the tall organizational structure can influence managers to use the F theory, that is management by *fear*. With pathological need for control as its basis, an authoritarian leadership style may, according to Marriner: ". . . become a defense mechanism through the use of power and fear strategies over subservients and enforcement of norms through arbitrary and rigid rules."[21] Manipulative use of rewards and punishment to elicit desired behaviors merely tends to alienate personnel.[22] Thus, the structure of an organization can change the way people interact.

Flat Structures

An example of a *flat* model organizational structure is presented in Figure 10–3. In contrast to the tall structure, the flat structure delegates or decentralizes power to positions very near the point where the nurse interacts with the clients. Not only does this structure facilitate open communication between all levels, but also decision making moves downward, and the span of control increases so that close supervision diminishes proportionately. Thus clinical nurses are able to participate in the decision-making process to a greater extent than in the tall structure. Clinical nurses have comparatively greater responsibility for maintaining quality nursing care. The flat structure offers opportunities for professional growth in knowledge, skill, and decision making.[23,24] According to Rowland and Rowland, the flat structure allows ease of flexibility, and it is more appropriate for the highly skilled technical and professional employees of health care agencies, since knowledge and credibility tend to be the major sources of power.[25] For those interested in moving up into management positions, however, limitation of opportunity may be a disadvantage. Since the number of managers is small, career ladders tend to be equally short. In some cases, unless someone resigns, one might have to wait for a manager to die before an administrative position becomes available. Those nurses who want management positions may have to move on to another health agency or organization.

Circular Structures

An example of the *circular* model organizational structure is presented in Figure 10–4. This example shows the governing board and hospital administrator at the center of the structure. The increasing larger circles about the center are indicative of the decreasing amount of delegated authority to each power center, and of the increasing distance from the center.[26] This conveys an egocentric perspective of upper management and a strict maintenance of hierarchical and status relationships, not unlike that of the tall structure. One might consider this kind of organizational chart appropriate if one has a systems theory perspective.

This is in contrast to the half-circle organizational structure presented in Figure 10–5. This is a functional and territorial organization of a hospital, and the theme is client-centered care. The increasingly larger circles indicate the amount of contact, accountability, and responsibility the administrators, technicians, professionals, and others have with the patient.[27] The chart conveys the power of the patient or client who is representative of society at large. It emphasizes a humanistic perspective of the patient as well as the need to satisfy the client by providing quality care, apparently the goal of the agency. It also clearly identifies who has the greatest opportunity and responsibility for speaking and acting as if a delegate for administrators—the clinical nurse. It presents the hospital as a nursing center where doctors practice occasionally and all other employees serve in a supportive capacity. Decades old, this model is seldom seen and rarely operationalized.

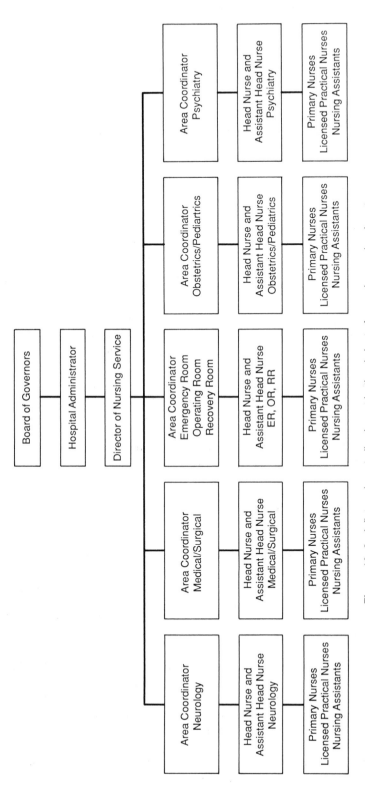

Figure 10–3. A flat or decentralized organizational chart of a nursing service department. Area coordinators are responsible for directing each major clinical nursing speciality, with head nurses and assistant head nurses providing unit management for days, evenings, and nights. Primary nurses are RNs, with LPNs, nurse aides, and orderlies providing assistance as needed.

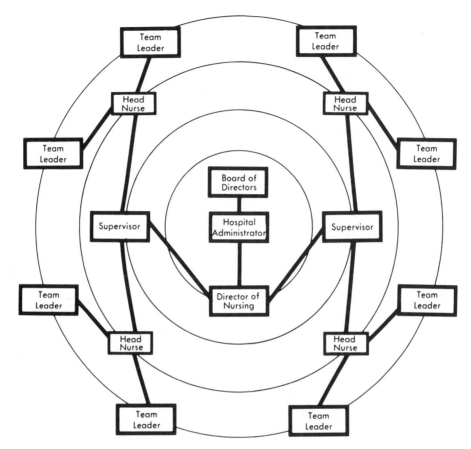

Figure 10–4. A circular organizational structure of a hospital, showing the distribution of power centers in line positions. The flow of authority moves from the center outward. *(Reproduced by permission from Marriner, A. Guide to nursing management (2nd ed.). St. Louis: The C.V. Mosby Co., 1980, p. 68.)*

Matrix Structures

The *matrix* model of organizational structure is a relatively recent development that provides a complex answer to complex organizations. The matrix organizational chart basically is a grid of rows and columns that displays both hierarchical, or authority, and lateral, or task, coordination (see Fig. 10–6A). Vertical or hierarchical authority follows the classic line and staff relationships. One can also plot and analyze the lateral coordination of patient care teams consisting of professionals, technicians, therapists, and others assigned to departments throughout the hospital.

Figure 10–6B can be used as an example for the matrix team. The patient care team leader (perhaps a BSN graduate as a primary nurse or a MSN graduate as a Clinical Nurse-Specialist) is indicated on the chart by a boxed x or [x]. Other personnel assigned to the team are indicated by another x located at the intersection of the lateral and vertical lines. According to this chart, the first patient care team consists of a nurse-leader, two members from the service department, one each from laboratories, physical therapy, and social work. In addition, each team has an assigned medical staff member.

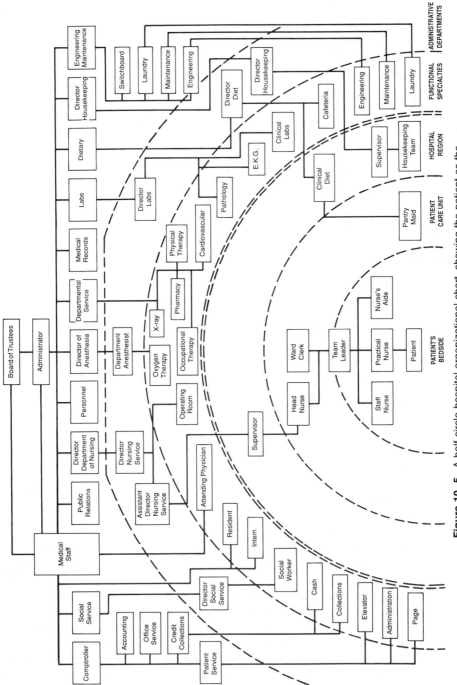

Figure 10–5. A half-circle hospital organizational chart, showing the patient as the central focus. The outward flow indicates the degree of functional and territorial social interaction hospital administrators and personnel have with the patient. (*From Mauksch, H.O. The nurse: Coordinator of patient care. In: J. K. Skipper, Jr., & R. C. Leonard, Social interaction and patient care. Philadelphia: Lippincott, 1965.*)

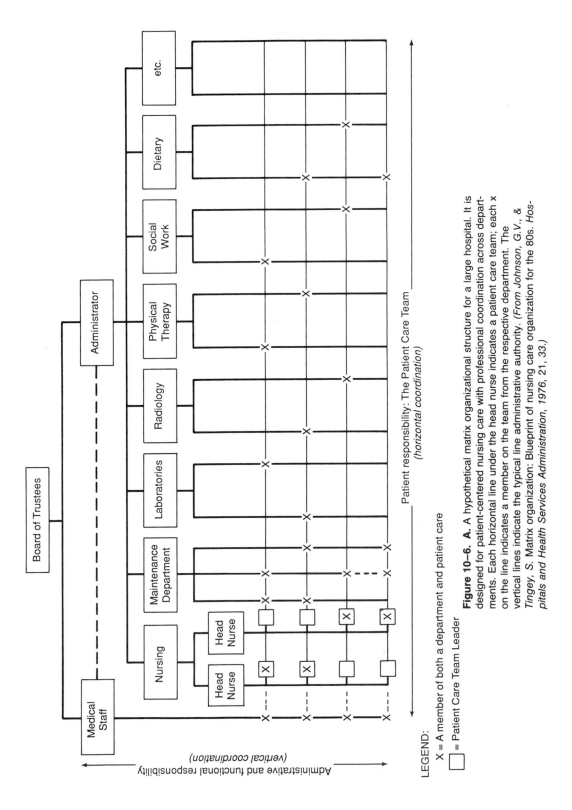

Figure 10–6. A. A hypothetical matrix organizational structure for a large hospital. It is designed for patient-centered nursing care with professional coordination across departments. Each horizontal line under the head nurse indicates a patient care team; each x on the line indicates a member on the team from the respective department. The vertical lines indicate the typical line administrative authority. *(From Johnson, G.V., & Tingey, S. Matrix organization: Blueprint of nursing care organization for the 80s. Hospitals and Health Services Administration, 1976, 21, 33.)*

LEGEND:

X = A member of both a department and patient care

☐ = Patient Care Team Leader

173

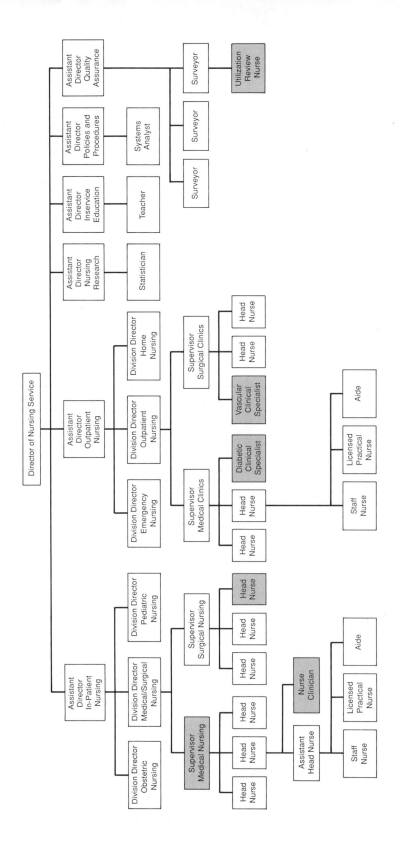

B. Application of the matrix organization concept in which a committee, task force, or project team is assigned the task of developing a teaching program for diabetic patients. The membership is indicated by the darkened block. This use of the matrix organization is more commonly used than for coordination of patient care. See *A*, above. *(From Gillies, D.A. Nursing management: A systems approach. Philadelphia: Saunders, 1982, p. 129.)*

The team members report administratively to their respective department managers, and they report to the nurse, who is the patient care team leader, about the therapeutic care plans and protocols for the team's patients. Upon admission, each patient is assigned to the one nurse-leader responsible for coordinating all efforts to that patient's best interest, not only the nursing care but also the care provided by other team members. Johnson and Tingey view the matrix nursing structure as being based on job enrichment and patient-centered nursing care; they propose it as an answer to task-oriented modes of organizing nursing care delivery.[28]

According to Rowland and Rowland, the advantages of coordination within the matrix structure include decreased confusion, decreased intrusion on patients' privacy, and increased effectiveness in utilization of nursing resources, skills, and interprofessional influence, as well as increased motivation and job satisfaction among the clinical nursing staff.[29] The management role of the nursing traditional supervisor, however, has to be changed to either a clinical resource or a division manager with an increased span of control; that is, this person is responsible for a larger number of patient care areas.[30] Another option is to delete the supervisory position, which is in accord with the current trend to eliminate middle management. In addition, instead of charge nurse, the title of assistant head nurse is used with the associated appropriate authority and responsibility; this provides staff nurses with a preliminary administrative experience under the mentorship of the head nurse.[31–33]

While the matrix structure is being used with apparent success in many hospitals, one needs to be aware of some reservations. One quickly noted is the potential problem of reporting to two leaders, and possibly more if one is assigned to several patient care teams. Evaluation of individual team members often requires input from numerous sources, and a person can get lost. For example, Judy was a young staff nurse in a matrix organization. After receiving her first six-month evaluation from her head nurse, Judy asked the head nurse how she had known what to say in the evaluation report. She went on to explain that she had been moved to so many patient care teams on different floors of the hospital, and worked briefly with so many different nurses, that she had only seen the head nurse on three occasions during the six months. Judy did not think anyone even knew her name. To Judy's dismay, the head nurse validated this speculation when she confessed that she did have to describe Judy several times as she inquired about Judy's performance. (After this alienating interview, incidentally, Judy moved on to another agency.)

Reporting on their research to identify characteristics of excellence in management, Peters and Waterman describe the matrix structure as their "favorite candidate for the wrong kind of complex response" to structural problems.[34] While the matrix structure does place emphasis on the point of delivery for nursing services,—the nurse-client contact—it is confusing. Not only do people not know what to report to whom; everything one does becomes so interrelated to everything else. This matrix idea originated at Boeing as a way of managing multiple teams assigned to projects. The Boeing personnel, however, operated in only two ways, either as a member of a discipline or a member of one project team. There was no confusion.[35] Peters and Waterman state the key to making the matrix or any other structure work is *clarity of values* and *simplicity of structure*.[36] Their discussion of future forms suggests other potential options in the organizational structure of hospitals.

Advantages and Disadvantages of Organizational Charts

There are some important advantages in making an chart of the organizational structure. It is helpful when planning structure changes, plotting communication networks (see the research by Bavelas in Chapter 6), and determining official relationships among units within the organization. The chart can also be helpful in locating problem areas. Rowland and Rowland list the following as rather easily located faux pas:

> Confused lines of authority.
> Overlap and duplication of functions.
> Dual reporting relationships.
> Overextended spans of management.
> Lack of intermediate supervisor.
> Lack of intermediate supervisory levels.
> Excessive levels of supervision.
> Gaps in function.[37]

These are a few of the common blunders, and more may become evident upon analyzing specific organizational charts.

For example, the organizational chart for a rather large hospital, presented in Figure 10–7, reveals several problems. It shows the line relationships with the usual solid lines, while dotted lines indicate coordination. The hierarchy is shown with the board of trustees as the primary power center, the hospital administrator next highest in power, and the associate administrators third highest. Below this level, the hierarchical sequence seems to change, since the boxes below the associate administrators identify some centers of equal power, yet the placement of some boxes is lower. According to the titles, all the boxes below the associate administrator of patient services appear to be equal in delegated power. In addition, the hierarchical sequence is *not* maintained for those power centers under the associate administrator of nursing. The assistant administrator for nursing special studies would seem more appropriately placed immediately under the associate administrator of nursing, along with the other assistant administrators. What about the medical staff? It is not even on the chart. One wonders whether the placement of some positions may be a reflection of someone's sense of interpersonal closeness, the level of credibility of individuals filling the positions, or the limitations encountered by the size of the paper used. This chart exemplifies some other faux pas one can make in developing an organizational chart.

In contrast, the organizational chart of a typical large private general hospital, shown in Figure 10–8, does present most of the departments necessary to provide services needed. While this appears to be a tall or centralized structure, it conveys more information about the roles expected of individuals in the management positions and the functions of each department or box. The hierarchical arrangement is consistently followed in placement on the chart of the power centers or positions on the chart. In addition, the relationship of the medical staff to other hospital personnel is also on this chart. One needs to be inquisitive about the organizational structure of any agency to validate interpretation. Generally, the organizational chart is supposed to communicate, not confuse.

Formal versus Informal Communication Networks

One significant aspect of organizational charts is that only planned, formal communication networks are shown, while informal communications are omitted. The formal networks within an organization usually include goals and objectives, policies and procedure manuals, job descriptions, annual reports, memos, and other forms of written communications. Verbal communication during conferences, meetings, and presentations is also considered formal.

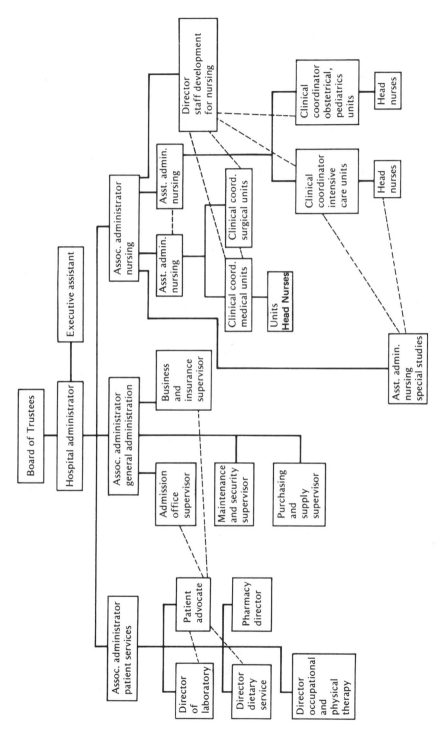

Figure 10–7. A typical organizational chart of a large hospital. *(From Langford, T. L. Managing and being managed: Preparation for professional nursing practice. Englewood Cliffs, N. J.: Prentice-Hall, 1981, p. 168.)*

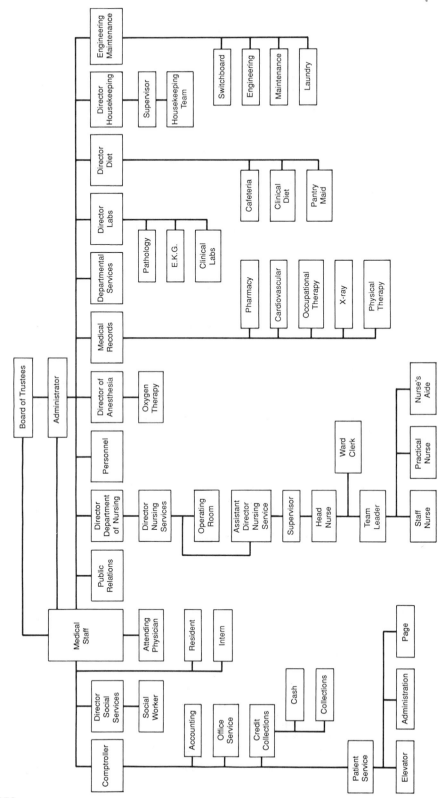

Figure 10-8. An organizational chart of a typical private general hospital, showing the medical staff and major departments in addition to the nursing department. (*From Mauksch, H.O. The Nurse: Coordinator of patient care. In J. K. Skipper, Jr., & R. C. Leonard (Eds.). Social interaction and patient care. Philadelphia: Lippincott, 1965, p. 254.*)

178

This network is established to flow downward, upward, and laterally. It exists by design to meet the needs of leaders in achieving the organizational goals.

The informal communication network, better known as the *grapevine,* is unplanned, developing according to people's preferences and friendships. According to Hagopian, it is probably just as important as the formal communication network in that it provides social values and cohesiveness; providing spice to break the monotony of work, the grapevine is accurate approximately three-fourths of the time.[38] It provides information about social attitudes, needs, mores, expectations, traditions, and history.[39] Kanter describes the power and control of secretaries of organizational leaders, which develops because of their unique position of centrality and access to information without official authorization to use the information. Consequently, administrative secretaries are in a unique position of influence and credibility.[40] This influence can be useful. For example, one administrator wanted to know how the hospital employees would react to the change in the parking system he was considering. He asked his secretary to casually mention it at her morning coffee break. By lunch, everyone had learned about his plan via the grapevine and was angry about it, and the administrator knew he could forget about his plan. In general, if one infringes upon some social value or breaks one of the unwritten rules, one will become very aware of the disciplinary force of the informal communication network. This influence, however, typically becomes a problem when the information is incomplete, of unknown source, or political and self-serving in nature. The resulting rumors can spread and cause needless anxiety among employees.

> Managers need to listen to the grapevine. It tells them what employees are excited about and what is important to them. It shows gaps in information and helps to pinpoint these with regard to certain departments or areas. It provides useful information to any manager who is trying to understand what is happening in an organization.[41]

Leaders can maintain some control over rumors and the grapevine by providing timely and sufficient information about those things that are of concern to their followers.

Structure Issues Unique to Health Agencies

There are several structural issues that appear to be unique to health agencies, particularly to hospitals and medical centers. Classic organizational structures that have been presented are commonly used in business, industry, government, and the armed services. The unique issues you will probably find in health care agencies center about (a) relationships with the medical staff, (b) communication networks in a dual authority situation, and (c) the location of the nursing unit in the administrative line of authority. In addition, there is a relatively new issue. While mergers and take-overs of smaller corporations by larger ones is common in the business world, when one hospital joins or takes over another, strange things seem to happen. The development of hospital chains or mega-hospitals, then, presents a fourth unique structural situation. Each of these presents issues for nursing to consider in relation to the unique influences upon the way nursing management and clinical practice is conducted.

The Medical Staff

Of particular interest is the position of the medical staff in relation to all others in the agency. Historically, the medical staff is not employed by the hospital, but is comprised of physicians in private practice who have been approved for membership on the agency's medical staff. Traditionally, private practice has been the primary way a physician maintains professional credibility. If salaried by the hospital, the physician cannot be in private practice; this would constitute a conflict of interest when voting on hospital policies. The conflict centers on voting priorities in that there may be a tendency for the physician employed part-time to support his or her own private practice, have an inappropriate competitive advantage in relation to other physicians in private practice, or support hospital interests.

To avoid this conflict, physicians maintain a unique relationship to the health agency, professional rather than administrative. Consequently, this is a dual authority within the hospital organizational structure. This violates the organizational principle of unity of command, mentioned earlier in this chapter. The line of authority of the medical staff often extends vertically over several administrative levels from a point midway in the hierarchy to a level equal to that of the administrator and/or governing board (see Figs. 10–5, 10–6, and 10–8). Medical staff members also usually have direct communication with members of the governing board, bypassing the chain of command.

> The role of the physician is a unique one in that he is an independent practitioner who has within his own confines the prerogative and the responsibility for one total function or process, namely that of cure. In view of this, he has a reciprocal relationship with the hospital, which places him on an equal level with the administrator and the board of trustees. Yet in the performance of his function he enters the hospital, he dons his white coat and he joins the workers of the front lines. Thus he not only may be within or outside the institution, but he is also in a sense privileged to move up and down across all levels . . . while [other members] are hierarchically fixed and therefore limited in their relationships.[42]

Thus the physician's relationship with the hospital is a uniquely influential one. It is compounded by the fact that it is the physician who decides patients' admission to and occupancy status in the hospital. Patients and third-party payers, such as insurance companies, are the primary source of revenue for health agencies.

Communication

There are several unique aspects of the way hospitals are organized and the way people in the various roles are required to interact that can lead to serious communication barriers. First, all lines of communication and authority focus on the head nurse. She or he serves as a front-line representative of nursing and of both authorities, the hospital administrator as well as the physician. Second, because the nurse comes to the patient care unit and stays, the dual system of authority between the hospital administrator and the medical staff, who visit the patient unit, focuses on the position of the head nurse. While all other departments within the hospital relate upward to the administrative authority, the head nurse must coordinate tasks performed by personnel of these other departments and coordinate the orders of doctors, interns, residents, and consultants. Nurses are in charge of the care structure. Each physician has no restrictions and hence no need to consider the implications of his or her orders and directives of other physicians upon the work load of the nursing staff. The head nurse has no formal administrative means of controlling the quantity of demands made upon staff for nursing services. He or she must draw upon personal power, persuasive appeals, and conflict resolution to influence this task variable.

Third, as a head nurse, one is expected to organize the staff and work load with minimal guidance concerning how to manage in the covert dual-authority, perhaps contradictory, directives of the physician's power and prestige on the one hand and the expectations of administrative officials on the other. Often this means reminding medical staff of hospital policies. Physicians who serve as clinical faculty often tell the head nurse to watch over the interns and not let them write inappropriate orders.[43] While the head nurse's immediate superior would normally be expected to provide guidance, successful approaches are more often a matter of an individual head nurse's attitudes and interpersonal communication skills.

Fourth, as a front-line worker *and* a nonemployee peer of the governing board, the physician may switch from side to side during debates and power struggles on policy issues. For example, one or more physicians initially may vocally support the development of a new service or the purchasing of unique and expensive equipment for the operating room advocated by representatives of nursing service. When approached by a member of the governing board known to be very conservative in relation to any budgetary issue, however, the physician may withhold support. The physician may even express doubt regarding the wisdom of any of the recommendations coming from the nurses if it is to his or her own advantage to do so. Clearly, nurses have been perceived by themselves and others as having limited bargaining power when negotiating with administrators, physicians, and governing boards. It remains to be seen whether this bargaining position is maintained or changed.

Fifth, employees are often involved in imposing administrative policy upon physicians. For example, the medical records librarian must impose policies regarding accuracy and timeliness of progress notes, and the pharmacist must impose policies regarding use of supplies and drugs, all to maintain the hospital's accreditation status. The laboratory chemist who is Director of the Laboratory may need to confront physicians who visit the laboratory seeking reports, and somehow begin directing and supervising the laboratory technicians.[44]

Finally, most employees are tied to individual departments by training and education, unable to become mobile like the physician. In order to advance, most must leave, acquire further education, and return to a position higher or different in the hospital hierarchy.[45] These unique aspects of health agencies, hospitals in particular, have been known for some time (as evidenced by very old references), and extensive effort on an interpersonal level by individuals and groups has made little impact. Pathological communication patterns have developed over the years, and unfortunately nurses continue to encounter communication problems, as suggested by Stein's "doctor-nurse games" and Hoekelman's "nurse-physician relationships."[46–48] Giving some practical and helpful guidance, Korner provides an in-depth analysis of the "political jungle" of working with physicians in health agencies.[49] It is probably only through major changes in the privileges society is willing to extend to physicians and a resulting revision of the hospital structure, eliminating some of these unique factors, that the communication barriers can be removed and collaborative relationships supported. Revision of medical education regarding consultation versus collaboration would also be helpful. (See the discussion of collaboration in Chapter 8.)

Location of Nursing Agency Organizational Structure

With the advent of Diagnosis Related Groups (DRGs), a competitive market for health care, a shortage of professional nursing personnel, and the oversupply of physicians, some changes in the placement of medical and nursing leadership positions are occurring in the organizational structure of many health agencies. One relatively new trend is the increase in the number of administrative positions for medical affairs. As the number of available physicians increases, physicians in private practice are finding part-time and even full-time employment a realistic attraction. This availability of physicians and the increasing complexity of health care administration has apparently prompted the development of vice-president or director of medical affairs (salaried) positions in health agencies.

The development of this position affects the role of the nursing administrator and ultimately the manner of conducting nursing practice. Structural placement of the medical administrative position is evolving into two commonly occurring types. In one, the placement is the same, but the vice-president or director of nursing is placed below, and reports to, the vice-president of medical affairs. In the second, the vice-president of medical affairs is placed on a level equal to other vice-presidents, including the vice-president of nursing (see Fig. 10–9 and Fig. 10–10). If the nursing leader is to participate in policy making as an equal, representing a discrete discipline and practice profession, then the nursing leader needs to be placed as a vice-president with delegated power (and salary, office, parking space, etc.) equal to that of all other vice-presidents, including vice-president of medicine. This placement ensures autonomy of both medical and nursing practice, each having equal authority in decision making for their respective responsibilities. According to Sheedy, national associations of both nursing and medicine have published statements supporting this position placement.[50]

> To add nursing as an additional responsibility to the vice-president of medical affairs is to underestimate the expertise nursing administration demands and the need of the institution to have medicine and nursing at the top level of decision making.[51]

By reporting to the vice-president of medical affairs, the nursing leader usually assumes a staff relationship position.

> The most common problem for nursing directors in the staff model is a lack of power. The chief and the program leaders have the option to confer power to the nursing director for a necessary task. For the most part, however, the director must rely on influence and professional respect within the facility to accomplish anything.[52]

Concrete suggestions are available regarding how people, particularly women, can increase their power in an organization.[53] There are significant implications, however, for the quality of nursing practice within an institution that depends upon whether or not the top administrative leader of nursing has power. (See the discussion of position power and cycles of change in Chapter 6 of this book.)

Megahospitals

Generally, as the turn of the century draws nearer, experts state the organizational structure of health care agencies needs to move toward decentralization and delegation of power in order

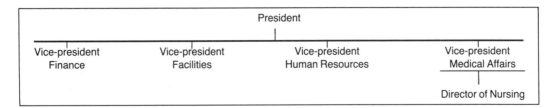

Figure 10–9. An administrative organizational structure, showing the vice-president of medical affairs as an equal with other vice-presidents, but with the head of the nursing unit reporting to the medical administrator. The nurse-administrators would tend to be loyal to the vice-president of medical affairs, who selects, evaluates, and fires. The vice-president of medical affairs would tend to have split loyalty among the institution, medicine, and nursing, probably in that order of priority. The influence and power of the nursing administrator within the institution would tend to diminish accordingly. *(From Sheedy, S.G. Vice-president of medicine/vice-president of nursing: Collaboration or conflict? The Journal of Nursing Administration, 1984, 14 (6), 40. With permission.)*

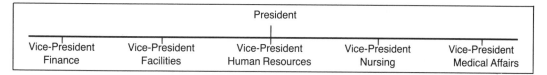

Figure 10–10. An administrative organizational structure, showing the vice-president of medical affairs and the vice-president of nursing as an equal with other vice-presidents. Both medicine and nursing have autonomy. *(From Sheedy, S.G. Vice-president of medicine/vice-president of nursing: Collaboration or conflict? The Journal of Nursing Administration. 1984, 14 (6), 40. With permission.)*

to meet the challenges expected. For example, Poulin describes the current and future health care system as:

> . . . being characterized by traditionalism, standardization, centralization, duplication, and, all too often, immobility and obsolescence . . . the organizational model of the future will be one . . . characterized by coordination, communication, integration, flexibility, dynamism interrelated with professional values and autonomy.[54]

Perhaps the matrix organizational structure is one means of achieving Level IV, holistic planning as proposed by Troub.[55] (See Chap. 9.) The organization structures and charts presented in this chapter are merely simplistic samples, because the trend had been established for some hospitals to unite into even more complex structures. This is in addition to the complex contractual relationships health agencies have with medical and nursing schools to provide clinical practice areas for students. Since the early 1900s, hospitals have been considered not only centers of care, but of research and education also. According to Rowland and Rowland, these organizational relationships facilitate integration of systems.[56] Hospitals are joining together to provide more diversified services to the community, eliminate duplication of services, and encourage effective utilization of specialized personnel and technology.

Rowland and Rowland report one such approach is *shared services*. This means several hospitals contract for services such as laundry, laboratory, or purchasing. The *consortium* is a second approach. This involves several health care agencies that develop a partnership and maintain full-time staff devoted to joint planning and program development for members of the consortium. Member health agencies may agree to provide one another specialized clinical services. One hospital in the community may provide x-ray and others oncological treatments, while still others may provide a burn center or cardiac intensive care units.

A third approach is the *megahospital systems* or corporations. National chains have developed with a central office for training and development of management personnel and systems, clinical teacher orientations and educational materials, purchasing and finance. These may be church-related or investor-owned. There is a tendency to adopt a single management approach and a system of services enabling reductions in costs. Development of facilities through realistic long-term planning and utilization of financial resources is another benefit, since the economic base usually is sound. Clinical and administrative personnel can be brought in-hospital to cope with internal problems or brought together to deal with external, systems concerns.

A fourth approach is *contract management*. The governing board hires a total management team and system to manage an investor-owned hospital. The management team usually includes the administrator and all the vice-presidents or equivalent, often including nursing and finance. The budget and major changes are approved by the governing board before being implemented by the management team. Rowland and Rowland state that through use of cost control statistics, centralized purchasing, and standardized evaluation procedures, services are maintained at an appropriate level. Many institutions can benefit from these megasystems managerial arrangements.[57]

As a nursing leader, it is necessary for you to have some basic awareness of organizational structure and the aspects unique to hospitals and health care agencies. While an underlying theoretical perspective often is deliberately selected, the way people communicate, with whom, how often, and with what degree of effectiveness is to some degree influenced by organizational structure. As a general principle, we suggest the following:

> *In order to be an effective leader, it may be necessary not only to know the overt policies and structure of an agency, but also to compensate for and work around organizational inadequacies until the organizational structure is revised.*

Next, the organizational structure within the nursing unit is discussed from a nursing leadership perspective.

STRUCTURE OF THE NURSING UNIT

The challenge of nursing leaders is to develop units (departments or divisions) of nursing services that can be characterized by "coordination, communication, integration" as predicted by Poulin.[58] You probably noted the formal organization of the nursing units coincidentally in discussions earlier in this chapter. (See Figs. 10–2, 10–3, 10–4, and 10–5.) By the time the vice-president or director of nursing arrives, the main organizational structure is already in place, and the nursing unit structure is expected to follow that of the total organization. Given Poulin's prediction (and she is probably correct), the nursing unit needs to be moved toward open communication and integrated groups. Even given the tendency toward tall, centralized structures, a system of committees can be developed within the nursing unit that have high potential for coordination, communication, and so on.

While the day-to-day task of providing nursing care is assigned to the nursing managers and staff, there are aspects of nursing practice and administration that are the responsibility of the total unit. These areas need to be either monitored continuously through a system of committee assignments or researched and developed by special task or project groups. According to Gillies, a nursing leader who wants to establish participative management can involve all assisting management and many nursing staff in committee assignments. Gillies states this is an major factor in developing leadership skills. It provides opportunities for nurses to meet and work from within nursing, to develop group leadership skills, and to gain confidence. By accepting committee assignments, nursing staff may increase the probability of promotion.[59]

There are several types of committees. First, the committee structure within the nursing unit usually includes an administrative executive council. This group typically consists of all nursing management or leaders within the nursing unit, that is, the director or Vice President of Nursing (VPN) and all assistant directors and supervisors. Meeting as often as once a week, this group plans and solves problems of daily operations, and they may make recommendations to the VPN or director for referral beyond the nursing unit.

A second category of committees may include nursing personnel representing both managers and nursing staff. These committees usually include a policy and procedures, a staff development, and a nursing care committee, as well as recruitment and quality assurance committees. A third type of committee may consist of nursing staff personnel. This type may include a committee on employee health and welfare, or one on patient education.

If quality circles, a form of participative management, are initiated, the problem-solving groups are developed according to the job similarities; one circle consists of staff nurses, another of head nurses, and so on. (See Fig. 10–11.) While participative management is time-consuming, it is known to produce a diversity of opinions and quality outcomes. Reports

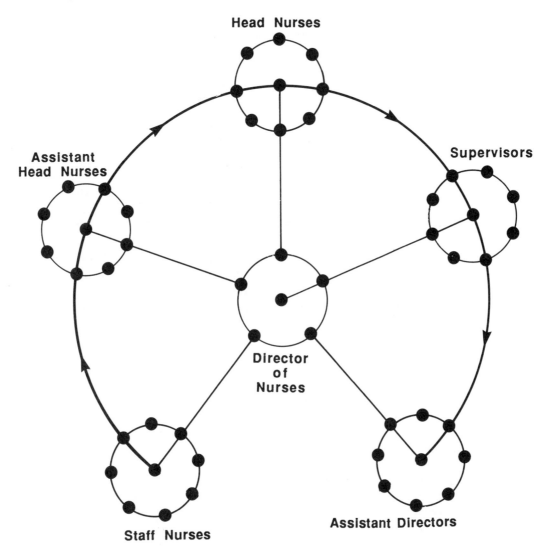

Figure 10–11. A suggested plan for development of quality circle groups, beginning with three circles and adding circles until all nursing personnel are members of a circle. *(From Strader, M.K. Adapting Theory Z to nursing management.* Nursing Management, *1987,* 18 *(4), 62. With permission.)*

1. Specify objectives for the meeting.
2. Build an agenda for the meeting, including all reports, discussion items, and action items, and the time allotted to each.
3. Decide who needs to come to the meeting, and give each person a copy of the agenda and any support documents needed for action and/or discussion items.
4. Make provision for appropriate space and for all supplies and resources (including people).
5. Begin and end the meetings promptly at the announced time.
6. Provide brief "group building" activities at the beginning ("coffee and conversation" time; small-group discussion) and time for summarizing and reflecting on the achievements of the meeting and planning the next meeting.
7. Continually look for ways to relate the work of the group to the purpose and goals of the organization.
8. Provide a short break for each hour or hour and a half of the meeting.
9. At the beginning of each meeting, always share the objectives and review the proposed agenda for possible revision. Try using newsprint for this purpose.
10. The size of the group affects how the group works together. If the task group is only four to six persons, then all group work can be done together. If there are more than four members, some group assignments could be done in subgroups.

Figure 10–12. Suggestions for planning and running nursing service department committee meetings. *(From Duldt, B.W., Giffin, K., & Patton, B.R. Interpersonal communication in nursing. Philadelphia: Davis, 1984, p. 163. With permission.)*

indicate that quality circles increase morale, decrease alienation, and provide incentives for productivity among nursing staff.[60] Strader stresses the process of moving from a Theory X to Theory Z orientation. This author also cautions nursing leaders to move slowly, and lists a set of steps involved in the quality circle process.[61] Sullivan and Decker describe yet another perspective you may want to consider.[62]

A third category consists of task forces charged with the research and development of a specific job; upon completion of the special assignment, the task force is disbanded. For example, task forces might be appointed to write the nursing department's sections of the hospital accreditation report, to research and develop a new service for oncology or cardiac rehabilitation, to select a nursing theory(ies) to serve as the basis of nursing care, or to investigate drug abuse among hospital employees. These temporary committees typically report to the director of nursing, making appropriate recommendations. If a new service is developed, such as an oncology unit, the chairman of the task force usually becomes the nurse-manager, that is, assistant director or head nurse, of the new unit.[63]

In addition, the internal committee structure is linked to a similar agency-wide system of committees. Nursing management and staff personnel may be asked to serve on the interdepartmental committees. As a general principle, the following is suggested:

To the same degree the director of nursing believes that communication is the lifeblood of an organization, this nursing leader will promote open communication among nursing personnel and support multiple memberships on both intra- and interdepartmental committees.

This strongly supports a holistic, humanistic, participatory management and leadership philosophy.

Membership to committee is usually based on nursing experience and expertise, and may vary in number. For small, hands-on working committees, limiting the membership to five people seems to be most conducive to effectiveness and productivity. Research shows that increasing the size of a group decreases the interaction potential of the membership; dominant members begin to take over as the quiet members participate less.[64-66] Another consequence of increased group size is the need for specific structure and regulation of behavior.[67] As groups increase in size, the number of ideas generated also increases in larger groups, but not in proportion to the increased number of members. Instead, some members tend to withhold ideas so that creativity is stifled.[68] In experimenting with groups of two to seven, Slater found the five-member groups expressed the most satisfaction; in groups of fewer than five, the members participated less due to fear of alienating the others.[69] Thus appointment of five-member committees or task forces has the highest probability of achieving success.[70]

While leadership initiative is taken by any member, provided all members of the group approve, it is the responsibility of the designated chairperson to facilitate group movement toward the goal. In addition to the discussions regarding facilitating found in Chapter 7, a more pragmatic guide is provided for planning and conducting committee meetings. (See Fig. 10–12.) For further information, it is suggested readers refer to texts that concentrate on social interactions and communication in small task groups.

SUMMARY

In Chapter 10, organizing as a concept was defined and its significance noted, and some principles of organization were stated in relation to the delegation of power and the cooperation extended to those individuals in positions or centers of power within an organization. There is no one best way to organize, so the concentration was on relating leadership theories to the models after which organizations are structured. The models, tall (centralized), flat (decentralized), circular, and matrix, have been discussed and presented in a rather pure form. Two examples of typical hospital organizational charts were shown for analysis, and common advantages and disadvantages of organizational charts were noted. In addition, the informal communication network was described as being potentially helpful or dangerous to management. Several unique aspects of hospitals and health institutions were considered. Organizational structure within the nursing unit itself has also been presented.

Historically, hospitals have been big business, and nursing has been in a servitude relationship with paternalistic hospitals.[71] Contemporary nursing is rapidly moving into a different role now. Nursing services delivers 90 percent of the patient care (product) provided by hospitals, and costs only 30 percent of the hospital's operating budget.[72] Since nursing is so valuable an asset to health care, leaders of nursing are well advised to study the organizational structure of the agencies in which they practice. Knowledge of the centers of power, the formal communication network, and the unique aspects of organizational structures seems to be fundamental information for any leader striving to achieve an integrated, dynamic, autonomous nursing department.

REFERENCES

1. Guralnik, D.B. (Ed.). *Webster's New World Dictionary* (2nd ed.). New York: Prentice-Hall, 1980, p. 1002.

2. Marriner, A. *Guide to nursing management* (2nd ed.). St. Louis: Mosby, 1984, p. 54.
3. Talcott, P. *Structure and process in modern societies.* Glencoe, Ill.: The Free Press, 1960, p. 17.
4. Etzioni, A. *Modern organizations.* Englewood Cliffs, N. J.: Prentice-Hall, 1964, p. 3.
5. Guralnik, *Webster's Dictionary,* p. 372–373.
6. Gillies, D.A. *Nursing management: A systems approach.* Philadelphia: Saunders, 1982, p. 115.
7. Stevens, B.J. *First-line patient care management* (2nd ed.). Rockville, Md.: Aspen, 1983, p. 49.
8. Gillies, *Nursing management,* p. 115.
9. Ibid.
10. Stevens, *First-line patient care management,* p. 49.
11. Lawrence, P.R., & Lorsch, J.W. *Organization and environment.* Homewood, Ill.: Irwin, 1969, pp. 11, 185–245.
12. Langford, T.L. *Managing and being managed: Preparation for professional nursing practice.* Englewood Cliffs, N. J.: Prentice-Hall, 1981, pp. 171–172.
13. Rowland, H.S., & Rowland, B.L. *Nursing administration handbook.* Germantown, Md.: Aspen, 1980, p. 67.
14. Weber, M. [*The theory of social and economic organization*] (A. M. Henderson & T. Parsons, trans.). New York: Oxford University Press, 1947, pp. 329–341.
15. Langford, *Managing and being managed,* p. 170.
16. Marriner, *Guide to nursing management,* p. 55–56.
17. Gillies, *Nursing management,* p. 115.
18. Drucker, P. *Management, tasks, responsibilities, practices.* New York: Harper & Row, 1973, pp. 231–245.
19. Langford, *Managing and being managed,* p. 170.
20. Marriner, *Guide to nursing management,* p. 58.
21. Ibid.
22. Ibid.
23. Ibid., p. 67–73.
24. Rowland & Rowland, *Nursing administration handbook,* p. 72.
25. Ibid.
26. Marriner, *Guide to nursing management,* p. 68.
27. Mauksch, H.O. The nurse: coordinator of patient care. In J. K. Skipper, Jr., & R. C. Leonard (Eds.). *Social interaction and patient care.* Philadelphia: Lippincott, 1965.
28. Johnson, G.V., & Tingey, S. Matrix organization: Blueprint of nursing care organization for the 80's, an alternative to the present system of task-centered care. *Hospital & Health Services Administration,* 1976, *21,* 27–39.
29. Rowland & Rowland, *Nursing administration handbook,* p. 72–73.
30. Ibid., 73.
31. Johnson & Tingey, Matrix organization, 27–29.
32. Lawrence & Lorsch, *Organization and environment.*
33. Neuhauser, D. The hospital as a matrix organization. *Hospital Administration,* 1972, *17,* 8–25.
34. Peters, T.J., & Waterman, R.H., Jr. *In search of excellence: Lessons from America's best run companies.* New York: Warner Books, 1982, p. 306.
35. Ibid., 307.
36. Ibid., 308–317.
37. Rowland & Rowland, *Nursing administration handbook,* p. 68.
38. Hagopian, G. The communication network. In J.L. Schweiger (Ed.). *Handbook for first-line nurse managers.* New York: Wiley, 1986, pp. 102–103.
39. Sheridan, D.R., Bnonstein, J.E., & Walker, D.D. *The new nurse manager.* Rockville, Md.: Aspen, 1984, p. 87.
40. Kanter, R.M. *Men and women of the corporation.* New York: Basic Books, 1977, pp. 96–97.
41. Davis, K. *Human behavior at work: Organizational behavior.* New York: McGraw-Hill, 1981, p. 342.

42. Mauksch, The nurse, p. 255.
43. Ibid.
44. Smith, H.L. Two lines of authority are one too many. *The Modern Hospital*, 1955, *84*, 59–64.
45. Ibid.
46. Stein, L. The doctor-nurse game. *American Journal of Nursing*, 1968, *68*, 101–105.
47. Stein, L. Male and female: The doctor-nurse game. *Archives of General Psychiatry*, 1967, *16*, 699–703.
48. Hoekelman, R. A. Nurse-physician relationships. *American Journal of Nursing*, 1975, *75* (7), 1151.
49. Korner, A.R. Working with physicians: The view from below. In *Really trying: A career guide for the health services manager*. Ann Arbor, Mich.: AUPHA Press, 1984, pp. 160–182.
50. Sheedy, S.G. Vice-president of medicine/vice-president of nursing: Collaboration or conflict? *The Journal of Nursing Administration*, 1984, *14*, 38–41.
51. Ibid., 40.
52. Rowland & Rowland, *Nursing administration handbook*, p. 69.
53. Stone, S., Firsich, S.C., Jordan, S.B., Berger, M.S., & Elhart, D. (Eds.). *Management for nurses: A multidisciplinary approach* (3rd ed.). St. Louis: Mosby, 1984, pp. 15–20.
54. Poulin, M.A. Future directions for nursing administration. *The Journal of Nursing Administration*, 1984, *14* (3), 37.
55. Troub, R.M. A general theory of planning: The evolution of planning and the planning of evolution. *Journal of Economic Issues*, 1982, *16* (2), 382.
56. Rowland & Rowland, *Nursing administration handbook*, p. 79–80.
57. Ibid., 81.
58. Poulin, Future directions for nursing administration, 37.
59. Gillies, *Nursing management*, p. 130–131.
60. Moore, R.C., et al. On the scene: Quality circles at Barns Hospital. *Nursing Administration Quarterly*, 1982, *6* (3), 23–46.
61. Strader, Adapting Theory Z to nursing management, 64.
62. Sullivan, E.J., & Decker, P.J. *Effective management in nursing*. Reading, Mass.: Addison-Wesley, 1985, pp. 190–194.
63. Langford, *Managing and being managed*, p. 173–174.
64. Bass, B.M. *Leadership, psychology, and organizational behavior*. New York: Harper & Row, 1960, Chapter 17.
65. Harnak, V., & Fest, T.B. *Group discussion: Theory and techniques*. New York: Appleton-Century-Crofts, 1964, pp. 241–242.
66. Bales, R.F., et al. Channels of communication in small groups. *American Sociological Review*, 1951, *16*, 461–468.
67. Hamblin, R.L. *An experimental study of the relationship of communication, power relations, specialization, and social atmospheres to group size*. Unpublished doctoral dissertation, University of Michigan, 1955.
68. Gibb, C. A. The effects of group size and of threat reduction upon creativity in a problem solving situation. *American Psychologist*, 1951, *6*, 324. (Abstract)
69. Slater, P. E. Contrasting correlates of group size. *Sociometry*, 1958, *21*, 129–139.
70. Patton, B.R., & Giffin, K. *Decision-making group interaction*. New York: Harper & Row, 1984, p. 73.
71. Ashley, J.A. *Hospitals, paternalism, and the role of the nurse*. New York: Teachers College Press, 1979, pp. 1–33.
72. Curtin, L. Who Says "Lean" must be "Mean"? (Editorial) *Nursing Management*, 1986, *17* (1), 7–8.

11

STAFFING, PART I: ASSESSING AND SELECTING

INTRODUCTION

The selection and placement of people in positions throughout the organization is the third task function of leadership, *staffing*. It can only be as effective as the preceding functions, planning and organizing, and it builds upon them. Staffing is the key to achieving the goals of the organization, and the leadership functions of directing and controlling can only be as effective as staffing.

Since staffing is a complex management function, the presentation has been organized into two chapters according to the following set of elements: Part I, assessing and selecting; Part II, scheduling and evaluating. In the introduction to Part I, staffing and its significance will be defined, and related standards, philosophy, and theory will be considered.

Decisions about staffing, to a considerable extent, are preceded by assessing values. Decisions must be made about which patient care system is used: Staffing arrangements and job descriptions differ according to whether one uses case, functional, team, or primary nursing systems. Methods of needs assessments and measurements used to forecast the amount of staffing needed are presented, whether for individual nursing units, divisions, or the entire hospital. In addition, selecting nursing staff will be discussed, including development of job descriptions, recruitment, screening, and orientation of staff. In the next chapter, Part II of Staffing, a variety of approaches to scheduling personnel are considered, noting the advantages and disadvantages of each. Personnel policies, selected issues, and variables are also included in this chapter. Finally, evaluating of staffing programs is considered in relation to standards, as well as such issues as productivity, cost-effectiveness, unions, and labor laws.

DEFINITION AND SIGNIFICANCE OF STAFFING

The dictionary defines *staff* as "a group of people assisting a chief, manager, president, or other leader."[1] Staffing is a process consisting of the following set of elements: assessment, planning, budgeting, scheduling, controlling, informing, and evaluating.[2] Stevens provides the following definition specific to nursing: "Staffing is the creation of a plan to determine how many nursing personnel, of what classifications, will be needed for a given nursing unit on each shift."[3]

While many business organizations maintain staffing for business hours from 8 A.M. to 9 P.M. for six days a week, the hospital is one organization that provides services around the clock throughout the year. This places a unique burden on decision making about staffing. In this respect, then, staffing hospitals and similar health agencies is comparatively more difficult administratively and less attractive to health personnel than that of other professions, businesses, and occupations.

> No other profession, not even medicine, is faced with such a demand for relentless, continuous service. DiVincenti cites staffing as one of the most persistent and critical concerns facing nursing service administration and indicates that there is not very much evidence of whether the problem is quantity, quality, or utilization (DiVincenti, 1977). It is likely to be all three.[4,5]

Variables that influence the staffing process are numerous. If only this old maxim were true: "A nurse is a nurse is a nurse." Just *any* nurse will not do. The diversity of educational preparation, specialization, certification, licensure, and experience of professional nurses is compounded by the increasing number of citizens seeking care for a corresponding variety of health problems. The purpose of staffing is to match the expertise of nurses with the health care services offered to meet clients' needs. This matching is the goal and the rub.

ASSESSING

In assessing staffing needs, we have selected three concepts that seem to include most of the factors considered of significance in determining the number of nursing staff and the staffing mix, or ratios of licensed and unlicensed personnel. One factor is *valuing*: The approach used, the standards met, and the quality of care reflect the values implemented. A second factor is *forecasting:* The accuracy of determining the number and mix of staff varies according to methods used to forecast needs. The third factor is *budgeting*: the realities of what one can actually afford must eventually be included in the process of assessment. Determining staffing needs for a nursing unit or an entire hospital can be viewed according to three major elements: valuing, forecasting, and budgeting.

Valuing
Valuing refers to the philosophical beliefs and opinions about the level of nursing care to be provided. (See the discussion of valuing in Chapter 9.) Historically, nursing has generally maintained a humanistic philosophical perspective of focusing on the client and meeting health care needs of individuals. The terms used to describe this nursing care have included *individualized, patient-centered, comprehensive, holistic,* and similar labels for personalized care. Philosophically, nursing is most compatible with a decentralized organizational structure and a humanizing leadership style.

The degree to which the philosophical perspective has been operationalized has depended, however, to a significant degree upon a number of variables. A primary variable has been the quantity and quality of trained or registered nurses available. Recruitment and retention of nurses has been a recurring issue, often in response to events and phenomena in the American society and, too often, in response to administrative errors and poor judgment in hospital personnel policies, staffing designs, and patient care assignment systems. Other variables have included, among others, the centralized organizational structure of hospitals, militaristic and religious organizations, and autocratic leadership styles.

The specific task of providing nursing care to patients or clients has been delegated by means of several control systems. (See also the discussion on structure of work assignment control systems in Chapter 6.) For example, prior to World War I, most nurses were private-duty nurses assigned to individual patients according to the case method system of scheduling.

By the late 1940s, the supply of nurses had decreased and the functional nursing system was common. Team nursing was introduced during the early 1950s as an alternative control system to achieve efficient utilization of the professional nurses' skills. These systems tended to place a variety of assisting personnel *between* the nurse and the patient. Recently, a full circle has been completed by returning to a system that again places the professional nurse in direct relation to the patient through the development of primary nursing.[6,7]

According to contemporary reports, a new and increasing shortage of professional nurses poses still another threat to quality nursing care.[8] The struggle to juggle philosophical beliefs and pragmatic reality will probably continue for some time. Rather than a single system of patient care assignments within one health care agency, a combination of systems may appropriately provide the desirable philosophical quality of care as a function of the complexity or intensity of clients' needs. Thus it is necessary that nurses know the four classic systems of patient care assignments. We recognize, however, that most nurses will find variations and mutations of each in practice. (See, again, the discussion of structure of work assignments control systems, in Chapter 6.)

The Case Method

Oldest of assignment systems, the case method is the assignment of one nurse to one patient or client for all nursing care needs of that individual (see Fig. 11–1). Historically, one nurse would contract to remain with the client continuously in the client's home until the need for nursing care ended. One nurse accepted total, 24-hour responsibility for the nursing care provided. Later the practice was to have one private duty nurse contract for each 8-hour period, each accepting responsibility for their respective period of duty. Independent practitioners of nursing, or private-duty nurses, still use variations of this system in a variety of settings, such as hospitals, rehabilitation centers, and clients' homes.

The case method is typically used today in teaching nursing in most educational programs. Although the responsibility of the assignment remains with the head nurse, an official employee of the agency, the nursing student delivers the nursing care required by selected patients under the direction of an instructor; patient cases are selected specifically to meet the student's learning needs and meet curriculum objectives. Second, this system is used in contemporary health care agencies to meet specific needs, as in the case of intensive care and isolation. If a patient suddenly becomes severely ill or psychotic, or similar critical situations develop, a head nurse may, for a brief period, use the case method system to assign a member

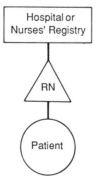

Figure 11–1. Organizational structure of the case method nursing care control system.

of the nursing staff to provide care until the patient is better, moves to an appropriate service, or dies. As a third example, the case method is still commonly used in community health agencies, but each nurse has a *case load* of a number of clients rather than only one.[9] The reader is probably able to think of other examples of the case method being used today as a control system in nursing practice.

This system, however, is seldom used to assign nursing assistants because of their limited qualifications and legal restrictions according to state nurse practice acts; nursing assistants are not prepared or licensed to give medications and treatments, make assessments, and be responsible for total care.[10] Continuity of care in the case method system can be a concern because, in a given period of time, the head nurse may assign different staff members to care for one patient.[11] Ideally, all aspects of the patient's care needs are met without omissions because one nurse knows all that is done; this may not realistically always be true.

Nevertheless, the case method is the forerunner of the primary care system. The case method is used today in a variety of ways, particularly in health agencies having an all-professional nurse staff.[12] A decentralized organization is the most appropriate structure to accommodate the degree of decision making required of nurses in the case method.[13] One futuristic organizational structure that presumes the case method was reported in testimony to the National Commission of Nursing. It described an independent practice of nursing, comparable to that of physicians, in which:

> nurses will apply for practice privileges, be in control of and accountable for their practice, be reimbursed on the basis of quality and quantity of care given, and be self-governing and self-disciplining.[14]

The case method is exceptionally useful in clinical nursing research to document extensive detail of patients' holistic responses to deviations from health. (See Appendix E for additional aspects of the case method and comparisons with other control systems used in nursing.)

We can state the following principle regarding use of the case method:

> *If you have a patient(s) presenting unique nursing care problems about which little is known, then the most effective control system for delegating patient care is to assign by case method those nurses who, other things being equal, are most accurate in providing humanistic care, yet most open and flexible in perception, assuming sufficient funding and a pressing need to develop a nursing knowledge base of the unique health problem.*

For example, in our society today, there is a pressing need to know how to deal with AIDS. Use of the case method might be the most appropriate way to provide, document, and potentially improve nursing care specific to those suffering from AIDS.

The Functional Method

During the depression in the 1930s, families were unable to afford having a nurse provide care in the home, so the nurses returned to the hospitals for employment. The functional method had evolved by the early 1940s before the shortage of nurses developed during World War II. At that time there was a pressing need for nursing services at home and abroad. The functional method provided a variety of helpers as a support to the registered nurse so that she (men rarely were nurses) might be relieved of those duties that could safely be delegated to others. The new classification of Licensed Practical Nurse was established to fill this need (see Fig. 11–2). These

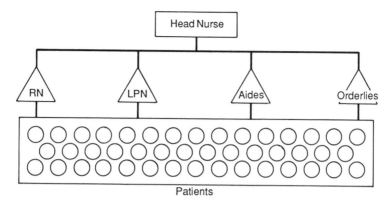

Figure 11–2. Organizational structure of the functional method nursing care delivery system.

helpers were assigned specific tasks to be performed for all patients on a unit, while the registered nurses performed only those nursing tasks that could not be delegated.[15]

> Thus, one registered nurse in the unit might be responsible for administering medicines to all patients in the unit, another for changing dressings and administering special treatments (such as postural drainage or warm compresses) for all patients in the unit, and another for predischarge teaching of all patients in the unit. One licensed practical nurse might be responsible for taking vital signs and recording intake and output of all patients in the unit, while another might be responsible for giving baths to all bedridden patients. An aide or attendant might be responsible for making beds for all ambulatory patients in the unit.[16]

Nurse aides were often assigned housekeeping duties such as delivering or "passing" meal trays and fresh water, feeding patients, running errands, delivering mail to the patients' rooms, and caring for their flowers. For the first time, nurses became a part of the chain of command, responsible for supervising the actions of others.[17]

> Emphasis is usually on "get the work done," and workers are judged by such things as how many baths they gave, beds they made, or medications they administered. The head nurse was responsible for direction and supervision of the entire staff and is the person to whom staff members must go with their questions and reports.[18]

This method fit the classic centralized organizational structure of most hospitals, civilian or military. Management behavior and attitudes tended to be congruent with this structure. (See Fig. 10–1.)

The advantages of the functional method parallel those of an industrial assembly line. The nursing and auxiliary staff become very skillful in performing a few tasks or nursing procedures for a large number of patients. Equipment is maintained in good repair, and the "experts" are even called to other nursing units to "perform" specialized care there. On first impression, the relatively high ratio of auxiliary or unlicensed staff to registered nursing staff in the functional method gives the appearance of being cost-effective.[19]

There are four major disadvantages, however, to the functional method. First, the registered nurses, particularly the head nurses, become deeply involved with the paperwork and administrative details associated with being responsible for a large number of patients. In some agencies, positions of ward secretaries or unit managers have been developed to relieve the registered nurses of these tasks. In some situations these positions function effectively, but too often only develop chaos.[20] "As chief of all [clinical] activities the charge nurse is barraged with input from all sides; physicians, nursing staff, students, patients/clients, visitors and the public."[21] Role stress often develops because of the dichotomy of clinical versus management expectations, so that nurses often feel inadequate; they tend to leave the agency for another— or just leave nursing.

Second, the care patients receive is fragmented and in illogical order; lacking coordination, the patient seldom knows who "my nurse" is. Third, the personnel soon tend to feel they are not being provided opportunities to perform to their educational potential. Too much of their nursing knowledge and skill remains unused and, consequently, is quickly lost. Indeed, in the functional method of delegating nursing care, the nurses seldom see the whole of nursing practice or the "whole" patient and, unless they ask, seldom know what happens to the patients, if they get well, have complications, or die.[22] Finally, the superficial interpersonal involvement with patients decreases opportunities for humanizing interpersonal experiences, and the emphasis on tasks tends to invite criticism and reduce to a minimum the needed support behaviors from registered nurse colleagues. Nurses become discouraged and experience decreasing job satisfaction.[23] (See Appendix E for additional aspects of the functional method in comparison with other control systems used in nursing.)

We can now state the following principle from our discussion of the functional method:

If the level of patient care is to be minimal and standardized, and if the productivity level needed (number of nursing tasks) is high with a limited number of qualified nurses, then the functional method tends to be the control system of choice, assuming the humanizing relationship needs of both nurses and patients are not to be given high priority.

The functional method of delegating patient care gets the work done and works well for a short time. You will probably want to use the functional method as little as possible, and if you do, you will want to plan something for your nursing staff in order to maintain morale, motivation, and job satisfaction at acceptable levels.

The Team Method

With the development of auxiliary personnel, the team approach was developed to more effectively utilize the talents of *all* staff members. The nursing team usually consists of a Registered Nurse serving as the team leader, a Licensed Practical Nurse, a nurses' aide, and maybe a second Registered Nurse. The number of patients assigned to each team is limited (10 to 20 for a team of 3 to 5 members), and the responsibility for nursing care remains with the registered nurses. The team leader delegates the nursing care and activities to the team members according to their capabilities or readiness—education, licensure and experience.[24] (See Fig. 11–3.) The heart of the team method is the communication system. A form of decentralization, the head nurse confers with the team leader, who provides direction for the team members. The head nurse role focuses on management, and the team leader role incorporates the dichotomy of clinical versus management expectations, providing direct care to critical patients plus providing assistance and direction to the team members. A significant part

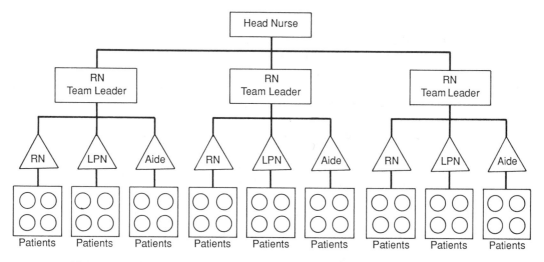

Figure 11–3. Organizational structure of the team method nursing care control system.

of this communication system is the team conference, which provides the opportunity for the team to develop patients' individualized care plans.[25]

The original research and development of team nursing was led by Eleanor Lambertsen and funded by a Kellogg Grant in the 1950s. Other early advocates were Dorothy Newcomb and Thora Kron. Team nursing is based on a philosophy that values the individual, recognizes the Registered Nurse as having the qualifications to control the nursing care plans, and acknowledges the need of people to develop to their potential. The project's goal was to develop a control system of delegating patient care assignments to replace the functional method. This system would increase the cost-effectiveness of nursing by utilizing nursing staff to the fullest and increasing job satisfaction of all staff.[25,26,27] Team nursing is designed to offer a new way for nurses to practice humanistic nursing and a way for nurses, themselves, to be treated in a manner that we are labeling humanistic.

There are several advantages of team nursing. First, all team members have an opportunity to become involved not only in a variety of nursing tasks, but also in the planning, implementation, evaluation, and revision of nursing care of a small number of patients. Since participation in decision making tends to increase group members' commitment to their decision, this provides job enrichment and job expansion.[28,29] Second, the nursing team members receive more supervision than is possible in the functional method, and the unlicensed members benefit from the instruction received from the team leader.[30] Third, the team conference recognizes the need to set aside a specific time for the team members to develop nursing care plans and solve patient care problems. There is ample opportunity for them to perform to their educational potential, decreasing team members' boredom from routines. In conducting the conference, the team leader can receive valuable experience in a leader role.[31] Fourth, the nursing care plan is formalized by using the Kardex to write a plan for each patient.[32] Fifth, from the patients' perspective, fewer people provide care, so that the care tends to be coordinated and individualized more than that of the functional method.[33]

In practice, however, nurses have noted a number of disadvantages in using team nursing. Marriner notes several problems. First, there is more opportunity for communication errors as orders and information move from the head nurse to team leader to team member; there is a greater than usual need to validate information. Second, the team members assigned to one team vary so much (due to days off, rotating shifts, vacations, and so on) that the team leader often has difficulty determining who is most capable of caring for specific patient needs. Third, the team conferences are frequently just omitted. Nursing staff members find it difficult to break away from patient care and come to the conference. When conferences are held, the focus frequently is on physician's orders, and the team leader checks with each member to make sure all tasks are completed. Consequently, the care becomes so routinized that it is difficult to distinguish from care provided in the functional method.[34] Fourth, Douglass cites increased costs as a disadvantage; there is an increased amount of nursing time used for administration of technical details and direction of the team members. Fifth, Douglass reports that some Registered Nurses would just rather not conduct the team conferences.[35]

Ultimately, the Registered Nurse (RN) team leaders came to be viewed as merely being responsible for medications, treatments, and new orders. These activities are also within the Licensed Practical Nurses' (LPNs') scope of practice, so it is now common for an LPN to be assigned to the team leader role. With all due respect to the LPNs and their qualifications, this implies that the Registered Nurse is not really required and thus diminishes the potential quality of team nursing.[36] This assignment practice has been the unfortunate source of contention between RNs and LPNs as individuals compare activities and salary. Where hospital workers' unions exist, the nonprofessional LPNs usually belong, but RNs typically do not. Where there are unions, the team nursing assignments frequently are an issue. Part of the philosophy of team nursing is based on the belief in "co-equal status with minimal hierarchical lines of demarcation between the leader and followers. . . ."[37] One is reminded of George Orwell's *Animal Farm:* "All animals are equal, but some are more equal than others."[38] Such is the downfall of team nursing.

From the above discussion of team nursing, we can state the following principle:

If a humanistic quality of patient care and humanistic treatment of nursing personnel is expected, then team nursing is a control system method of choice, assuming adequate resources (people, time, and funding) are available to support initial and concurrent orientation, instruction, and supervision for both nursing followers and leaders.

Apparently sound theoretically and based on an appropriate research-and-development approach to problems in nursing practice, team nursing, as it is operationalized, has helped achieve humanistic nursing care in some ways. Where the original philosophy and methods of operationalizing team nursing have been violated, however the problems of nursing care delivery have merely been compounded. (See Appendix E for additional aspects of the team method in comparison with other control systems used in nursing.)

Primary Nursing
A second method of assignment control systems based on research and development is *primary nursing*. This system is defined as follows:

> The performance of clinical nursing functions by professional nurses with minimal or no delegation of nursing tasks to others. Nurses who are individually responsible for patients' comprehensive nursing care are able to enter into a collegial relationship with physicians who provide the patients' medical care.[39]

While there are many definitions of primary nursing, it may be less confusing if the twelve key concepts Zander identifies are used as the conceptual basis for the development and operationalization of primary nursing:

1. Accountability	7. Commitment
2. Advocacy	8. Collaboration
3. Assertiveness	9. Contracting
4. Authority	10. Coordination
5. Autonomy	11. Communication
6. Continuity	12. Decentralization[40]

Primary nursing, like team nursing, is as much a philosophy of nursing as it is an assignment control system (see Fig. 11–4).

To avoid confusion, we need to distinguish between *primary nursing* and *primary care*. *Primary* (health) *care* refers to a client's first contact with the health care system, usually occurring in clinics based in hospitals or community centers in which a broad range of health care services are offered by a variety of professional care providers. The emphasis of primary care is on health promotion and maintenance, primary prevention of illness and disability, and counseling, guidance, and referral services. The provider may be a nurse, physician, dentist, psychologist, and so on, functioning as an individual practitioner or as a member of a primary care team.[41]

Primary nursing is designed for the primary nurse, a Registered Nurse (RN), to assume full responsibility for a small number of patients. It is most congruent with the decentralized organizational structure. The matrix structure is particularly preferred if the patient's care requires a team of a variety of professionals comprising a patient care team for which the primary nurse serves as leader. (See Chapter 10, Fig. 10–6, and the related discussion.) Usually the nurse is assigned four to six patients to whom he or she provides direct nursing care during the time "on duty." Since this RN is not expected to be present at all times, other RNs

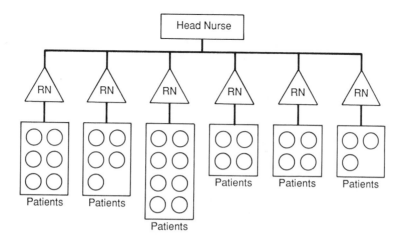

Figure 11–4. Organizational structure of the primary nursing method of nursing care control system.

serve as associate nurses, providing care at other times. The original RN, in turn, may serve as the associate nurse in caring for the patients of other primary nurses. Thus the primary nurse may expect to have four to six patients, plus serve as associate nurse in caring for a few patients assigned to other primary nurses. The patient assignment begins upon the patient's admission, and continues until the patient is discharged.[42]

Like the physician's, the primary nurse's presence is not required continually, but the responsibility continues on a 24-hour basis. The primary nurse conducts the health (and physical) assessment upon admission, identifies the nursing diagnosis, and writes nursing orders. These orders are not to be changed by the associate nurses unless the primary nurse concurs. Consequently, it is understood that all other nurses respect the decisions made by another nurse, an idea new to typical nursing practice. Traditionally, the nurse who is "there" decides, ignoring previous nurses' decisions. When nursing has limited autonomy, authority, and collaboration, this is what happens. In this control system, however, the primary nurse initiates and maintains the written nursing care plan, personally provides most of the care, and shares the plan with the associate nurses with the expectation that this plan will be followed. The primary nurse continually evaluates the effectiveness of the plan in terms of the patient's responses, and revises it when convinced by an appropriate data base that a change is appropriate. Any teaching or discharge planning is conducted by the primary nurse.[43]

There are numerous important advantages of primary nursing. First, the number of people involved in the patient's care is decreased, and the chain of communication required in arranging for care is also reduced; thus, the number of errors is also reduced. All communication about the individual patient is directed to the primary nurse responsible for that patient's care.[44]

Second, the primary nurse can identify the effects of his or her nursing interventions and see the results of his or her efforts. By making all nursing decisions, the primary nurse is more committed to the patient and experiences increased job satisfaction. The patient's complaints are significantly reduced because the patient knows he or she can talk about concerns with "my nurse."[45] The frequent interpersonal communication and contact between the same nurse and patient enables the primary nurse to get to know the patient and family as individuals. The nurse begins to perceive the patient in a holistic and humanistic manner, and can become a true advocate of the patient when the elements of the health care system itself present problems to the patient.[46]

Third, only primary and associate nurses provide care to the patients; there are no nursing aides or assistants between the nurses and the patients. According to Ganong and Ganong, the associate nurses may be Licensed Practical Nurses.[47] Since most nurse practice acts require LPNs to function under the direct supervision of a Registered Nurse, this does not provide legal congruence in assignments and scope of practice. According to Zander, however, the associate nurse title should be dropped because it is "impossible" to implement. Instead, Zander suggests the primary nurse consult with the nurse-manager for off-duty coverage for patients.[48] An all-RN staff tends to be highly recommended by most authors. Thus a shift to primary nursing from functional or team methods poses a threat to the LPN. Nurse aides continue to be assigned housekeeping, dietary, and messenger duties; usually one aide is assigned to two primary nurses in all-RN staffing.[49]

Fourth, the emphasis is on professional clinical practice. This includes the use of the nursing process, problem solving and decision making, and similar processes of abstract thinking expected of members of an academic discipline and professional practice. The focus is on the patient's needs or maladaptive responses to stress or illnesses rather than on getting routine tasks done.[50]

Fifth, research has shown that primary nursing, with its required all-RN staffing, is cost-effective. Fagin summarizes several examples of research findings indicating a reduction in the number of hospital days required and in the incidence of complications for patients receiving care from primary nurses in comparison with patients receiving the traditional (functional or team) methods of nursing care control systems. For example:

> Jones's evaluation of the postoperative adaptation of renal transplant patients indicated a reduction of three weeks in hospital stay and significantly fewer complications suffered by the patients receiving primary nursing. The actual savings for one year for this very small group of patients was more than $51,000.[51]

Again:

> Dahlen found that an all-RN staff in a 99-bed acute care hospital in Oregon cost less than staff at two other comparable hospitals with traditional staffing patterns. . . . [and a study] at the Mainland Division of the Atlantic City [N.J.] Medical Center showed that in one year, it cost $96,516 less to staff Mainland Division's nursing units than it did at 33 other hospitals using team nursing. Fewer nursing care hours, made possible by an all-RN staff practicing primary nursing, accounted for the reduced costs.[52]

Agencies that have used the primary nursing method of assignment control system include the Loeb Center and Rush-Presbyterian.

Primary nursing provides advantages in promoting interprofessional collegial relationships and collaborative communication. As the physician consistently contacts the same primary nurse about the same patient, interpersonal trust can be established, and the communication patterns move through the Situational Leadership styles: telling, selling, participating, and delegating. As dialogue develops, each comes to respect the other's competencies and commitment to patient care. This relationship is supported by the integrated patient records system, which is based on a problem-oriented approach to the patient's health care. Since both the physician and the nurse write progress notes on the same pages of the chart, this provides documentation of opportunities to share information and ideas about the patient's nursing and medical plan of care and progress, and to coordinate both plans.[53]

There are disadvantages to primary nursing, too. First, the expertise and talents of one outstanding nurse are limited in availability to the few assigned patients. If a nurse is not outstanding, the nurse and the patient both may be at a disadvantage: neither one has immediate access to other nurses' perspectives and influence, as in the functional and team methods.[54]

Langford states there are difficulties in implementing primary nursing, particularly when attempting to move from the functional or the team methods. The major problem she cites centers about personnel. Since many agencies have a nursing staff consisting of a large number of LPNs, it is difficult to determine where to place the LPNs. Terminating them is not an acceptable answer. Langford also believes that, where there is an inadequate source of registered nurses, it is not appropriate even to attempt primary nursing.[55]

Zander states that lack of consistency in definition and practice have caused the difficulties encountered in attempts to research and implement primary nursing. In fact, according to

Zander, primary nursing has really been quite successful. After a decade of research, it has been found that quality patient care is given by satisfied registered nurses.[56]

In 1972, the National Joint Practice Commission (NJPC) was established by the American Nurses' Association and the American Medical Association to study physician–nurse relationships and roles in hospitals and to make recommendations for improving the nurses' role. By 1977, the NJPC had identified five areas for further study: primary nursing, the integrated patient record, support for nurses' decision making, a joint practice committee, and joint care review.[57] In the 1981 interim report, nurses' testimony to the NJPC showed strong support for primary nursing, but research findings were conflicting.[58]

One covert strength of primary nursing is its effect of revealing unsuspected problems of nursing practice. One long-standing problem that nurses have had to work around has been the failure of other departments in the hospital to support the nursing role.

> One point about primary nursing deserves further emphasis: the nurses do nursing. Ancillary personnel do not perform nursing functions, and neither do nurses perform non-nursing chores. They do not function as clerks, secretaries, messengers, escorts, or housekeepers. What actually happens, however, is that if the escort service is busy or ancillary personnel aren't available, the nurses take on their chore. If a nursing unit needs an item quickly, the messengers will not interrupt their routine to get it. The nurse does. There is very little effort to have 24-hour coverage by support sources.
>
> Many administrators do not understand the inadequacy of most ancillary services, and one reason is nursing's ability to be subversive. Despite inadequate delivery systems, nurses will always manage to get what they need. They hoard supplies, borrow from each other, take more than they need and hide the extras, and keep emergency stashes in unlikely places. Most pharmacists and hospital engineers would cringe in horror if they knew how much medication gets stored under the sink in the medication area next to the condenser for the ice maker. But nurses are not helping themselves with such tactics. By circumventing the old dinosaur delivery system, nurses keep administration convinced that the system works.[59]

It has been typical for nurses to be assigned duties of dietary, pharmacy, laboratory, and other hospital departments during the nights and on weekends. With the development of primary nursing, this practice stops, and each department must make arrangements with its own staff to provide services at all hours.

Nurses will not only need to eliminate subversive behaviors, but other behaviors as well. In providing leadership for primary nurses, the head nurse cannot be a high controller and militaristic authoritarian, but needs to function as a coach or facilitator of the nurses and be a clinical specialist as well.[60] Ganong and Ganong distinguish between the *nurse*–manager and the nurse–*manager* in a manner similar to the description of humanistic nursing leadership we provide in Chapter 3, and they suggest this kind of leadership is crucial for primary nursing to be successful.[61]

In addition, it is crucial to the successful implementation of primary nursing that the registered nurse be willing to accept total responsibility, accountability, and authority for the care provided. Some nurses may not want or may not have the personal and professional commitment, competence, or maturity to be primary nurses. Some find the 24-hour continuous responsibility for the patient attractive or satisfying. Skills in problem solving and decision making are required for the primary nurse role, as well as experience in writing nursing care plans. The nurse needs to be competent in analyzing a data base derived from his or her own assessment (health history and physical examination) of the patient; this is necessary to the development of a realistic nursing care plan. Humanistic attitudes and interpersonal sensitivity to others, both patients and colleagues, is also necessary in the broad scope of practice required of the primary nurse role.

From the description and evaluation of primary nursing, we believe the following principles can be stated:

> *If a humanistic and holistic quality of patient care and humanistic treatment of nursing personnel is expected; in a practice assignment system that supports nurses' continuous autonomy, authority, and credibility; and in an interpersonal climate that supports intra- and interprofessional collaboration and coordination of care; then primary nursing is the control system method of choice, assuming adequate resources are available to support an all-RN staff, and also to support initial and concurrent orientation, education, and facilitation of the primary nurse.*

The humanistic philosophical perspective of focusing on patients' needs can be focused, through careful and wise leadership, on nurses' and nursing's needs as well by choosing primary nursing. (See Appendix E for additional aspects of primary nursing in comparison with the other control systems.)

This concludes the review of the four classic systems of patient care assignments. You must choose from these which one system, or variation thereof, is most congruent with your own beliefs and values. If you choose from the perspective of values and beliefs, you may be able to avoid some errors of past leadership and management efforts. For example, in the past few decades, nursing has had numerous difficulties, which we believe are basically due to management error. The following quote presents consequences of these errors and reality-oriented implications.

> Turnover has been and is costly. The American Hospital Association estimates a current shortage of 100,000 nurses, and this number is growing. . . . Impact: Nursing represents the single most critical area for hospital cost containment. . . . Each time an experienced nurse leaves a hospital, it costs from $4,000.00 to 6,800.00 to recruit and train a replacement. . . . When it cannot fill beds and must close a unit because of insufficient nursing staff, the hospital will lose approximately $10,000 per day in revenues. . . . Labor pool shrinking: Of the 1.4 million licensed nurses in the U.S. 414,000 have stopped working . . . only 69% of the RNs in the U.S. are actually working in their profession.[62]

Given the discussions about philosophical beliefs and values in relation to selecting a patient assignment control system, we can state the following principle, which we hope will assist you in prioritizing your own beliefs:

> *To the same degree that registered nurses' assignment involves direct nursing care, there is a comparable probability that humanistic nursing care, communication, and leadership will tend to occur.*
>
> *To the same degree that registered nurses' assignment involves direct nursing care, there is a comparable probability that the nurses will tend to engage in inter- and intra-professional collaboration.*
>
> *To the same degree that registered nurses' assignment involves direct nursing care, that nurses are afforded autonomy and increased participation in decisions and policy develop-*

ment relating to patient care, there is a comparable probability that the nurses' job satisfaction and nursing staff retention will increase.

In addition to the information and principles presented, there are sets of criteria available from important professional groups that you need to consider also. For example, the American Nurses' Association publishes *Nursing Staff Requirements for In-Patient Health Care Services.*[63] Similar statements of requirements may be available from accrediting and licensing agencies associated with your own agency, and you may want to ask about these. In addition, you may have to participate in developing precise statements of the kind and quality of care the agency is to provide. These statements will tend to reflect philosophical perspectives that you will want to read carefully and compare with your own beliefs.

Forecasting

The second element of assessing staffing needs is *forecasting,* a method of determining the future based on current trends. As suggested by Toffler and Naisbitt, several alternative futures can be identified so that you can choose your preferred future and plan, increasing its probability.[64,65] In health management, forecasting is a way of identifying alternative economic futures that tend to influence the health care industry. Apparently applying Lewin's change theory[66] (see Chapter 6 and Chapter 9), Strasen cites the following steps in forecasting:

1. Identify the organization's present position.
2. Identify the organization's weaknesses and strengths.
3. Identify the driving trends in the environment that could be threats or opportunities for the organization.
4. Construct possible alternative future scenarios based on the driving trends in the environment.
5. Identify the desired future for the organization.[67]

Futures research, a relatively new discipline, is being used in a few health care agencies to identify future scenarios. Scenarios are stories about alternative futures from which a preferred future can be selected.[68] For example, the ten trends John Naisbitt has identified for society can be used as a basis of scenario development.

1. Information society
2. High tech/high touch
3. World economy
4. Long-term perspective
5. Decentralization
6. Self-help
7. Participatory democracy
8. Networking
9. Southern migration
10. Multiple options[69]

Working from these ten trends, health care futurists Mitchell, Cloner, and Coile have identified the following four socioeconomic scenarios for the health industry:

1. Continued growth or boom
2. Competition or conglomerates

3. Decline and stagnation
4. Voluntary simplicity or transformation[70]

Like Naisbitt, Mitchell, Cloner, and Coile have identified 10 major trends or "driving forces" of the 1980s for the health care industry:

1. Aging
2. Competition
3. Conglomerates
4. New consumer
5. Corporate practice
6. Diversification
7. Information/telecommunications
8. Shifting dollars
9. Technopush
10. Changing values[71]

The chart has been developed showing the ten driving forces, the four scenarios, and the economic implications of each for health care in the United States. (See Table 11–1.)

We have included this material because we believe as a nurse-leader and manager you need to have some basic knowledge and understanding of the national health care trends for comparison purposes. You may wish to compare the philosophy and objectives of the hospital with which you are associated to the information in Table 11–1. Institutional objectives usually are not changed and have a direct relationship to the quality and quantity of services offered and the operating budget. Some health agencies, however, are finding a need to revise their philosophy and objectives to meet contemporary needs because technology, programs, services, and economic trends have changed quickly.[72]

As a manager of a nursing unit, you will be expected to meet the institution's objective and keep the institution's operating budget at your unit level. The task portion of your performance evaluation will depend to a great extent on how well you are able to forecast patient and staff needs and to administer the resources under your control.

As a general principle, to the degree to which you are able to accurately forecast patient occupancy rates, acuity mix of patients, technological changes, and changes in medical or nursing practice, you will be able to effectively plan the utilization of institutional resources, which includes the budget.

There is some basic terminology with which you, as a nurse-leader, need to be familiar. Most businesses are primarily concerned with profits or the amount of money or revenue after all expenses. In health care agencies, however, the break-even point is of primary concern (see Fig. 11–5). There are certain expenses or overhead involved in maintaining a health agency; these expenses are labeled *fixed costs* because these cannot be changed. *Variable costs*, however, do fluctuate according to the productivity or amount of service provided by a nursing unit. Fixed and variable costs, when added together, provide the *actual cost* of maintaining the nursing unit and providing nursing care. The amount paid by the patient, third-party payers, such as health insurance companies and the federal government health programs (social security, Medicare, Medicaid), or both, should be an amount greater than the actual costs of maintaining the nursing unit and providing nursing care. A *profit* is made if these charges exceed actual costs; if charges are less than actual costs, a *loss* is incurred.[73]

TABLE 11–1. THE TEN DRIVING FORCES IDENTIFIED FOR THE HEALTH FIELD, THE SCENARIO AFFECTED, AND THE ECONOMIC IMPLICATIONS FOR HEALTH CARE AS IDENTIFIED BY MITCHELL, CLONER, AND COILE.

Driving Force	Affected Scenario	Health Care Implications
1. Aging	1, 2, 3, & 4	There will be increasing numbers of elderly consumers demanding specialized services. The need for chronic degenerative disease and organ transplantation services will increase, because of longer life expectancy. The market for an entire line of geriatric services will expand (*e.g.,* life care concept). Aggressive treatment modalities will be utilized in individuals much older than is now the case. Middle-aged persons will be 60 to 80 years old.
2. Competition	1, 2, & 3	Health care advertising will increase. Hospitals will compete with physicians and other health professionals for market. Increased numbers of hospitals and services will merge into conglomerates for strength. Health care consumers will shop around for services and price. Institutions will compete through pricing.
3. Conglomerates	1 & 2	The trend will be toward multi-hospital systems to accomplish economies of scale and increase power base. There will be a trend toward vertical integration, rather than full-service institutions. Health care institutions will "unbundle" services and diversify into other areas (*e.g.,* providing hotel services and rooms for visitors and community). There will be a trend toward joint venturing with competitors, physicians, nurses, and the public sector.
4. New consumer	1, 2, & 4	Consumers will be healthier, more price conscious, better educated, and informed about treatments and alternatives to maintaining their health. Consumers will take more responsibility for their own health and well-being. They will seek professional services less frequently than in the past. More books and audio and video recordings will be marketed, allowing the consumer to treat himself. The consumer will question the health care provider more frequently about the service and will demand more efficiency and greater quality.
5. Corporate practice	1, 2, 3, & 4	Diagnosing will be done by more cost effective and accurate computers. Cost and oversupply of physicians will motivate them to unite for economic security and power. They will create corporations to provide health care services in competition with hospitals. Physicians will attempt to regulate health care policy by increasing lobbying activities. Physicians will become more generalist-minded to maintain clients. They will return to making house calls and be more sensitive and in-tune with consumer needs as a result of economic pressures.
6. Diversification	1, 2, & 4	There will be a great increase in the development of health care products (*e.g.,* vitamins, food, education, etc.). There will be a trend toward "unbundling" of hospitals ser-

TABLE 11–1. (Continued)

Driving Force	Affected Scenario	Health Care Implications
		vices and creating for-profit corporations (e.g., incorporating the printing department and selling service to the community).
		There will be an increasingly broad re-definition of the "health care" business. The business will include services that improve the quality of life, rather than just treating illness.
		Joint ventures with physicians and nurses, and for-profit and public sector will increase. In the "information age," health information will be a business. Health information will include software to diagnose illness and prescribe treatment.
7. Information/telecommunications	1, 2, & 4	Diagnosis and prescription will be done by computers. Software for home personal computers will be available for sale.
		There will be the potential for a health care corporation to serve the world rather than a single community.
		Health care will become more a business of health information rather than actual hands-on care.
		All health care services will be capable of being delivered to the individual consumer's home.
8. Shifting dollars	1, 2, 3, & 4	The uncertain economic environment will create a three-tier health system:
		Public beneficiaries
		Middle class
		Wealthy
		The consumer will be willing to take more risk and responsibility for his own health. He will pay less for health care insurance by assuming a larger deductible.
		More health care institutions will become for-profit.
		There will be an increased demand for outpatient, home health services, etc.
		There will be decreased health care services available for the poor.
9. Technopush	1 & 2	Life expectancy, productivity, and population will increase.
		The cost of health care will increase because of increased cost of research and development and increased number of people to care for.
		The number and complexity of ethical issues will increase as a result of high technology. The high tech aspect will be balanced by a corresponding development of high touch technology.
		Health care policy will be unable to keep up with the demands placed on it.
		Legal implications will become very complex in this high tech environment.
10. Values	1, 2, & 4	The complexity of bioethical issues will increase.
		There will be an increased number of arbitrations necessary among doctors, families, lawyers, and patients.
		Resource allocations may be determined on the cost-effectiveness of various health programs based on years of additional life provided.
		Many conflicts based on values will arise because of the diversity of ethnic groups in the United States.

From Strasen, L. Key business skills for nurse managers. *Philadelphia: Lippincott, 1987, p. 30.*

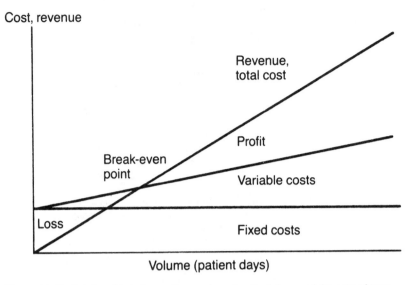

Figure 11–5. Relationship between the number of patient days and the cost of nursing care, showing the break-even point of the loss and profit line intersecting with fixed, variable, and total costs. *(From Strasen, L.* Key business skills for nurse managers. *Philadelphia: Lippincott, 1987, p. 145. With permission.)*

It is important for you as a nursing manager to know exactly where the *break-even point* is in order to avoid incurring a loss. The break-even point is that point on the chart (see Fig. 11–5) where the profit line crosses the actual (fixed and variable) cost line. Generally, as the number of patient care days increases, variable costs, such as the number of nurses on duty, go up along with profit. When below the break-even point, or when the unit has a reduced census (number of patient days), however, the unit is functioning at a loss. In order to maintain appropriate staffing standards, a minimum level of staffing must be maintained for that unit. When the census drops very low, then you as the nursing manager with the supervisor or area coordinator, and other nurse-managers may consider closing one unit for a while. A decreased census of a number of nursing units might be combined to maintain one of the nursing units at capacity.[74] This means losses are cut by moving patients from low-census units to another unit, thus creating a high-census unit operating above the break-even point. Since over 90 percent of the nursing service operating budget is allocated for personnel (salaries and benefits or variable costs), the way you, the nurse-manager, handle staffing represents a significant aspect of your role.[75] The process of forecasting provides a justification for your recommendations about how to spend or allocate institutional resources at the level of the nursing unit.

In forecasting nursing staff requirements, a variety of factors need to be considered, and only a few will be considered here. Table 11–2 lists many factors that influence forecasting. Basically, there are several steps that you will need to understand in order to forecast patient census or occupancy rate. First, there are a number of systems or formulas in the literature for estimating daily, monthly, or annual patient census. For example, the New Britain General Hospital System provides a one-year forecast of the daily census.[76] Second, each system has a patient acuity classification system that indicates the patient's degree of illness and the number of nursing hours required to provide care at the desired level. One example of such a system is shown in Table 11–3. Third, a standard number of nursing hours is identified for each classifica-

TABLE 11–2. FACTORS INFLUENCING THE FORECASTING OF NURSING STAFF REQUIREMENTS

Government, Federal and State
  Regulations and policies
  Labor laws
  Nurse Practice Act
  Social Security; Diagnostic Related Groups (DRG)
  Medicare, Medicaid
  Tax Equity Fiscal Responsibility Act (TEFRA)
  Licensing and credentialing

Professions
  Codes of ethics
  Accreditation criteria
  Educational requirements
  Scope and modes of practice, that is, private, group, and so on.
  Specialization

Community
  Demography of population
  Number, education, & experience of nurses available
  Business and Industry investment in health promotion programs
  Educational facilities; community college, university, medical and nursing school, and so on.
  Labor unions
  Philanthropic contributions and similar funding available
  Research activity in health care
  Image of nursing

Health Agency
  Size of agency, that is, bed capacity, number of services, clinics, and programs
  Philosophy, goals, mission, objectives
  Revenue
  Marketing
  Capital investments
  Physical plant; size, maintenance, expansion, and allocation of space
  Administrative expertise
  Personnel policies and benefits
  Organizational structure
  Size of medical staff; number of specialists; intern program
  Research involvement: grants, traineeships
  Educational affiliations; medical, nursing, social work, pharmacy, physical occupational therapy, and so on.

tion of patients; this number is then multiplied by the number of patients in each classification to identify the total nursing hours required per day. Fourth, depending on the assignment control system used (case, functional, team, or primary nursing), personnel available, institutional standards, and so on, the staffing mix is decided, that is, the number of RNs, LPNs, and aides needed to provide the nursing care. Fifth, the cost of care for the 24-hour period can be determined by multiplying the hourly pay rate of each staffing mix category by the number of nursing staff in each category. Finally, to convert this to monthly or annual figures, simply multiply the nursing hours of care or the cost of care for 24 hours by the number of days in the month or the year.[77–80]

This information may be available if a centralized staffing system is being used, or you may have to do the calculations yourself, using formulas to arrive at the patient and staff forecasts. If the staffing system is centralized, it is probably calculated by using one of several

TABLE 11–3. A PATIENT CLASSIFICATION SYSTEM RELATING THE DEGREE OF ILLNESS AND AN ESTIMATE OF THE REQUIRED NURSING CARE IN NUMBER OF HOURS PER DAY. THE DAILY STANDARD IS 4.3 NURSING HOURS. FOR EXAMPLE, CATEGORY 1 REQUIRES ONLY 65 PERCENT OF THE STANDARD DAILY HOURS, OR 2.8 NURSING HOURS PER 24 HOURS.

I. (65%) A PATIENT WHO REQUIRES ONLY MINIMAL AMOUNT OF NURSING CARE (An average of 2.8 nursing hours per 24 hours)

Examples
- A patient who is mildly ill (generally termed convalescent).
- A patient who requires little treament and/or observation and/or instruction.
- A patient who is up and about as desired; takes his own bath or shower.
- A patient who does not exhibit any unusual behavior patterns.
- A patient without intravenous therapy or many medications.

II. (100%) A PATIENT WHO REQUIRES AN AVERAGE AMOUNT OF NURSING CARE (An average of 4.3 nursing hours per 24 hours)

Examples
- A patient whose extreme symptoms have subsided or not yet appeared.
- A patient who requires periodic treatments and/or observations and/or instructions.
- A patient who is up and about with help for limited periods; partial bed rest required.
- A patient who exhibits some psychological or social problems.
- A patient with intravenous therapy with medications such as IV piggybacks every six hours.
- A newly admitted patient, either surgical or medical, who is a routine admission and not necessarily acutely ill.

III. (135%) A PATIENT WHO REQUIRES ABOVE AVERAGE NURSING CARE (An average of 5.8 nursing hours per 24 hours)

Examples
- A moderately ill patient.
- A patient who requires treatments or observations as frequently as every two to four hours.
- A patient with significant changes in treatment or medication orders more than four times a day.
- An uncomplicated patient with IV medications every four hours and/or hyperalimentation.
- A patient on complete bed rest.

IV. (200%) A PATIENT WHO REQUIRES MAXIMUM NURSING CARE (An average of 8.6 nursing hours per 24 hours)

This classification is most often used in intensive care areas.

Examples
- A patient who exhibits extreme symptoms (usually termed acutely ill).
- A patient whose activity must be rigidly controlled.
- A patient who requires continuous treatment and/or observations and/or instructions.
- A patient with significant changes in doctor's orders, more than six times a day.
- A patient with many medications, IV piggybacks, and vital signs every hour and/or hourly output.

The total amount of time required to care for each patient determines his classification.

From Rowland, H.S., & Rowland, B.L. Nursing administration handbook (2nd ed.). Rockville, Md.: Aspen, 1985, p. 153.

computer programs available. Marriner believes centralized staffing provides advantages in that it is consistent, objective, and applies the standards and policies impartially.[81] A disadvantage is that a computer expert is usually necessary to interface or communicate between the computer and the administrators and managers. Nevertheless, the head nurse or nurse-manager, are relieved of long hours of calculating and dealing with the data. It is still necessary, however, to gather and provide the correct information to the computer. When staffing is decentralized, the head nurse or nurse-manager is directly responsible for all decisions involving forecasting. While critics of computerized and centralized systems complain about the lack of accuracy and effectiveness of the system, the same can be true for the decentralized method. Some nursing staff acquire or demand individual and special requests that violate policies and can be disruptive to nursing staff morale and relationships. It is easier to deal with only one small unit rather than an entire agency, but it still requires long hours of work, often on off-duty time.

Basically, the process just described is the way to forecast the patient census and the number of nursing staff hours needed to provide resources for the level or quality of care stated in the agency's goal or mission statement. You now have the fundamental information to begin building the unit budget.

Budgeting

The third element of assessing staffing needs is budgeting, or developing an estimate of the costs for operating the nursing unit for a specified period. Usually a unit budget is prepared for a year in advance, but monthly and quarterly reports are usually provided for analysis so there is opportunity to make necessary adjustments.

Operating budgets are usually developed for one *fiscal* year, with monthly and quarterly reports to all managers. By reviewing the budgets each month, you, as the manager, are able to plot trends and make adjustments if the budget varies more than the established variance norm. The difference between the budgeted funds and the actual expenditures is the *variance*. Using this flexible budget approach, many institutional business managers or controllers establish the *variance norm,* which may mean an 8 to 10 percent variance in expenditures from the budgeted amount is acceptable; variances beyond 10 percent are examined very closely. As manager, you decide either to make an intervention or to allow the variance to continue as a *managerial exception.*[82] A closely monitored budget tends to reduce the incidence of brush-fire or reactive management; putting out "fires" of unexpected events tends to consume an inordinate amount of managerial time better spent in planning.[83]

The following principle can be derived from the above discussion:

If you monitor the budget on a monthly basis by analyzing the percentage of variance versus the variance norm and make appropriate and timely interventions, then there is a high probability you will be successful in maintaining the budget in the acceptable range if not above the break-even point, assuming you have established unit goals that are congruent with institutional goals and have followed your plans to meet these goals.

Some agencies use a *continuous budget*: this means a 12-month budget is always in place, dropping last month's and adding a new 12th month as each month passes.[84] Often this budget is reviewed annually, requiring additions to be justified. Other health agencies may however use a *zero-base* budget.[85] This means that each fiscal year, you, as the nurse-manager, would have to justify (present arguments and data to support) each line item on the unit budget. According to Sullivan and Decker, this means some basic questions are asked: "Why does this activity or department exist?" and "What should the objectives be?"[86] This means you as the manager must be prepared to justify each line item on your budget.

While you will need to become familiar with a specific form, a few aspects can be identified that can be expected to appear on most agency reports or computer printouts of monthly, quarterly, or annual budgets. Figure 11–6 is an example of a monthly budget report form. One budget category is allocated one line, and is generally referred to as a *line item.* There are usually some unwritten rules in working with budgets, which will need to be determined. For example, moving funds from one line to another, that is, from one category to another, is usually not allowed without special authorization from the controller or administrator. This is particularly true in regard to funds allocated for "salaries" being moved to "travel" or "repairs and maintenance." Another example is that funds must be spent within the period of time indicated on the budget. If you neglect having repairs made or purchasing equipment by the end of the fiscal year,

Item	Expenditure	Budget	Variance
Variable Costs			
Salaries			
Head Nurse			
RN			
LPN			
Aides			
Orderlies			
Unit secretary			
Total Wages			
F.I.C.A.			
Benefits			
Health insurance			
Life insurance			
Pension and retirement			
Workmen's compensation			
Sick Leave			
Overtime (time and half)			
Staff Development			
Travel			
Dues			
Subscriptions			
Workshops			
Books			
Unit Supplies			
Pharmacy			
Central supply			
Office supplies			
Instruments & equipment			
Repairs & maintenance			
Depreciation on equipment			
Rental, equipment			
Subtotal			
Fixed Costs			
Overhead			
Utilities			
Telephone			
Other			
Subtotal			
Total Expenses			

Figure 11–6. An example of a nursing unit monthly budget report form. *(Reproduced with permission from Douglas, L.M. The effective nurse: Leader and manager [2nd ed.]. St. Louis: The C.V. Mosby Co., p. 192.)*

the funds remaining in that line item will revert to the health agency's central budget; you will lose the funds for that year. If this occurs too often, the agency's business manager or controller will probably tend to question your credibility as you attempt to justify new expenditures in the future. You will soon find yourself being more attentive to your nursing unit budget than you are to balancing your personal checking account.

The degree to which you will be expected to participate in the budgetary process will depend to a great extent upon the organizational structure and leadership style. In some agencies having the participatory management style, everyone in the agency is expected to have input to the development of the budget. In the organizations having centralized management with authoritarian management styles, however, the final budget is often distributed to the vice-presidents by the administrator with the expectation that everyone will function within it; input is not expected or sought.

In either case, it is important to you for your development as a manager and leader to seek some information about budgetary matters. Often there is a time frame or schedule for budget development, such as the one shown in Figure 11–7. If you are to have input into the budgetary process, whether expected or not, you need to know the time frames and deadlines for the

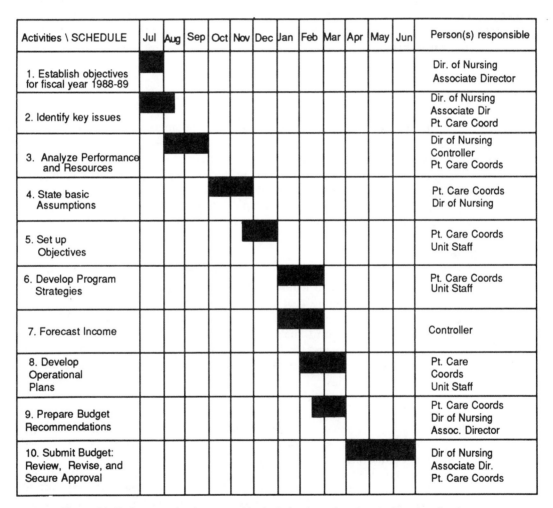

Figure 11–7. An example of an annual budget plan for a department of nursing, fiscal year July 1, 1988 to July 30, 1989. This monthly plan indicates which budget development activities are to be completed and by whom. *(Adapted from Ganong, J., & Ganong, W. Annual budget plan for nursing administration.* Journal of Nursing Administration, *1973, 3 (3), 6.)*

various stages of budget development so that you can develop your suggestions and plan to present them to the appropriate person at the right time and place.[87] As a general principle, we suggest the following:

> *If you need to obtain funding for implementing your plans within the next fiscal year, then you will need to develop and submit an itemized budget and a rationale justifying the request according to the organizational budgeting process time schedule, assuming your plans are congruent with management's fiscal year goals.*

At this point, assume that you have adequately assessed the staffing needs for the unit by (1) identifying the assignment control system that will provide the quality of nursing care desired, (2) forecasting the patient care needs and the number of nursing staff necessary to meet these needs, and (3) budgeting sufficient funds to cover anticipated costs. The next step is selecting the nurses to deliver the nursing care.

SELECTING

The second element in staffing is selecting nursing staff members or personnel. This can be viewed as a process involving four elements: describing, recruiting, screening, and orienting. *Describing* refers to a written definition of a job in order to communicate its classification, role, and functions. *Recruiting* is actively seeking nurses to fill vacant positions in a health agency. *Screening* refers to the process of reviewing credentials, interviewing candidates, and selecting specific individuals who apply for vacant positions. *Orienting* refers to the process of familiarizing new nursing staff members to the specific job as well as the entire agency.

Describing

The written description of a job is designed to communicate to a variety of groups, and for this reason, is an important document. It needs to provide complete information about what each person does according to each position or group of positions identified on the organizational chart of the health agency. (See Chapter 10 for diagrams of organizational charts.) Job descriptions are usually based on a careful analysis of two aspects: the tasks, responsibility, and authority associated with the job, and the knowledge, skills, and attitudes of the person filling the position. These aspects are closely associated with the range of salary and benefits allocated for each position. (See Figs. 11–8 and 11–9 for examples of job descriptions.) Gillies states:

> In analyzing any job it is customary to study the following aspects: procedures to be executed, equipment to be used, subject matter to be dealt with, problems to be handled, scope and responsibility associated with the job, amount of discretion allowed in making decisions, standards of job performance, magnitude of workload, number and type of supervisory and reporting relationships, length of training period required, working conditions and hazards, and promotional opportunities associated with successful job performances.[88]

One job description is necessary for each job classification or level within the organizational structure and may include one, several, or a large number of positions. For example, there is usually one job description for "staff nurse," which applies to all first-level staff nursing

POSITION DESCRIPTION	POSITION TITLE Staff Nurse	CLASSIFICATION 1
HOSPITAL	DEPARTMENT Nursing Service-Medical and Surgical	PAGE 1 of 1
IMMEDIATE SUPERVISOR Head Nurse		

JOB SUMMARY

Under the supervision of the head nurse, give medications, treatments and routine care to patients. Assist doctors, maintain records, and assist in maintaining sterile and other supplies.

SPECIFIC DUTIES

As assigned, give hypos, check doctors' orders for preoperative patients admitted during night, check visible record card or order sheet for each patient, and prepare schedule for and administer hypos to assigned group of patients. If assigned to give medications, set up medication schedule using schedule cards and make new schedule cards for orders given during shift. Administer medications and make all necessary entries on patients' charts.

Give routine care to assigned patients, including taking temperatures, giving baths and making beds. Serve meals to patients after verifying name and type of diet to be provided on each tray. Feed patients when necessary. Collect used trays and stack on tray cart. Note quantities eaten and record on chart if necessary.

Accompany doctors on visits to patients when requested and assist in changing dressings, administering treatments, and other procedures ordered by doctors.

As assigned by head nurse, perform any of the following duties: preparing list of drug charges, charge slips and requisitions; posting new orders on patients' visible file cards; cleaning utility rooms and equipment; operating autoclave to replenish sterile supplies and stock dressing cart; checking narcotic supplies and register; and performing other duties related to the operation of the unit. May be assigned to substitute for head nurse in her absence.

QUALIFICATION REQUIREMENTS

Education

High school graduation, plus graduation from approved school of nursing and R.N. licensure.

Experience

None beyond that required as student nurse.

Physical Requirements

Job requires considerable walking. Some lifting required in moving patients.

Figure 11–8. Example of a job description for a staff nurse position. *(Reprinted with permission from Steinle, J.G.* Hospital cost management. *Englewood Cliffs, N. J.: Prentice-Hall, 1982, p. 4325.)*

positions throughout the agency, regardless of clinical speciality or service. In contrast, there may be only one position having the job description for "medical-surgical nursing area coordinator." Clearly stated and thoughtfully designed job descriptions are helpful in preventing unnecessary frustration and conflict among personnel; careful analysis can eliminate overlapping, that is, the same tasks' being assigned to two or more job descriptions.[89]

Traditionally, overlapping has been a common problem in nursing because of the overlap-

POSITION DESCRIPTION	POSITION TITLE Operating Room Supervisor	CLASSIFICATION 11
HOSPITAL	DEPARTMENT Nursing Service—Operating Room	PAGE 1 of 1

IMMEDIATE SUPERVISOR

Director of Nursing Service

JOB SUMMARY

Under general direction, schedule use of operating rooms, prepare work and on-call schedules for operating room personnel, make daily work assignments, supervise and instruct operating room personnel, train new personnel, and supervise the maintenance of adequate stocks of sterile and nonsterile supplies, instruments, and equipment.

SPECIFIC DUTIES

Schedule operations in one minor and two major operating rooms at request of doctors. Estimate time required for operation specified and reach agreement with doctor on time allotted. Arrange for services of nurse anesthetist upon request.

Prepare work, time off, and on-call schedules for operating room personnel. Assign subordinate nurses to specific jobs for each case. Observe work of nurses while surgery is in progress and give instructions and assistance as necessary. Serve as circulating nurse.

Assume responsibility for the maintenance of adequate supplies of sterile and nonsterile supplies and instruments. See that setups for scheduled operations are completely and promptly made and are protected from contamination. Supervise clean-up and sterilization processes to see that procedures and standards are observed. Prepare daily drug orders and prepare supply orders twice weekly. Confer with administrator on purchases of operating room supplies.

Prepare or check charge slips prepared for operating room, anesthesia, laboratory work, and other charges and submit to business office.

Train new personnel in preferences of doctors and in procedures. Conduct periodic meetings of staff to demonstrate new equipment or procedures and to maintain awareness of standards.

QUALIFICATION REQUIREMENTS

Education

Graduation from approved school of nursing. BSN required; MSN preferred. R.N. licensure.

Experience

Three years' experience as an operating room staff nurse.

Physical Requirements

Work involves almost constant walking and prolonged standing. Much of work is done in overheated areas. Some personal hazard from explosion.

Figure 11–9. Example of a job description for an operating room supervisor position. *(Reprinted with permission from Steinle, J.G. Hospital cost management. Englewood Cliffs, N. J.: Prentice-Hall, 1982, p. 4326.)*

ping of functions within the education and licensure of the RN and the LPN. To a large degree, these are problems of role definition, competencies, licensure, and credentials yet to be resolved within the profession of nursing. To a degree, however, one nursing unit within an agency can develop sufficient distinctions in nursing job descriptions so that overlapping is minimized, respecting the integrity and dignity of each nursing staff member.

It is also helpful to look at job descriptions from the perspective of Mead's role theory.[90] In actual practice, roles are perceived from a number of perspectives, such as that of the patient, other nurses, nursing leaders, physicians, and society in general. Each of these has expectations of the person functioning in the role of a nurse. The job descriptions primarily provide the perspective and expectations of the organization in which the nurse functions. In a sense, a person who takes on the role of the nurse plays multiple roles in meeting the needs and expectations of others and of the organization.

According to Mead, a symbolic interactionist theorist, the meaningfulness—significance, purpose, or importance—of roles is found in the communication and interaction between the individual or *self* and the *significant other*. *Role ambiguity* develops when role expectations are communicated vaguely and are poorly defined; the person does not have a clear idea of how to behave. *Role strain* occurs when expectations of colleagues and of the organization are incongruent, resulting in internal feelings of distress arising from receiving the mixed and conflicting messages about role expectations. *Role stress* occurs when it is difficult or impossible to meet role demands and expectations.[91] The job may require too much to accomplish in the time allotted, so that the nurse is continually working overtime to catch up, such as charting after reporting off. It is also important to clarify the roles of leaders and followers.[92] There are numerous statements describing nursing characteristics and the roles that nurses are prepared to assume, statements such as those provided by the National League for Nursing.[93,94] Such statements provide excellent guidelines in writing, revising, or interpreting job descriptions. When you participate in job analysis, evaluation, orientation, and development of members of your nursing staff, it may be helpful to study the individual nurse's situation from the perspective provided by role theory. In writing job descriptions, you need to consider the potential for role ambiguity, role strain, and role stress so that the job you design is for *success*. A major function of the job description is *role clarification*.

A job description speaks to a variety of people and is useful in several ways. It provides a written record of what tasks, roles, and functions a nurse is to perform when filling a particular position. The nurse can refer to it for specific guidance. The nurse-manager or leader who supervises the nursing staff's activities often refers to it for recruitment, orientation, evaluation, and promotion purposes. The agency controller or business manager refers to the job description when administering salary policies and procedures, and the agency personnel manager and staff refer to it in administering personnel policies.

Because of the process of change, planned and unplanned, every few years the vice-president for nursing needs to assign a committee to analyze all job descriptions and make recommendations for needed adjustments and updating. Aside from accreditation criteria expectations, job descriptions need to be current, accurate, and realistic in terms of agency resources and of the way nurses experience being in the job.[95]

Recruiting

Although recruiting new nurses may be primarily delegated to a nurse-recruiter, it truly is the responsibility of all nursing leaders and managers to restore and maintain their nursing staff so that there are sufficient numbers of qualified nurses to provide the quality and quantity of nursing care desired. The agency nursing budget usually needs to have a line item allocated specifically for recruitment, a variable cost. As a nursing leader, you may participate in a task force or committee to develop long-term strategies for recruitment, as suggested by several authors.[96-98] Or you may be involved simply by talking to individuals you know, suggesting they submit a résumé and application. Your primary role, however, is to develop a positive interpersonal and working climate among your current nursing staff so that they are satisfied with their job and speak well of you, their administrators, and the agency.[99] Whatever your degree of involvement in recruitment, it is a continuous concern in agencies having high turnover rates or areas experiencing a shortage of nurses.

In the health professions generally and nursing in particular, there has been a history of unequal distribution in relation to population and needs for health services. Hospitals and health care agencies located near medical centers and schools of nursing, usually in metropolitan areas, tend to have a continuous source of potential nursing staff. The primary problem is not a source of supply, but that of marketing with a theme that will attract and retain nursing staff. In contrast, small hospitals, without a nurse-recruiter and located in more remote areas, may have a stable core of nursing staff members, but must recruit replacement staff and nursing leaders from outside the area.

The guidelines of affirmative action must be followed so that recruitment and hiring practices will be nondiscriminatory. A sufficient number of applicants will need to be recruited in order to develop the required pool of qualified applicants. All applicants are to be treated equally, and the same standards used to evaluate each. All recruitment materials need to carry the agency's equal-opportunity, nondiscriminatory statement.

There are certain decisions that need to be made in the process of developing a plan of recruitment. In view of the job description and qualifications, it may be appropriate to recruit from within the agency, or necessary to recruit from outside at the local, regional, state, or national level. Generally, it is preferable to recruit from within; this tends to build cohesiveness and commitment among staff members and supports career ladder policies. Many, however, favor recruiting outside the agency for top leadership positions; sometimes a talented person is least appreciated by people in his or her own home town.

There are hospitals that are unusually unsuccessful in attracting qualified nursing staff. To solve this problem, some agencies collaborate to recruit nurses from other nations, but at considerable effort and expense. This is not a viable, long-term solution, since most nurses go home after a year or two.* A similar result tends to occur when a hospital offers a bounty of from $200 to $1000 to its own nurses for each new nurse recruited, if the recruited nurse stays for at least a year. In addition, when the bounty program is withdrawn, the nurses tend to stop all recruiting efforts, which is detrimental in terms of long-term staffing. In many such incidents, administrators have ignored nurses' low job satisfaction, attributing their high annual turnover rates to nurses' being young and unsettled, marriage, children, the economy, and so on. Fortunately, administrators are beginning to collect data about nurses' job satisfaction and morale. If an agency's administrators attempt to solve these problems and concern themselves with retention of nursing staff, then turnover rates tend to decrease.[100]

It is important to know your own staff and agency. The nurse-recruiter or person(s) responsible often develops a staff profile. This consists of the number of nurses on staff, their

---

*This statement is based on one of the author's direct experiences. These nurses have had difficulties with passing state nurse licensure examinations, using the English language and medical and nursing terminology, and adjusting to the contemporary high technology of nursing.

ages, and the nursing schools from which the staff graduated. Also included might be the number of nursing staff attending local colleges, average length of employment, annual turnover rate, and areas of specialization or certification.[101] In developing your presentation to prospects, you need to know the salary scales, clinical specialties, and areas in which positions are available, staffing hours, health and retirement plans, as well as other benefits.[102]

There are numerous ways to contact nurses for recruitment purposes. Placing advertisements in newspapers, nursing journals, and on television are rather typical approaches. Some agencies hold "career day" events at which nursing staff from each unit in the agency set up a recruitment booth so that invited guests, new graduates, inactive nurses, and others might have an opportunity to speak directly with the staff. One agency invites the senior nursing students from each nursing school in the area to dinner at the local country club, where members of the nursing department make presentations, answer questions, and provide brochures. The most successful recruitment seems to be through personal contacts and seeking nurses who live locally. Head nurses and their staff have direct contact with nursing students while they are still in the nursing program; being supportive and helpful while the student is in the process of becoming a nurse is particularly successful.

From previous discussions, we believe the following principles can be stated:

As the number of nurses available exceeds the demand for additional nursing staff, the recruitment of nurses tends to become more selective, and recruitment efforts tend to be reduced.

If certain aspects of a competing institution tend to be more attractive than the same aspects of your agency, then you need to identify and emphasize some other aspects of your agency that may be even more attractive to prospective recruits, while avoiding commenting in a negative manner about the competing institution.

If you are truthful in describing the agency you are representing, then the nurses you recruit will tend to have a realistic expectation of job requirements, and they will tend to experience job satisfaction with minimal turnover.[103] Nurses recruited through informal, personalized contacts tend to remain with an agency longer than those recruited by formal, impersonal contacts.[104]

Generally, we advocate an individualized, humanistic approach to recruitment programs.

Once a pool of qualified applicants are recruited for the vacant positions on your nursing staff, you will need to screen each applicant, the next step in selecting nursing staff.

Screening

Once you have a pool of applicants, the screening process begins. All of the information needs to be reviewed carefully. Your objective is to select the applicant who has the highest probability of being successful in the position to be filled. Errors in judgment at this point can be expensive, not only in terms of your budget, time, and efforts to meet your unit's staffing needs, but also in terms of the applicant's career development, time, and perhaps preventable distress if unsuccessful. It is crucial for you to select the appropriate person for the job.

Of all the information gathered about each applicant, certain *predictor* data are often selected as being particularly relevant to successfully matching the person and position. As manager, you will probably have access to applications, letters of reference, transcripts of academic records, personal information, Social Security numbers, and health records. In some agencies, personality or interest tests are required. For nurses, a copy of the Registered Nurse or Licensed Practical Nurse license is expected, too; this needs to be verified by contacting the state board of nursing. You probably will have more information than you need. If the job description is based on adequate job analysis, you probably will be able to describe key task skills and personal characteristics required for the position. For example, you would expect nurses to be trustworthy, dependable, interested in clients, and capable; traits such as these might serve as guides in reviewing the applicants' files.

Validity of predictor data satisfies legal requirements. One validation practice is for two or three nurse-managers to interview applicants and provide written documentation of their impressions; they validate one another's impressions. Screening, selecting, and hiring practices, as well as employee selection processes for training programs, performance appraisal results, termination, benefits, and so on, must be conducted in a nondiscriminatory manner. Documentation of the screening and selection process is required since the enactment of Title VII of the Civil Rights Act of 1964, the Equal Pay Act of 1963, and the Age Discrimination Act of 1967. The Equal Employment Opportunity Commission (EEOC) is charged with enforcing and interpreting the Civil Rights Act.[105] This commission has provided Uniform Guidelines on Employee Selection Procedures, which state specific methods for validating predictors. This means you can expect to receive information and direction from the agency's personnel director, who is primarily responsible for assuring all personnel selection processes in the agency adhere to these guidelines.[106]

These federal laws prohibit employment decisions based on sex, race, color, religion, national origin, and handicap. This means questions that might be posed to one sex and not the other must be avoided. For example, questions about marital status and children are considered discriminatory, since they are usually asked of women and not of men. Asking a man how he feels about having a woman as a supervisor or asking an older person about having a younger supervisor is also discriminatory. The handicapped are to be judged only on their ability to perform, and non-task-relevant questions are illegal. Questions about arrests are discriminatory, but it is all right to ask about convictions; convictions are matters of public record.[107]

If these federal laws are not followed, you and your institution can suffer consequences.

> An institution can face serious penalties for violations of civil rights laws. Fines may be assessed against the employer. If the organization receives federal funds, those funds may be cut off or, more seriously, a federal contractor may be debarred, preventing it from applying for future federal contracts as well. Institutions which are successfully sued by individuals or classes of individuals claiming their civil rights have been violated face substantial costs to cover back pay, lost benefits, attorney's fees, and punitive damages. In addition to institutional cost liabilities, responsible individuals may be fined, found criminally responsible, or held liable. . . . The costs of litigation and legal assistance for civil rights violations are often expenses that can be avoided by the use of adequate procedures or receipt of competent advice before a complaint is filed. Civil rights disputes also tend to be time consuming. Many violations have occurred because organizations failed to spend a few hours to learn compliance requirements, only to spend hundreds of person hours over 2 to 3 years in resolving a complaint.[108]

As the manager, you need to rely on the agency's personnel director and legal counselor for specific interpretation of these laws for the selecting task in which you participate.

A review of the application and letters of reference may eliminate a number of applicants. Incomplete applications are usually disregarded. Letters of reference from previous employers occasionally are not available because the former supervisor or teacher cannot be located;

keeping records in a placement center can simplify obtaining reference letters. It is important to contact former employers or supervisors by phone to ask some specific questions. For example, a number of inferences can be made based on responses to questions about the applicant's duty attendance record, health status, and record of transfers within the agency.

Applicants' files are reviewed only after the advertised date for the search to end. All documents are assembled. Incomplete files are eliminated from consideration prior to interviewing. The purpose of the job interview is to gather more information from the applicant and to amplify and clarify the job description. The applicant needs to know what is expected of a person filling this position. Any questions the applicant may have are answered. There are certain questions that cannot be asked an applicant if one is to avoid discrimination. See Table 11-4 for examples of both lawful and unlawful questions. Conducting this kind of interview has been developed to an art and a science by some authors, and, for further information, we suggest some references the reader may find helpful.[109-112]

It is important that the interviewing process be standardized; all interviewers consistently need to follow a similar interview schedule or outline for all applicants. (See Fig. 11-10 for a sample interview schedule.) Unstructured interviews often fail to produce consistent, comparable information when interviewers do not ask the same questions.[113] Either all or none of the applicants need to be interviewed; to interview some and not others could be interpreted as discrimination. If there are a large number of applicants, however, criteria can be developed to use in selecting a limited number for interviewing. Interviewing is expensive. It takes at least an hour per interview for preparing, conducting, and documenting. If there are 15 applicants to interview by 3 nurse-managers for an hour each (15 applicants × 3 interviewers × 1 hour), this would take a total of 45 hours of nurse management time. Interviewing selectively is a cost-effective practice.

After all of the information has been assembled, Gillies suggests it is helpful to develop a chart summarizing the predictor data in tabular form. (See Table 11-5 for a sample chart.) You can more easily make comparisons and identify strengths quickly. Gillies states that there is less chance of important details being overlooked in the comparison process.[114] The person most qualified for the position can be selected from the pool of applicants.

Finally, Ganong and Ganong state that an evaluation of the total recruitment and screening effort provides information helpful in your future planning. You need to note the time spent in recruiting, the expenses incurred, and the methods of recruiting used. Then note the number of applications received, the number of offers you made, and how many applicants accepted or rejected the position. Notice how many nurses were hired, and keep a record of their progress during their period of employment. When these nurses leave, record the length of service.[115] Information gathered during exit interviews (interviews conducted when an employee leaves the agency) needs to be considered along with all your notations. By studying these things, you may come to some conclusions about, for example, which recruitment method produced the most applicants, which can be helpful as you revise and improve recruitment plans.

Once the applicants have been selected to fill vacant positions, the next step in the process of staffing is the orientation of new staff members.

Orienting

The process of orienting new employees is defined by Gillies as:

> An individualized training program intended to acquaint a newly hired employee with job responsibilities, workplace, clients, and coworkers, so as to enable her to relate effectively to her surroundings and identify her niche in the organization.[116]

TABLE 11–4. GUIDELINES FOR LAWFUL AND UNLAWFUL QUESTIONS POSED TO APPLICANTS IN PREEMPLOYMENT INTERVIEWING.

Subject	Lawful Pre-Employment Inquiries	Potentially Unlawful Pre-Employment Inquiries, Statements, Requirements
Name	What is your full name? Have you ever worked for this company under a different name? Is any additional information relative to a different name necessary to check your work record? If yes, explain.	Has your original name been changed by court order or otherwise? What is your maiden name?
Address or duration of residence	How long have you been a resident of this state or city?	Do you own a home?
Birthplace		What is your birthplace? What is the birthplace of your parents, spouse, or other close relatives? Requirement that applicant submit birth certificate, naturalization, or baptismal record.
Age	Are you 18 years old or older?*	How old are you? What is your date of birth?†
Religion or creed		Inquiry into an applicant's religious denomination, religious affiliations, church, parish, pastor, or religious holidays observed. An applicant may not be told. "This is a Catholic, (Protestant or Jewish) organization."
Race or color	Indicate race and/or ethnic group‡	
Photograph		Requirement that an applicant for employment affix a photograph to an employment application form. Request that an applicant submit a photograph, at his or her option. Requirement for photograph after interview but before hiring.
Height		Inquiry regarding applicant's height.
Weight		Inquiry regarding applicant's weight.
Marital status		Requirement that an applicant provide any information regarding marital status or children. Are you single or married? Do you have any children? What are the ages of your children? Is your spouse employed? Spouse's occupation? What is your spouse's name?
Sex		Mr., Miss, or Mrs., or an inquiry regarding sex. Inquiry as to the ability to reproduce or advocacy of any form of birth control.
Health	Do you have any impairments, physical, mental, or medical, which would interfere with your ability to do the job for which you have applied? Inquiry into contagious or communicable diseases that may endanger others. If there are any positions for which you should not be considered or job duties you cannot perform because of a physical or mental handicap, please explain.	Do you have a disability or handicap? Have you ever been treated for the following diseases? Do you use any adaptive device or aid? Requirement that women be given pelvic examinations.

TABLE 11–4. (Continued)

Subject	Lawful Pre-Employment Inquiries	Potentially Unlawful Pre-Employment Inquiries, Statements, Requirements
Citizenship	Are you a citizen of the United States? If not a citizen of the United States, do you intend to become a citizen of the United States? If you are not a United States citizen, have you the legal right to remain permanently and to work in the United States? Do you intend to remain permanently in the United States?	Of what country are you a citizen? Are you a naturalized or a native-born citizen? Can you produce naturalization papers or first papers? Are your parents or spouse naturalized or native-born citizens of the United States; when did your parents or spouse acquire citizenship?
National origin	What languages do you speak and write fluently?	Inquiry into applicant's (a) lineage; (b) ancestry; (c) national origin; (d) descent; (e) parentage, or nationality. What is the nationality of your parents or spouse? What is your mother tongue? How did you acquire the ability to read, write, or speak a foreign language?
Education	Describe your academic, vocational, or professional education. What public and private schools did you attend?	What is the religious affiliation of the education institutions you attended?
Experience	Describe your work experience. What countries have you visited?	
Arrests	Have you ever been convicted of a crime? If so, when, where, and nature of offense? Are there any felony charges pending against you?	Have you ever been arrested?§
Relatives	Are any of your relatives already employed by this company? Their names?	
Notice in case of emergency	What is the name and address of *person* to be notified in case of accident or emergency?	What is the name and address of the *nearest relative* to be notified in case of accident or emergency?
Military	Inquiry into an applicant's service in particular branch of United States Army, Navy, etc. Inquiry into applicant's military experience in the Armed Forces of the United States or in a State Militia.	Inquiry into an applicant's general military experience in other countries.
Organizations	Inquiry into the organizations of which an applicant is a member excluding organizations, the name or character of which indicates the race, color, religion, national origin, or ancestry of its members.	List all clubs, societies, and lodges to which you belong.
References	Who suggested that you apply for a position here?	

From Poteet, G.W. The employment interview: Avoiding discriminatory questioning. The Journal of Nursing Administration, *1984, 14 (4), 40. This table first appeared in "Nurse staffing after hospitals merge," by Elsie A. Schmid, in* Nursing Administration Quarterly, *2(1) 75, fall 1977. Reprinted with permission of Aspen Publishers, Inc., 1984.*

*This question may be asked only for the purpose of determining whether applicants are of legal age of employment.

†Unlawful unless accompanied by statement such as federal and state laws that prohibit discrimination because of age, then OK to ask.

‡Lawful inquiries if used only for statistical reporting.

§Generally illegal unless it can be justified by business necessity.

Source: Developed by G. Poteet using Federal Register. Uniform Guideline on Employee Selection Procedures *43(166) 1978.*

1. Nursing license number _____
   (Applicant's license must be seen by interviewer)
   Copies of reference letters attached
2. How did the applicant learn of the position? _____
3. Reason for applicant's interest in the position _____
4. Basic nursing education
   Name and location of school _____
   Type of program _____
             diploma   associate   baccalaureate
   Year of graduation _____
5. Education following graduation from basic nursing program _____
   School(s) _____
   Certificate(s) or degree(s) _____
   Date(s) of completion _____
6. Employment history, proceeding in chronological order backward from present date (include part time employment).

Dates From-To	Institution	Job Title	Duties and Responsibilities

7. Professional organization membership _____
8. Continuing education courses completed during the past year _____
9. Current enrollment in college courses _____
10. Publications _____
11. Research _____
12. Short-range career goals _____
13. Long-range career goal _____
14. Which shifts applicant is available to work: 7–3   3–11   11–7
15. Date applicant would be available to start work _____
16. Job posting or advertisement reviewed with applicant
17. Description given of   nursing department   division   unit
18. Job description discussed with applicant   yes   no
19. Performance standards reviewed with applicant   yes   no
20. Information given regarding:
    work schedules   shift rotations
    tour hours   vacation schedules
    weekends off   holiday schedules
21. Discussion of personnel benefits:
    salary range for position   tuition reimbursement
    paid holidays   uniform laundry
    paid vacation   pension fund
    paid convention days   continuing education
    health insurance   orientation
    life insurance
22. Further steps to be taken by candidate in making application for employment

Figure 11–10. An example of a standard preemployment interview outline. *(From Gillies, D.A. Nursing management: A systems approach. Philadelphia: Saunders, 1982, p. 201, with permission.)*

TABLE 11–5. AN EXAMPLE OF A SUMMARY OF PREDICTOR DATA FOR FIVE APPLICANTS FOR THE POSITION OF RECOVERY ROOM SUPERVISOR. MS. B. WAS SELECTED FOR THE POSITION.

Applicant	Undergraduate Education	Graduate Nursing Experience	Surgical Nursing Experience	Recovery Room Experience	Credits or Degrees Since Graduation	Relevant Continuing Education Courses Completed in Past Two Years
Ms. A	BSN	11 years	9 years	8 years	0	0
Ms. B	Diploma	10 years	8 years	8 years	BSN, MA in psychology	6 weeks, critical care nursing
Ms. C	BSN	9 years	5 years	1 year	MBA	0
Ms. D	ADN	6 years	6 years	0	BSN	0
Ms. E	Diploma	13 years	7 years	6 years	0	6 months, family nurse practitioner

From Gillies, D.A. Nursing management: A systems approach. *Philadelphia: Saunders, 1982, p. 202.*

Objectives of an orientation program include enabling the new employee to become adjusted to the new environment so that he or she becomes productive as quickly as possible and fostering the belief that he or she is a welcome and needed addition to the nursing staff of the unit you supervise.

Contemporary orientation programs are based on principles of adult education. Knowles states that an adult's survival, personal growth and development, and basic competences depend upon the ability to learn without instruction.[117] The adult learner is characterized by the ability to diagnose his or her own learning needs and identify subject matter that is particularly relevant to his or her own needs and expectations. Thus an effective orientation program for the nurse who joins your staff needs to include opportunities for the nurse to identify personal needs and to participate in the development of an individualized orientation program. As a general principle:

To the same degree that the new nursing staff member has opportunity to identify his or her own learning needs and participate in the development of an individualized orientation program, the new member will tend to learn quickly with minimal dependency upon the nurse-leader and the other nursing staff members.

As the nurse-leader, it becomes your responsibility to establish between the new nurse, you, and your current nursing staff an interpersonal climate that is conducive to learning. While there are many descriptions of a climate or environment conducive to learning, we believe the humanistic attitudes identified in Duldt's Humanistic Nursing Communication theory are appropriately applied here. (See Chapter 2.) In addition, the developmental cycle of Situational Leadership is also appropriately applicable to the process of orienting a new nursing staff member. (See Chapter 1.)

Essentially, there are three aspects of the orientation program. The first aspect consists of the standard centralized orientation program and process for all new employees of the agency, usually established and conducted by the personnel department staff. The second aspect consists of developing an individualized orientation to the specific role and functions of the position as expected of a new nursing staff member. The third aspect (perhaps it really should be first) involves the preparation of present nursing staff members so that they will favorably anticipate the new colleague and greet him or her warmly.

Centralized Orientation Program

This program is based on the assumption that the individuals know nothing about the agency, and a "telling" leadership style is used. It is required of all new employees of all disciplines and administrative units within the agency. Content often includes a tour of common facilities, such as the administrative offices, dining facilities, library, and chapel. Policies, procedures, rules, and regulations required of all employees are also included, such as duty hours, identification badges, parking, educational programs, health and insurance benefits, grievance processes, and pay checks. Typically new employees experience information overload and cannot be expected to remember everything presented in one or two days. Each employee usually receives an employee handbook that documents all of this and additional information as well. As a rule, a presentation is made about the history of the institution, its customs, significant events, accomplishments, and goals.

Individualized Orientation Program

After the centralized program is completed, the individualized orientation program for your new nurse becomes your responsibility as immediate supervisor. If there are a large number of new nurses joining the agency, some of this orientation may be coordinated by the director of nursing in-service education and that director's teaching staff. This is particularly true when a large group of new graduates join the nursing department staff. To the extent possible, checklists of policies, procedures, and skills may be reviewed by the new nurse to identify those areas of nursing practice that are his or her strengths or weaknesses, and to proceed accordingly. Moving from these self-identified learning needs, the new nurse's orientation plans can be developed.

Other Types of Programs

Orientation programs can take several forms. Some agencies use a buddy system, which involves another relatively new nursing staff member serving as an authorized but informal source of information, advice, and support. Other agencies have a mentor system in which a nurse who has been on the staff for some time serves in a role similar to the buddy, but focuses to a greater extent upon development of the new nurse's capabilities. Both of these systems attempt to meet the new nurse on an individualized and interpersonal level. Internships are sometimes used, not only to orient the new nurse, but also to meet professional needs by providing opportunities to develop specialized skills or to provide the enriching experience of rotating through a variety of nursing service units. The internship programs often provide an educational theme with a strong clinical emphasis by including regularly scheduled classroom lectures and perhaps clinical grand rounds with nurses, physicians, and other health care professionals in the agency. The health care agency does not have to be a large medical center to provide excellent internships; small, private, specialty hospitals, such as the Children's Hospital and St. Jude Hospital in Memphis, Tennessee, do provide unique and specialized programs for their nurses. The orientation period can range from one month or three months to six months. Most internship programs are one year in length. Given the high turnover rate of nursing staff and the increasing shortage of nurses, nursing leaders have experimented extensively with their orientation programs in an attempt to increase staff retention and job satisfaction, while reducing reality shock, burnout, and the incidence of those who are so discouraged that they "just quit and stay," that is, quit trying but stay anyway.

The Preparation of Nursing Staff

Just as parents need to prepare their children for the arrival of a new baby, so you, as the nursing leader, need to prepare your nursing staff for the arrival of a new staff member. Initially, it is helpful to share information with your nursing staff about the vacancy, the advertisements, and the search process. As a general principle, we believe the following statement tends to be true:

> To the same degree the nursing staff has an opportunity to participate in the recruiting, screening, and orientation processes, the nursing staff will tend to develop and maintain a humanizing attitude toward the new staff nurse, assimilating him or her into the group and maintaining an interpersonal climate that facilitates orientation.

We believe the concepts of communication, motivation, initiating, facilitating, and integrating—the five people-oriented functions of the nursing leader—are to be carefully considered and applied to the new nurse joining the staff. For example, watch for Gibb's defensive behaviors and act quickly to intervene and change the communication mode to supportive behaviors.[118] (See also Chapter 4 and Chapter 7.)

With a few exceptions—such as enlisting in the armed services, for example—the new nurse is *voluntarily* joining the nursing staff group. Research has shown that as long as an individual's personal goals can be achieved through membership in a particular group, the individual will remain a member of the group.[119] If, however, the cost of this membership is too much in terms of the group's unwarranted controls (expected behaviors and group norms) over the individual's behavior, then the individual may decide a bad bargain has been made.[120] You need to take note of the expected behaviors and group norms as received by your new nurse. Perhaps these need to be changed or eliminated. It is important that you, as the nursing leader, do not hesitate to intervene so that the new nurse, as well as the rest of your nursing staff, will continue to perceive working together as attractive and voluntarily stay a long time.

SUMMARY

In this chapter, staffing has been defined as a plan to determine specifically the number and kind of nursing staff needed to provide nursing care to a target population of patients or clients. Initial aspects of staffing, assessing the staffing needs has been emphasized. Depending upon individual values and beliefs, as well as organizational structure and management behavior, one of the classic assignment control systems is selected to organize the delivery of nursing care; case, functional, team, or primary nursing. The process of forecasting the number and mix of nursing staff needed has been presented, and some basic information about the nursing leader role in budgeting has been provided.

Selecting individuals to serve in the vacant nursing staff positions is the second focus of this chapter. First, describing the job itself is an important task with many practical, communication, and legal aspects to be considered. Recruiting potential candidates to fill the nursing staff positions and screening each individual has been described in considerable detail. Finally, orienting new nursing staff members has been considered from the perspective of the total agency and the individual nursing unit. The preparation of current nurses to appropriately receive the new appointee has also been considered.

This chapter serves as the first half of the total consideration of staffing. The second half is presented in Chapter 12, in which scheduling staff members' duty time and evaluating the total staffing program is considered. Throughout both chapters, we emphasize the role and function of the nursing leader responsible for arranging the staffing program for the nurse staff followers.

REFERENCES

1. Guralnik, D.B. (Ed.). *Webster's New World Dictionary* (2nd ed.). New York: Prentice-Hall, 1980, p. 1384.
2. West, E. M. *Manpower control system for the nursing division.* Unpublished manuscript, Nashville, Tennessee: Hospital Affiliates International, Inc., 1979, pp. 3, 6, 7, 127.
3. Stevens, B.J. *First-line patient care management* (2nd ed.). Rockville, Md.: Aspen, 1983, p. 143.
4. DiVincenti, M. *Administering nursing service* (2nd ed.). Boston: Little, Brown, 1977, p. 125.
5. Ganong, J.M., & Ganong, W.L. *Nursing management* (2nd ed.). Rockville, Md.: Aspen, 1980, p. 231.

6. Marriner, A. *Guide to nursing management* (2nd ed.). St. Louis: Mosby, 1984, p. 117.
7. Ashley, J.A. *Hospitals, paternalism, and the role of the nurse.* New York: Teachers College Press, 1979, p. 43–45, 70–74.
8. Selby, T.L. RN shortage threatens quality of care. *The American Nurse,* 1987, *19* (3), 1,11,14.
9. Langford, T.L. *Managing and being managed: Preparation for professional nursing practice.* Englewood Cliffs, N. J.: Prentice-Hall, 1981, p. 176.
10. Douglass, L.M. *The effective nurse: Leader and manager* (2nd ed.). St. Louis: Mosby, 1984, p. 87.
11. Marriner, *Guide to nursing management,* p. 117.
12. Kron, T. *The management of patient care: Putting leadership skills to work* (5th ed.). Philadelphia: Saunders, 1981, p. 74.
13. Langford, *Managing and being managed,* p. 176.
14. National Commission on Nursing. *Initial report and Preliminary recommendations.* Chicago: The Hospital Research and Educational Trust, 1981, p. 17.
15. Devereaux, P. McN. Essential elements of nurse–physician collaboration. *The Journal of Nursing Administration,* 1981, *11* (5), 20.
16. Gillies, D.A. *Nursing management: A systems approach.* Philadelphia: Saunders, 1982, p. 173.
17. Langford, *Managing and being managed,* p. 176–177.
18. Kron, *The management of patient care,* p. 74.
19. Langford, *Managing and being managed,* p. 177.
20. Yura, H., Ozimek, D., & Walsh, M.B. *Nursing leadership: Theory & process* (2nd ed.). New York: Appleton-Century-Crofts, 1981, p. 9.
21. Douglass, *The effective nurse,* p. 89.
22. Langford, *Managing and being managed,* p. 177.
23. Ibid.
24. Yura, Ozimek, & Walsh, *Nursing leadership: Theory & process,* p. 8–9.
25. Douglass, *The effective nurse,* p. 89–91.
26. Newcomb, D. *The team plan.* New York: Putnam, 1953.
27. Kron, T., & Gray, A. *The management of patient care: Putting leadership skills to work* (6th ed.). Philadelphia: Saunders, 1987.
28. Ibid., 91.
29. Marriner, *Guide to nursing management,* p. 118–119.
30. Yura, Ozimek, & Walsh, *Nursing leadership: Theory & process,* p. 8–9.
31. Marriner, *Guide to nursing management,* p. 118–120.
32. Ibid.
33. Langford, *Managing and being managed,* p. 178–179.
34. Marriner, *Guide to nursing management,* p. 120.
35. Douglass, *The effective nurse,* p. 91.
36. Langford, *Managing and being managed,* p. 179.
37. Douglass, *The effective nurse,* p. 89.
38. Orwell, G. *Animal farm.* New York: Harcourt Brace Jovanovich, 1946.
39. National Commission on Nursing. *Report of the final survey of innovative programs and projects.* Chicago: Hospital Research and Education Trust, 1984.
40. Zander, K.S. *Primary nursing: Development and management.* Germantown, Md.: Aspen, 1980, p. 5.
41. Ibid., p. 282–283.
42. Marriner, *Guide to nursing management,* p. 120–121.
43. Ibid.
44. Ibid.
45. Ibid.
46. Zander, *Primary nursing: Development and management,* p. 22.
47. Ganong & Ganong, *Nursing management,* p. 104.

48. Zander, *Primary nursing: Development and management,* p. 27.
49. Ibid., 23.
50. Ganong & Ganong, *Nursing management,* p. 104.
51. Fagin, C.M. The economic value of nursing research. *American Journal of Nursing,* 1982, *82* (12), p. 1844.
52. Ibid.
53. Porter-O'Grady, T., & Finnigan, S. *Shared governance for nursing: A creative approach to professional accountability.* Rockville, Md.: Aspen, 1984, p. 198.
54. Marriner, *Guide to nursing management,* p. 120–121.
55. Langford, *Managing and being managed,* p. 180.
56. Zander, *Primary nursing: Development and management,* p. 23.
57. Steinle, J.G. *Hospital cost management.* Englewood Cliffs, N. J.: Prentice Hall, 1982, p. 4413.
58. National Commission on Nursing. *Initial report and preliminary recommendations,* p. 20–21.
59. Devereaux, Essential elements of nurse–physician collaboration, p. 20.
60. Gillies, *Nursing management: A system approach,* p. 176; Kron, *The management of patient care,* p. 224.
61. Ganong & Ganong, *Nursing management,* p. 25.
62. Steinle, *Hospital cost management,* p. 4301.
63. American Nurses' Association. *Nursing staff requirements for in-patient health care services.* Kansas City, Mo.: ANA, 1977.
64. Toffler, A. *Future shock.* New York: Random House, 1970, pp. 485–486.
65. Naisbitt, J. *Megatrends: Ten new directions.* New York: Warner Books, 1982.
66. Lewin, K. Frontiers in groups dynamics: Concept, method, and reality in social science: Social equilibria and social change. *Human Relations.* 1947, *I* (1), 5–41.
67. Strasen, L. *Key business skills for nurse managers.* Philadelphia: Lippincott, 1987, p. 27.
68. Ibid., 262.
69. Naisbitt, *Megatrends.*
70. Mitchell, F., Cloner, A., & Coile, R. Multiscenario forecasting and health management in the 1980s. Presented at the Third International Symposium on Forecasting in Philadelphia, June 6, 1983.
71. Ibid.
72. Strasen, *Key business skills for nurse managers,* p. 132.
73. Ibid., 145–146.
74. Sullivan, E.J., & Decker, P.J. *Effective management in nursing.* Menlo Park, Calif.: Addison-Wesley, 1985, p. 367.
75. Ibid.
76. Rowland, H.S., & Rowland, B.L. *Nursing administration handbook.* Rockville, Md.: Aspen, 1985, pp. 150–152.
77. Ibid., 127–165.
78. Langford, *Managing and being managed,* p. 183–187.
79. Marriner, *Guide to nursing management,* p. 130–133.
80. Sullivan & Decker, *Effective management in nursing,* p. 367–376.
81. Marriner, *Guide to nursing management,* p. 123.
82. Sullivan & Decker, *Effective management in nursing,* p. 363.
83. Ibid., 362–363.
84. Ibid., 366.
85. Anderson, D.N. Zero-based budgeting: How to get rid of corporate crabgrass. In Berger, M.S., et al. (Eds.). *Management for nurses: A multidisciplinary approach* (2nd ed.). St. Louis: Mosby, 1980, pp. 215–228.
86. Sullivan & Decker, *Effective management in nursing,* p. 366.
87. Tappen, R.M. *Nursing leadership: Concepts and practice.* Philadelphia: Davis, 1983, p. 368.

88. Gillies, *Nursing management: A systems approach,* p. 138.
89. Marriner, *Guide to nursing management,* p. 92.
90. Mead, G. H. *Mind, self and society.* Chicago: University of Chicago Press, 1934.
91. Hardy, M.E., & Conway, M.E. *Role theory: Perspectives for health professionals.* New York: Appleton-Century-Crofts, 1978; Langford, *Managing and being managed,* pp. 13–18.
92. Corona, D.F. Followership: The indispensable corollary to leadership. In Hein, E.C., & Nicholson, M.J. (Eds.) *Contemporary leadership behavior: Selected readings.* Boston: Little, Brown, 1982, pp. 85–89.
93. National League for Nursing, Council of Baccalaureate and Higher Degree Programs. *Characteristics of baccalaureate education in nursing.* New York: National League for Nursing, 1978.
94. National League for Nursing, Council of Baccalaureate and Higher Degree Programs. *Characteristics of graduate education in nursing leading to the master's degree.* New York: National League for Nursing, 1979.
95. Gillies, *Nursing management: A systems approach,* p. 137–138.
96. Ibid., 192–193.
97. Filoromo, T., & Ziff, D. *Nurse recruitment: Strategies for success.* Rockville, Md.: Aspen, 1980.
98. Rowland & Rowland, *Nursing administration handbook,* p. 387–396.
99. Sullivan & Decker, *Effective Management in Nursing,* pp. 249, 252.
100. Gillies, *Nursing management: A systems approach,* p. 196.
101. Ibid., 191.
102. Ibid., 192.
103. Sullivan & Decker, *Effective management in nursing,* p. 253.
104. Ibid.
105. 43 Federal Registry, 38290-315(1978).
106. Sullivan & Decker, *Effective management in nursing,* p. 273–277.
107. Poteet, G.W. The employment interview: Avoiding discriminatory questions. *Journal of Nursing Administration,* 1984, *14* (4), p. 38–42.
108. Grier, M.W. Affirmative action and nondiscrimination. In Stone, S., Firsich, S.C., Jordan, S.B., Berger, M.S., & Elhart, D. (Eds.) *Management for nurses: A multidisciplinary approach* (3rd ed.). St. Louis: Mosby, 1984, pp. 292–293.
109. Ibid., 265–268.
110. Langford, *Managing and being managed,* p. 107–110.
111. Gillies, *Nursing management: A systems approach,* p. 197–204.
112. Duldt, B.W., Giffin, K., & Patton, B.R. *Interpersonal communication in nursing.* Philadelphia: Davis, 1984, pp. 245–258.
113. Sullivan & Decker, *Effective management in nursing,* p. 261.
114. Gillies, *Nursing management: A systems approach,* p. 200–204.
115. Ganong & Ganong, *Nursing management,* p. 245–247.
116. Gillies, *Nursing management: A systems approach,* p. 471.
117. Knowles, M.S. *Self-directed learning.* New York: Association Press, 1975.
118. Gibb, J. Defensive communication. *Journal of Communication,* 1961, *11,* 141–148.
119. Harnack, R.V., & Fest, T.B. *Group discussion: Theory and technique.* New York: Appleton-Century-Crofts, 1964, p. 169.
120. Ibid., 168–169.

12

STAFFING, PART II: SCHEDULING AND EVALUATING

INTRODUCTION

In the previous chapter, staffing was defined and the first two of its four essential elements were presented: *assessing* and *selecting*. In this chapter, the discussion of staffing is continued by considering the other two elements, *scheduling* and *evaluating*. Scheduling will be discussed according to three factors: *selecting, planning,* and *perceiving*. Evaluating is presented according to *standardizing, analyzing, appraising* and *reporting*.

SCHEDULING

Scheduling of staffing is a major management task in nursing practice. Generally, there are two approaches, centralized or decentralized. The approaches often are consistent with the organizational structure of the agency. As a practical matter, however, a bit of both is often found in most agencies. Table 12–1 provides a comparison of each approach. Typically, the scheduling is developed as follows:

> The traditional plan is for head nurses or their counterparts at the lower or first level of management to develop a schedule for their units as far as they can; then they depend upon the supervisor (middle level) to supply any vacant spots from their wider number of units. The staffing person in the director of nursing services office (top level) allocates any additional personnel necessary, drawing on nurses from other units, the float list (if one exists), part-time nurses who will work on call, or outside agencies. Regardless of the staffing system in effect, a master plan for the entire facility is maintained for overall control.[1]

Whether the staffing plan is centralized or decentralized, a master schedule for the entire nursing department's staff needs to be maintained in the nursing service office for purposes of communication and control. Although extensive effort is made in planning, changes in patients' acuity level or census, nurses' absence due to illnesses or other needs, and emergency situations (such as floods, tornadoes, and freeway pileups) that require changes in the number of staff on duty commonly require daily adjustments.

Selecting
Scheduling the round-the-clock and calendar duty time offers your nursing personnel a variety of possibilities today, and it provides you and other nursing leaders more opportunities to meet the variety of individual nurses' needs in juggling personal and professional time. The options

TABLE 12–1. CENTRALIZED VS. DECENTRALIZED DEVELOPMENT OF SCHEDULING NURSING STAFF DUTY HOURS.

Centralized	Decentralized
Advantages:	
1. Controlled at the vice-president of nursing service level in centralized organizations	1. Controlled at the unit level by the head nurse in decentralized agencies
2. Well-defined policies fairly and consistently implemented by computerized system	2. Head nurse is responsible for scheduling decisions and process; provides more individualized flexibility (which may seem unfair to some). Must adhere to agency policies, however.
3. Relieves unit head nurses of the time-consuming duty of arranging schedules	3. Easier and less complicated to work out staffing for a small area instead of the whole agency
4. Computerized programs take into consideration many of the variables influencing staffing needs, so that a variable or cyclical staffing pattern can be developed for full-time personnel for weeks or months in advance. Daily adjustments for over- and understaffing are still necessary.	4. Head nurse knows patient needs as well as staff capabilities, thus is better able to match needs and skills.
5. Head nurses and nursing staff may participate in the development of staffing patterns.	5. Head nurses may form support group to share problems and solutions.
6. Use of computerized scheduling is cost-effective because it reduces the need for clerical help and relieves nursing unit managers of a non-nurse function; but still needs monitoring.	6. Schedule can be rearranged quickly to meet daily over- and understaffing.
7. Enables the monitoring of data such as patient acuity, costs of staff, quality of care according to staffing mix	7. Head nurse has option to learn to use computerized program on mainframe or microcomputer, providing many of the advantages of centralized computerized scheduling.
Disadvantages:	
1. Resistance because it withholds power of head nurses to reward staff	1. Head nurse may misuse power by using preferred weekends, days off, or shifts as punishment or reward.
2. Denies head nurse the right, experience of making staffing decisions	2. Less effective utilization of resources
3. Minimizes direct contact with staff and nursing leaders	3. Cost containment becomes more difficult in relation to control of staffing.
4. Limits options for personalized, individualized scheduling to meet specific needs, interests of staff	4. Staff more inclined to make special requests
5. Limits knowledge of patient care needs in each nursing unit	5. Time-consuming; a continuous issue to be resolved daily
6. Match of patient needs and nursing staff skills may be less than desirable.	6. Difficult to make adjustments for understaffing

Developed by the authors from the following: Ganong, J. M., & Ganong, W.L. Nursing Management, (2nd ed). Rockville, Md.: Aspen Corporation, 1980, p. 255; Douglass, L.M., The effective nurse: Leader and manager (2nd ed.). St. Louis: Mosby, 1984, p. 83; Marriner, A. Guide to nursing management. (2nd ed.). St. Louis: Mosby, 1984, p. 123.

of shift hours from which you and your nurses select are presented in Table 12–2, with some of the advantages and disadvantages of each. Scheduling policies govern the selection of options, and a checklist of the policies that need to be in place in a typical nursing service department are presented in Figure 12–1. You will need to develop staffing patterns that take into consideration and are consistent with the budget, patient classifications and census forecasts, and personnel policies, and other factors to provide RN staff coverage of the nursing unit 24 hours a day, 7 days a week.

A recommended pattern is the *cyclic* staffing pattern, which provides repetition of a sequence of duty hours, days off, and rotations to days, evening, and night shifts for one, two, or three months in advance. This allows nursing staff to know their schedule well in advance. The pattern needs to take into consideration holidays, vacations, absenteeism, staff development, and unique needs of individual staff members. Figure 12–2 shows an example of a cyclical staffing pattern that can be repeated for an entire year, if adjustments are made for holidays, vacations, educational needs, and so on.

There are several advantages of cyclical staffing noted by Gillies. First, the "preferred" and "not preferred" shifts and days off are shared equally with all personnel. Second, institutional need for RN coverage and and the nurses' personal goals are balanced so that there can be a higher probability the nursing staff will be satisfied. Third, the nursing staff can have input in developing a cyclical pattern that meets most of their needs, and the pattern can be well publicized and implemented so that everyone knows what is expected. Fourth, as staff members of one unit, the group can begin to perceive themselves as one whole team rather than three groups of nurses, each on a particular shift. Fifth, each staff member can anticipate his or her schedule sufficiently to be able to take care of responsibilities and needs in private or personal life.[2] One common problem, however, is over- and understaffing due to changes in the patient census or acuity levels.

Another approach is *variable* staffing, which takes into account the fluctuations in the patient census. The number and mix of nursing staff is determined as a base staffing level. As the number of patients increases, the number of full-time-equivalent (FTE) staff is increased according to a predetermined formula that takes into consideration the patient acuity and all the other variables needed. According to Gillies, variable staffing is cost-effective in that it tends to adjust with need, avoiding over- or understaffing.[3]

Most nursing service departments maintain a list of extra nurses who can be called upon to fill in vacant shifts as necessary. A *float list* consists of those nurses who may be full-time or part-time nursing staff, and who have sufficient experience and expertise that they can easily move from one service (obstetrics, pediatrics, medical-surgical, and so on) to another within the same agency with minimal difficulty. In addition, some nurses prefer to work on a part-time basis, often because they are enrolled for a higher degree or because of family responsibilities or other interests. These nurses may prefer to be on the float list or to fill in as needed on a specific service or unit. Because of the pressing need for nursing staff, some hospitals have turned outside their own organization to the temporary manpower service agencies to meet emergency staffing needs.

We suggest the following as a general principle for consideration:

The degree to which float, part-time, and temporary manpower services can safely *provide nursing care to patients within an agency tends to fluctuate in relation to the degree of orientation. Concurrent staff development is possible to maintain these nurses' familiarity*

TABLE 12–2. OPTIONS FOR SCHEDULING STAFFING SHIFTS. WEEKEND DAYS ARE SATURDAY AND SUNDAY, AND THE WEEK BEGINS ON SUNDAY UNLESS INDICATED OTHERWISE.

Option	No. Days/Hours	Shift	Advantages/ Disadvantages
1. Regular	5/40	7 AM–3:30 P.M. 3 P.M.–11:30 P.M. 11 PM–7:30 A.M.	Dominant pattern: A ½ hr. lunch and ½ hr. overlap of shifts for reporting, etc. Weekends off every 2–3 wks. Regular full-time staff may choose permanent D, E, or N, or may rotate shifts. Problems: safety of RNs leaving, arriving at night. Disruptive tension develops between staff on 3 shifts.
2. Four-day week	4/10	7 A.M.–5:30 P.M. 1 P.M.–11:30 P.M. 9 P.M.–7:30 A.M.	Every other weekend off; cyclical schedule with 14 hrs off between shifts; 4-day weekend every 6 wk very attractive. Saves travel expense. Problem with fatigue.
3. Two-week cycle; 2 days on, 2 off; 3 on, 2 off; 2 on, 3 off, etc.	2/10 & 1/5 (or 1/6)	7 A.M.–5 P.M. 5 P.M.–10 P.M. 9 P.M.–7 A.M. (or 7 A.M.–5 P.M. 5 P.M.–11 P.M. 11 P.M.–7 A.M.)	Two sets of staff groups can cover one unit. Evening hrs. attractive to inactive RNs. Problem with fatigue & filling absences on 10-hr. shifts. Poor communications between RNs & MDs. Poor continuity of care.
4. Seven-Seventy (Paid for 80 hrs.)	7/70 & 7/0	6:45 A.M.–5:15 P.M. 12:45 P.M.–11:15 P.M. 9:15 P.M.–8:45 A.M.	Two sets of staff alternate Tues.–Mon. No rotations; all permanent D., E., or N. No holidays; no vacation pay. Shifts overlap, so increased continuity of care, esp. on weekends, quality of care and job satisf. Requires more staff, but reduces cost of personnel. Staff have more weekends off. More staff on duty at busy times; better lunch, dinner coverage. Staff able to attend classes, conferences, programs; have more time together so can work on projects, committees. Decreased sick leaves and staff turnover. Problems: some fatigue at end of a 7/70 week. Safety concern for RNs leaving at night.
5. Twelve-hr. shifts Variation Baylor plan	7/36 2/12 on wk.ends. or 5/8 M–F	7 A.M.–7 P.M. 7 P.M.–7 A.M.	Paid for 36 + 4 overtime with variable pattern. Fewer staff required. Improved patient care and communication. Less reporting on, off; less confusion. No overtime pay until 80+ hrs/2 wks. Total time off increased. Less travel and safer travel hrs for RNs. Less supervisory personnel needed. Baylor plan paid for 24 + 4 overtime. Some fatigue problems; personal life disrupted during week working.
6. Thirteen Hr. shifts	2/13, 1/14, & 4/0	Varied	Staff designed; morale increased, decreased absenteeism and turnover.

Developed by the author and derived from the following: Marriner, A. Guide to nursing management *(2nd ed.). St.Louis: Mosby, 1984, p. 127; Rowland, H.S., & Rowland, B.L.,* Nursing administration handbook *(2nd ed.). Rockville, Md.: Aspen, 1985, p. 180.*

Employee Categories
1. Full-Time
   1.1 Hours worked per week
   1.2 Weekends worked per schedule
   1.3 Benefits calculation
2. Part-Time
   2.1 Hours worked per week
   2.2 Weekends worked per schedule
   2.3 Benefits calculation
3. Float Pool
   3.1 Hours worked status
   3.2 Weekends worked per schedule
   3.3 Scheduling pattern
   3.4 Assignment method
   3.5 Line of authority
   3.6 Salary and benefits paid
   3.7 Differentials paid
   3.8 Orientation provided
4. On-Call Pool
   4.1 Availability requirements
   4.2 Weekends worked per schedule
   4.3 Assignment method
   4.4 Line of authority
   4.5 Compensation calculation
   4.6 Orientation provided

Scheduling
1. Authority and Responsibility
2. Length of Cycle Rotation
3. Posting Time
4. Reporting Responsibility

Assignments
1. Placement Determination
2. Basic Care Requirements

Days Off
1. Rotation Pattern/Service
2. Weekend Rotation
3. Special Requests
   3.1 School schedules
   3.2 Change status

Weekends
1. Definition
2. Family Member Schedules

Scheduling Requests
1. Request/Response Procedure
2. Weekend Requests
3. Educational Days
4. Emergency Leave
5. Failure to Report when Scheduled

Trade Procedure
1. Acceptable Trades
2. Request/Response Procedure

Vacations
1. Request/Response Procedure
   1.1 Time to submit
   1.2 Place to submit

2. Approval Guidelines
   2.1 Seniority Preference
   2.2 Who Decides
   2.3 Number limitations
3. Change Request
4. Extended Vacations

Holidays
1. Paid Holidays
2. Request/Response Procedure
3. Approval Guidelines
   3.1 Granting criteria
   3.2 Number limitations
4. Unexcused Absence on a Holiday
5. Vacation During Holiday Period

Illness
1. Notification Procedure
2. Extended Days
3. Illness on Duty

Leave of Absence (LOA)
1. Request/Response Procedure
2. Paid Leave Time Interface

Failure to Report to Work
1. Consequences

Transfers
1. Request/Response Procedure
2. Approval Guidelines

Temporary Reassignment
1. Who Will Float
2. Refusal Consequences
3. Equitability

Absenteeism
1. Percentage Acceptable
2. Days Absent Patterns
3. Disciplinary Action

Tardiness
1. Percentage Acceptable
2. Disciplinary Action

Irregular Hours Worked
1. Report/Return Home
2. Called After Shift Begins
3. On-Call Availability

Low-Census Procedures
1. Selection Process
   1.1 Sequence followed
   1.2 Patient care safety levels
2. Benefits Accrued
3. Paid Hours

Overtime
1. Payment Guidelines
2. Availability

Family Policy
1. Family Member Assignment
2. Time Off Policy

Figure 12–1. This staffing checklist provides a convenient way of evaluating the completeness of a nursing department's staffing policies. *(From West Coast Medical Management, Inc., Westlake Village, Calif., 1980)*

238

Figure A — Group A, Jan 1 – Feb 11 (weekday row: S M T W T F S, repeating)

	1	2	3	4	5	6	7	8	9	10	11	12	13	14	15	16	17	18	19	20	21	22	23	24	25	26	27	28	29	30	31	1	2	3	4	5	6	7	8	9	10	11
Day	S	M	T	W	T	F	S	S	M	T	W	T	F	S	S	M	T	W	T	F	S	S	M	T	W	T	F	S	S	M	T	W	T	F	S	S	M	T	W	T	F	S
Ms A	X	X						X	X						X	X						X	X						X	X						X	X					
Ms B			X	X						X	X						X	X						X	X						X	X						X	X			
Ms C					X	X						X	X						X	X						X	X						X	X						X	X	
Ms D	X						X	X						X	X						X	X						X	X						X	X						X
Ms E		X	X						X	X						X	X						X	X						X	X						X	X				
Ms F				X	X						X	X						X	X						X	X						X	X						X	X		
Ms G						X	X						X	X						X	X						X	X						X	X						X	X
Ms H	X	X						X	X						X	X						X	X						X	X						X	X					
Total on duty	5	5	6	6	6	6	6	5	5	6	6	6	6	6	5	5	6	6	6	6	6	5	5	6	6	6	6	6	5	5	6	6	6	6	6	5	5	6	6	6	6	6

Figure A — Group A, Feb 12 – Mar 25 (weekday row: S M T W T F S, repeating)

	12	13	14	15	16	17	18	19	20	21	22	23	24	25	26	27	28	1	2	3	4	5	6	7	8	9	10	11	12	13	14	15	16	17	18	19	20	21	22	23	24	25
Day	S	M	T	W	T	F	S	S	M	T	W	T	F	S	S	M	T	W	T	F	S	S	M	T	W	T	F	S	S	M	T	W	T	F	S	S	M	T	W	T	F	S
Ms A			X	X						X	X						X	X						X	X						X	X						X	X			
Ms B					X	X						X	X						X	X						X	X						X	X						X	X	
Ms C	X						X	X						X	X						X	X						X	X						X	X						X
Ms D		X	X						X	X						X	X						X	X						X	X						X	X				
Ms E				X	X						X	X						X	X						X	X						X	X						X	X		
Ms F						X	X						X	X						X	X						X	X						X	X						X	X
Ms G	X	X						X	X						X	X						X	X						X	X						X	X					
Ms H			X	X						X	X						X	X						X	X						X	X						X	X			
Total on duty	6	6	5	5	6	6	6	6	6	5	5	6	6	6	6	6	5	5	6	6	6	6	6	5	5	6	6	6	6	6	5	5	6	6	6	6	6	5	5	6	6	6

Figure B — Group B, Jan 1 – Feb 11 (weekday row: S M T W T F S, repeating)

	1	2	3	4	5	6	7	8	9	10	11	12	13	14	15	16	17	18	19	20	21	22	23	24	25	26	27	28	29	30	31	1	2	3	4	5	6	7	8	9	10	11
Day	S	M	T	W	T	F	S	S	M	T	W	T	F	S	S	M	T	W	T	F	S	S	M	T	W	T	F	S	S	M	T	W	T	F	S	S	M	T	W	T	F	S
Ms A	X				X				X					X	X				X				X					X	X				X				X					X
Ms B		X					X	X			X					X					X	X			X					X					X	X			X			
Ms C				X			X	X				X						X			X	X				X						X			X	X				X		
Ms D	X			X					X					X	X			X				X						X	X			X				X					X	
Ms E	X					X			X					X	X					X			X					X	X					X		X					X	
Ms F		X					X	X					X			X					X	X					X			X					X	X					X	
Ms G	X					X			X		X				X					X			X			X			X					X		X			X			
Ms H			X				X	X				X					X				X	X					X				X			X	X	X					X	
Total on duty	4	6	7	6	7	6	4	4	6	7	6	7	6	4	4	6	7	6	7	6	4	4	6	7	6	7	6	4	4	6	7	6	7	6	4	4	6	7	6	7	6	4

Figure B — Group B, Feb 12 – Mar 25 (weekday row: S M T W T F S, repeating)

	12	13	14	15	16	17	18	19	20	21	22	23	24	25	26	27	28	1	2	3	4	5	6	7	8	9	10	11	12	13	14	15	16	17	18	19	20	21	22	23	24	25
Day	S	M	T	W	T	F	S	S	M	T	W	T	F	S	S	M	T	W	T	F	S	S	M	T	W	T	F	S	S	M	T	W	T	F	S	S	M	T	W	T	F	S
Ms A	X				X				X					X	X				X				X					X	X				X				X					X
Ms B		X					X	X			X					X					X	X			X					X				X	X			X			
Ms C				X			X	X				X						X			X	X				X						X			X	X				X		
Ms D	X			X					X					X	X			X				X						X	X			X				X					X	
Ms E	X					X			X					X	X					X			X					X	X					X		X					X	
Ms F		X					X	X					X			X					X	X					X			X					X	X					X	
Ms G	X					X			X		X				X					X			X			X			X					X		X			X			
Ms H			X				X	X				X					X				X	X					X				X			X	X	X					X	
Total on duty	4	6	7	6	7	6	4	4	6	7	6	7	6	4	4	6	7	6	7	6	4	4	6	7	6	7	6	4	4	6	7	6	7	6	4	4	6	7	6	7	6	4

Figure 12–2. An example of cyclical scheduling using two patterns. Group A nurses have consecutive days off and change schedules every six weeks. Group B nurses have every other weekend and no more than four consecutive days on duty. The "X" indicates a day off. *(From Gillies, D.P., Nursing management: A systems approach. Philadelphia: Saunders, 1982, p. 216, with permission.)*

with services, resources (especially equipment), communication systems, and administrative policies.

For example, in very busy specialty areas, such as a unit for postcardiac surgical patients, it tends to be difficult, and even dangerous, for temporary nurses from manpower service agencies to function. In such a unit, all nurses are expected to be able to participate effectively in cardiac arrest teams; a regular schedule of testing is usually conducted to maintain this capability. Float, part-time, and temporary manpower service nurses may be able to function effectively in such critical situations, but this needs to be verified before placement. Sometimes it is difficult for these nurses to participate in staff development programs while on duty. Often administrative policies are such that these nurses must attend on personal or off-duty time, and after a while it becomes difficult for individuals to maintain the motivation and initiative to do this without specific administrative support.

Other options used by some agencies are *flex-time* and *job-sharing*. Flex-time allows nurses to choose their own hours, provided they are available during certain core hours that are typically very busy periods. The range may extend from 7 A.M. to 7 P.M., with a "core" period perhaps from 10 A.M. to 2 P.M. Job sharing, which probably grew out of the feminist movement, consists of two nurses' sharing one job. Two nurses may agree to a permanent day schedule, with one on duty the first four hours and the other nurse on the last four hours. The nurses' schedule may fit times when children might be attending a nursery school, or may enable the nurse to be at home when children come home from school. While attending a university, two nurses known to the author shared the position of director of nursing in a nursing home; each was on duty three weekdays, alternating every other weekday off. Both were on duty one of the weekdays, overlapping hours for planning, presenting in-service programs, evaluating personnel, and so on. This worked very well for the nurses and provided a professional level of nursing supervision in a health care setting that typically, in that region, has difficulty finding RNs to fill these positions.

No one can expect a schedule to work well all of the time. There will be occasions when it is necessary to fill a vacancy and none of the nurses who usually fill in are available. Then the tendency is to pull a nurse already on duty from one unit and place that nurse on another unit or in another service. A nurse may even be asked to work two shifts back to back, as 7 to 3:30 and 3 to 11 shifts. This is dangerous, however, not only because of jeopardizing patient safety, but also because of jeopardizing the nurses' trust of management and staff morale generally. As a guideline, we suggest the following principle:

As there is an increasing frequency with which nursing staff are pulled from the nursing unit or service to which they are assigned and expected to go to another unit or service with which they are unfamiliar in order to fill vacancies or temporary understaffing, there will tend to be comparable effects in four areas: an increase in errors, a decrease in the nurses' trust of you as a nursing manager, a decrease in the nurses' job satisfaction, and an increase in annual turnover rates of nursing staff.

People usually like to work in a specific place with people they know. This is true for nurses, too. It is disruptive for an individual nurse to report off in midshift, leaving her assignment to be completed by another staff member who already had a full assignment. The quality and continuity of patient care tends to decrease in the process. Nurses' attitudes can become negative and expressions of anger are not uncommon. For you, as a head nurse, to do this occasionally usually is understandable; to do this frequently is ultimately judged as just poor management, poor planning, and poor leadership. In fact, your nurses may refuse.

An increasing number of nurses are refusing to accept traditional unsafe staffing assignments on ethical and legal grounds. Taking a firm stand on this issue, the North Carolina Nurses' Association (NCNA) has developed "Guidelines for the Registered Nurse in Giving, Accepting, or Rejecting a Work Assignment."[4]* The typical situations at issue are described as follows:

> A labor and delivery nurse is pulled to the oncology unit to give chemotherapy.
> Because of a lack of nursing staff, an evening supervisor feels forced to pull a psychiatric nurse to the coronary care unit.
> A Community Health Nurse, usually assigned to the Family Planning Clinic, is reassigned to provide home care to a patient receiving total parenteral nutrition.
> Due to a decrease in the average daily census, the nursing administrator has had to reduce assigned budgeted positions in the critical care unit. The CCU census has risen and there is no additional qualified staff available.
> A nurse, who recognizes her fatigue and its potential for patient harm, is required to work an additional shift.[5]

The ethical dilemmas raised by these situations are cited as follows:

> . . . the right of the patient to receive safe professional nursing care at an acceptable level of quality;
> the responsibility for and appropriate utilization and distribution of nursing care services when nursing becomes a scarce resource;
> and the responsibility for providing a practice environment that assures adequate nursing resources for the agency while meeting the current socio-political reality of the shrinking health care dollar.[6]

The NCNA document lists a set of principles for deliberation and action.

There are four legal issues identified in the NCNA document that could lead to disciplinary action by the Board of Nursing (such as suspending a head nurse's RN license for two years) and malpractice litigation initiated on behalf of the patient. Briefly, these four issues involve: (1) practicing beyond the scope of the state's Nurse Practice Act; (2) abandonment or neglect of patients; (3) failure to supervise those who, by licensure, are only to practice under supervision, such as the Licensed Practical Nurse; and (4) delegating professional responsibilities to a nurse, knowing she is unqualified by training, licensure, or experience.

> . . . the issue of abandonment or neglect has thus far proven the most legally devastating. Abandonment or neglect has been legally defined to include such actions as insufficient observation (frequency of contact), failure to assure competent intervention when the patient's condition changes (qualified physician not in attendance), and withdrawal of services without provision for qualified coverage. Since nurses at all levels most frequently act as agents of the employing agency, the agency shares the risk of liability with the nurse.[7]

These actions can be taken against you as the nurse-manager delegating assignments, or against the nurse who accepts such an assignment.

---

*This statement was adopted by the Board of Directors of NCNA in February 1986.

In some states, as in North Carolina, hospitals have established legal precedents for the right to dismiss nurses at will. This continues to happen to nurses who refuse to accept assignments that are unsafe, unethical, and illegal. The NCNA guidelines suggest this whole issue needs to be discussed prior to employment or as soon as possible after you decide to refuse to give or take an assignment. You need to anticipate and decide what you are willing to do, when you are a head nurse, for yourself, your patients, nursing staff, and the agency regarding these issues.

There are many arrangements possible, and workable options for scheduling can be developed, assuming adequate planning, effective communication, and a mutually trustful relationship between you and your staff. Study the staffing options, and select those that best match the needs at your agency. Do not expect any of the options to be perfect or to work the first time. Learn to negotiate and work with your staff to develop a program designed just for them. Providing a range of options from which nurses can select a preferred shift schedule is basic to recruiting and retaining nurses. Cooperative attitudes and relationships are to a considerable degree dependent upon people being on duty when *they* choose.

Planning

Since developing staffing schedules involves such a large number of variables, you as a nursing leader need to set aside a considerable amount of time for planning. We suggest that you may want to briefly review the discussion of planning in Chapter 9.

One factor to consider in planning scheduling programs is the Fair Labor Standards Act or labor laws governing hour and wage regulations. In reference to overtime pay, there are two constraints for hospitals employees:

1. Overtime can be paid within one week for duty time above 40 hours per week; and
2. Overtime can be paid within a two-week period for duty time above 8 hours in one day or above 80 hours in a two-week period.[8]

Nursing staff, as employees, must agree in advance to scheduling arrangements. Of course, schedules need to be planned in such a manner that they are within budget allocations and the need for overtime pay is minimal.

Union contracts may also need to be considered in the development and implementation of staffing policies and programs. Gillies defines a union as: " . . . an organization through which employees deal with the employer concerning grievances, disagreements, and terms and conditions of work."[9]

Earlier in this century, labor unions were formed to protect industrial workers from unfair, inhumane treatment by managers. Violence was not uncommon in the confrontations and strikes that occurred in those early years. In recent years, automation has decreased the number of industrial or blue-collar workers, and the number of union members as well. Consequently, union leaders have sought new sources of members among clericals or white-collar workers. As health care became big business, the unions have rapidly established strongholds in the ranks of ancillary and clerical workers in hospitals and health care agencies.[10]

Many nurses belong to a union, particularly since some of the state nurses' associations became involved in collective bargaining and representing its members in contract negotiations and in resolving grievances. Collective bargaining is defined as: " . . . a legal process in which employees, acting as an organized unit, negotiate with their employer about working conditions and economic issues such as wages, hours, and fringe benefits."[11] This process is based on the democratic principle involving everyone's right to organize. Nurses were excluded from this right until the 1974 Health Care amendments to the Taft-Hartley Act.[12] See Table 12–3 for a list of some other significant and historical events that have influenced the nurses' acceptance of unionism. Essentially, unions protect employees from unfair labor practices. See Figure 12–3 for a list of unfair labor practices that you, when you are a head nurse, need to be able to identify and avoid. Some nurses still believe it is unprofessional to belong to a union and be so concerned about salaries and working conditions. In Figure 12–4 is a description of what can happen when management fails to recognize a union; this is a good argument for having a union. Gillies notes, however, that once a contract that provides for collective bargaining and processes for grievance and arbitration is adopted, strikes in health agencies tend to become less frequent.[13]

If there is a union in the health organization in which you serve as a first-level nursing

TABLE 12–3. HISTORICAL REVIEW OF SIGNIFICANT LAWS AFFECTING UNIONS, COLLECTIVE BARGAINING AND ARBITRATION.

1935 The Wagner Act or National Labor Relations Act (NLRA): required employers to bargain with employees and established the National Labor Relations Board (NLRB) for its administration to eliminate unfair labor practices.

1946 American Nurses' Association (ANA) began the Economic Security Program to set up national guidelines for nurses' salaries.

1947 Taft-Hartley Act: Nonprofit organizations (including hospitals) do not have to bargain with their employees; an employer need not bargain with a union containing supervisory personnel.

1962 Taft-Hartley Act amendment: federal employees, including nurses, have the right to bargain collectively.

1967 NLRB given jurisdiction over employer–employee disputes in hospitals and nursing homes.

1968 ANA canceled its no-strike pledge to enable use of strikes in supporting nurses' demands. Nurses bargained successfully in the next decade, and salaries rose rapidly.

1974 Health Care Amendments to the Taft-Hartley Act: granted employees of nonprofit facilities the right to bargain collectively; specified that union must give 10 days' notice before striking a health agency; both parties required to give 90 days' notice (60 days required of all other industries) before terminating or modifying a collective bargaining agreement.

1975 NLRA amended to cover employees of nonprofit hospitals.

1982 NLRA recognizes the following as bargaining units in health care facilities: doctors, excluding house staff; RNs and working nurses with licenses pending; all other professionals; technical workers, including Licensed Practical Nurses and Licensed Vocational Nurses; service and nonskilled maintenance employees such as ward clerks, nursing assistants, aides, and orderlies; skilled maintenance employees, such as plumbers; and business clerical staff.

(From Potter, D.O. [Ed.]. Practices: Nurse's reference library Springhouse, Pa.: Springhouse Corporation, 1984, p. 302; Gillies, D.A. Nursing management: A systems approach. Philadelphia: Saunders, 1982, p. 454, with permission.)

Recognizing Unfair Labor Practices

Like other employees, you have a legal right to participate in union activities. If your employer infringes on that right—through interference, domination, discrimination, or refusal to bargain—you can charge your employer with unfair labor practice. What's an unfair labor practice? Read the following examples to find out.

Interference includes:

* unilaterally improving wages or benefits during a union campaign to influence employees to vote against the union.
* making coercive statements about participation in union activities.
* threatening to close down the facility if a union is elected.
* questioning employees about union activities
* spying on—or implying the possibility of spying on—union meetings.

Domination includes:

* paying a union's expenses
* giving union leaders special compensation or benefits
* taking an active part in organizing a union.

Discrimination includes:

* discharging, disciplining, or threatening an employee for joining a union or for encouraging others to join.
* refusing to hire anyone who belongs to a union
* refusing to reinstate or promote an employee because she testified at a National Labor Relations Board hearing
* enforcing rules unequally between employees who are involved in union activities and those who aren't.

Refusal to bargain includes:

* taking unilateral action that affects any employment conditions either covered in an existing contract or included among legally mandated areas of bargaining
* refusing to meet with a union representative
* refusing to negotiate a mandatory issue
* demanding to negotiate a voluntary issue

Figure 12–3. Learning to recognize unfair labor practices. *(From Potter, D.O. (Ed.). Practices: Nurse's reference library. Springhouse, Pa.: Springhouse Corporation, 1984, p. 299.)*

The Perils of Not Bargaining

Can a hospital avoid collective bargaining by refusing to recognize its staff's union? Of course not. The law—strengthened by court-case decisions—requires a hospital to bargain in good faith with duly elected unions. Here's a key court case, *Eastern Maine Medical Center v. NLRB* (1981), that illustrates this principle:

Nurses at Eastern Maine Center voted 114 to 110 to be represented by the Maine State Nurses' Association, the state's largest nurses' union. In response, the hospital administration adopted a strong anti-union stand, refusing to meet with the nurses for collective bargaining talks. Moreover, the administration gave substantial wage-and-benefit increases to nonunion employees and withheld the increases from the union nurses.

The administration's policy of not bargaining with the union made the union nurses bitter and frustrated. And the union filed unfair labor practice charges against the hospital administration.

The National Labor Relations Board (NLRB) concluded that the hospital had violated the National Labor Relations Act by refusing to bargain in good faith and had discriminated against the union nurses. The board directed the hospital administration to negotiate with the union and to pay the wage-and-benefit increases withheld from the union nurses.

In upholding the board's actions, an appeals court ruled that the hospital's refusal to negotiate violated the nurses' collective bargaining rights.

Figure 12–4. The perils of not bargaining. *(From Potter, D.O. [Ed.]. Practices: Nurse's reference library. Springhouse, Pa.: Springhouse Corporation, 1984, p. 306.)*

manager, then the contract probably includes mandatory staffing policies that you must follow. For example, one unit of 360 RNs won the following:

> . . . the hospital cannot require a nurse to work more than a regular workday except in cases of emergency, which includes acts of God and unplanned staffing shortages. . . .
>
> . . . the hospital must first seek volunteers, such as float nurses or per diem nurses, to fill a position before it requires an on-duty nurse to work overtime. . . .
>
> . . . if the hospital is unable to fill the position on a voluntary basis, then an on-duty nurse may be required to work overtime up to one-half the nurse's normal shift. . . .
>
> . . . the hospital must give the nurse two hours notice of an overtime assignment and must provide the nurse working overtime at least 10 hours off between the overtime assignment and the nurse's next scheduled shift. . . .
>
> . . . establishment of a staffing committee, comprised of nurses, nursing administrators and hospital administrators . . . [to] meet monthly to review and make recommendations on such issues as recruitment and retention, staff-patient ratios and patient classification systems. . . . [14]

If you assign a nurse in a manner that breaks the contract, then the nurse can, as a union member, file a grievance against you. Employees frequently file grievances against their supervisors for dispensing discipline inconsistently, showing favoritism, or treating employees unfairly. In turn, management often files grievances against employees who allow personal problems to disrupt their jobs, fail to perform their assignments, show poor work habits (tardiness and unreliability), and maintain an antagonistic attitude toward management when representing the union in labor relations.[15] To maintain relationships, you need to be knowledgeable about union and management relationships and contracts, incorporating these into your planning.

There are three other major categories of factors that need to be considered in planning staffing schedules and programs: a patient classification system and time standards for giving nursing care (both were discussed in Chapter 11; see Table 11–3), plus staffing formulas. There is a lot of information to consider all at once. This is where computers can be helpful.

Unlike most nurse managers, the computer can balance all of this information even for the largest units. Further, because the computer can consider the needs for personnel beyond any one unit, it can evaluate opportunities for sharing of personnel with other units to improve the efficiency of nursing coverage. Finally, the computer can handle the complexities associated with flextime and split shifts that are almost impossible to consider by hand and thereby increase the desirability of working in the unit.[16,17]

In time, it is anticipated that computers will be available to nursing managers in most agencies to assist in planning and developing centralized staffing schedules. A primary use of computer data-base programs is to quickly arrange a large amount and variety of data into a form that can be understood and used. The amount of data and the number of variables involved in developing a staff scheduling program certainly matches this description. Since programming is a difficult and specialized computer skill, you will probably be sufficiently effective to just purchase a staffing program and become skillful in its use rather than try developing one specific to your agency. A computer search of your library will provide current information about what programs are available and what the programs will and will not do. Ultimately, you will probably want to depend upon your own analysis of your needs in order to decide what hardware (equipment) and software (programs) to purchase. You may find it very helpful to invest in two or three site visits to learn what nursing leaders and managers in other agencies are doing.

Recently a common topic of discussion is the term *computer competency,* and what this means. People can become intimidated by computers quickly. Computer programmers strut about with their data cards and track paper, creating a mystique, speaking only to themselves in "computerese." As a practical matter, we believe all you need to know to be computer competent as a nurse-manager is how to use two programs: a data base program for scheduling and a word processing program. As in learning anything new, this is simply a matter of getting started, proceeding at your own pace, and continuing to try. As in driving an automobile, you really do not have to know *everything* about a computer to get it to do the things you need.*

---

*Knowing the material about computers is quickly outdated, we do refer our readers, however, to the following two texts, which provide excellent overviews regarding computers in nursing: (1) Sullivan & Decker, Using computers in health care. In *Effective Management in Nursing,* p. 205. This chapter presents a good discussion of computer basics as well as applications to patient monitoring, histories and medical records, staff scheduling, and staff training and evaluation; bibliography is extensive. (2) Rowland & Rowland, Computers in Nursing. In *Nursing Administration Handbook,* p. 206. This chapter presents a nursing management perspective, including advice about what the computer can do in nursing administration, dealing with vendors, costs and benefits, and common errors. In addition, our readers are encouraged to consult the journal, *Computers in Nursing,* which covers computer applications to administration, practice, research, and education in nursing.

Figure 12–5. A description of how one nursing unit manager followed a formula to determine the number of nurses needed per day to provide a particular level of nursing care. FTEs = Full-time equivalent. Fixed FTEs = all indirect care positions, such as managers, clerks, secretaries, etc. Direct FTEs = positions for direct, hands-on patient care. Productive FTEs = hours paid and worked. Nonproductive FTEs = hours paid and not worked, as vacations, holidays, and sick days. *(From Kirk, R., Nursing quality and productivity: Practical management tools. Rockville, Md.: Aspen, 1986, p.21. Reprinted with permission of Aspen Publishers, Inc., 1986.)*

Unit A has documented the need for 4.0 nursing care HPPD through collection, compilation, and validation of patient classification data from the past fiscal year. The budget committee approved the standard, 4.0 direct care hours per each of the projected 15,000 patient days, and the resulting 36.0 FTEs were budgeted:

$$\frac{15{,}000 \times 4.0}{2080} = 28.8 \text{ Direct FTEs}$$

$$28.8 \text{ Direct FTEs} + 3.8 \text{ Fixed FTEs}^* = 32.6 \text{ Productive FTEs}$$

$$\frac{32.6 \text{ Direct FTEs} \times 216 \text{ (avg. benefit hrs.)}}{2080} = 3.4 \text{ Nonproductive FTEs}$$

$$32.6 \text{ Productive FTEs} + 3.4 \text{ Nonproductive FTEs} = 36.0 \text{ Total FTEs}$$

* 2.0 clerks + .4 day off relief for both + 1.0 Manager = 3.8 Fixed

The approved figure of 36.0 was used to develop a daily staffing pattern and make decisions about staff ratios of RN, LPN, etc. Due to the anticipated daily census of 41 patients (15,000 ÷ 365) the pattern showed a daily staffing compliment of 20 or 21 staff members, giving direct care for each 24 hour period (41 × 4.0 HPPD = 164 hours ÷ 8-hour shifts = 20.5 staff members on duty daily). Daily staff members were broken down by position category to ensure that hiring and prescheduling of staff would follow the same pattern.

One of the things the computer can do for nurse-leaders is the computations used in staffing. For example, Kirk uses a formula to hand calculate the number of personnel needed to provide nursing care for one unit (see Fig. 12–5). Next, this same formula can be calculated by a computer for an entire agency. Finally, the information is translated into a scheduling pattern, and you can appreciate the difficulty of doing this by hand compared to using a computer. Often questionnaires, such as the one shown in Figure 12–6, are used to obtain information about the nursing staff's preferences. It is also helpful to establish some orderly system and forms so that your nursing staff may submit well-in-advance requests for particular days off and for vacations; six weeks prior to posting the schedule may be sufficient time for you to incorporate requests into your computerized scheduling plans. Special holidays, such as Christmas and New Year's Day, can be alternated among staff on an annual basis; on duty this Christmas, off the next. If you use management by objectives (MBO) or a similar process in evaluating staff and planning with them the staff development and career ladder options needed, this information also needs to be considered in planning staffing.

Eason, Spickerman, and Lee suggest developing guidelines to help you compile this scheduling task as quickly as possible, yet accurately.[18] The following situation is provided by these authors:

Develop a time schedule for RNS for a three weeks period using the following requirements and constraints. The head nurse is not included.

1. The employees are 16 staff nurses who work 12 hours shifts either [7 A.M. to 7 P.M.] or [7 P.M. to 7 A.M.].
2. The maximum number of hours anyone may be scheduled in a two weeks time period is *84 hours*.
3. The maximum number of workdays anyone may be scheduled without a day off is *3 days* (36 hours).

4. No one is ever scheduled to work 24 consecutive hours.
5. There must be 4 RNs on duty at all times.
6. The week starts on Sunday and ends of Saturday.
7. All employees have off a three day weekend every other week.[19]

This is an assignment the authors give to their baccalaureate nursing students in the leadership course. The answers are provided in their article.

As a general principle, we propose considering the following statements:

The farther into the future you can plan the staffing schedule, the more opportunity you and your nursing staff will tend to have to discuss, negotiate, adjust, and incorporate the many needs and variables into the schedule, and the more satisfied you, your staff, and your nursing leader (supervisor) will tend to be with the result.

However:

The length of time you invest in planning the staffing schedule tends to have no relationship to the degree of satisfaction expressed by your nursing staff.

But:

The degree to which you listen to expressions of dissatisfaction with the staffing schedule and respond appropriately (by telling, selling, participating, or delegating in a humanizing manner) will tend to increase your staff's expressions of satisfaction with duty hours.

You need to be able to explain the logic behind the decisions you make and to interpret the policies to your staff. If your nurses continuously express dissatisfaction with a staffing policy, you need to bring this to the attention of your nursing leader or supervisor. It may be a concern of others, and you may be able to initiate a needed change in the policy. It is important that you understand the personal significance of the staffing schedule to each individual staff member. The perfect schedule is the one with which everyone is perfectly happy, everyone appears at their post at the appointed time, at readiness level IV, with no absenteeism, tardiness, or turnover. This is seldom achieved.

Perceiving

Perspectives or opinions of those who associate with you and your nurses are indicative of the image of nursing presented, the way you are perceived by one another and by others. This indirectly has an influence on scheduling that often is neglected, but worthy of consideration.

First, it is important that your staff and others in the hospital administration trust you as a nursing leader. In previous discussions of the development of workable options in scheduling, we have assumed a mutually trustful relationship between you and your staff. One earns others' trust, however; it does not just happen.

This perceived trustworthiness is achieved by consistency in your behavior, particularly in relation to scheduling. Fairness in distributing preferred and nonpreferred days off and in application of the personnel policies is another way to develop trust. Being attentive and responding to appropriately submitted special requests for days off, shift rotations, and so on is being respectful of the individual and of his or her rights as an employee. In contrast, use of

Employee Data Form for Shift Scheduling

1. Name _____ Blank, L _____ 2. Employee Number _____ 10886 _____

3. Classification _____ 1 _____ (1-head nurse, 2-assistant head, 3-RN, 4-LPN, 5-NA/ORD, 6-Sec.)

4. Unit Number _____ 215 _____

   Number of Shifts to be Assigned Weekly:
   5. Minimum _____ 3 _____   6. Desired _____ 5 _____   7. Maximum _____ 8 _____
8. Number of weekends can work between weekends off _____ 1 _____

   Length of work stretch (consec. days):
   9. Min. (usually 2) _____ 2 _____   10. Max. (usually 6) _____ 6 _____
11. Shift Rankings (1: beg–7 am; 2: beg.–3 pm; 3: beg.–11 pm)

    (If hired for straight shifts, specify first choice only)
    First Choice _____ 1 _____   Second Choice _____ 3 _____   Third Choice _____ 2 _____
12. Allocate 10 aversion points among choices of shift (aversion points must *increase* in value from 1st to 2nd to 3rd choice—let first choice aversion be 9999 if on straight shifts).
    First Choice .   Second Choice   Third Choice
    Aversion _____ 0 _____   Aversion _____ 5 _____   Aversion _____ 5 _____
13. Indicate preference for the first day off in a week prior to a weekend off.
    (2=Mon.; 3=Tues.; 4=Wed.; 5=Thurs.; 6=Fri.)

First	Second	Third	Fourth	Fifth
Choice _2_	Choice _3_	Choice _4_	Choice _6_	Choice _5_

14. Indicate preference for the second day off in a week following a weekend off.

First	Second	Third	Fourth	Fifth
Choice _6_	Choice _2_	Choice _4_	Choice _3_	Choice _5_

15. Indicate preference for day-off pairs midweek. [Usual alternatives are (2,3), (3,4), (4,5), (5,6), (2,5), (2,6), (3,6).]
    First Choice Pair _3, 4_ ; Second Choice _2, 3_ ; Third Choice _4, 5_ ; Fourth Choice _5, 6_ ; Fifth Choice _2, 6_ ; Sixth Choice _3, 6_ ; Seventh Choice _2, 5_
16. Cumulative number of holidays due _____ 0 _____
17. Cumulative number of vacation days due _____ 0 _____
18. Current value of shift aversion index _____ 5. _____
19. Current value of day-off aversion index _____ 2. _____
20. Number of times shifts worked to date:
    Shift 1 _____ 0 _____   Shift 2 _____ 0 _____   Shift 3 _____ 0 _____
21. Shift worked on last day of previous month _____ 1 _____
22. Number of weekends worked since last weekend off _____ 1 _____
23. Last day off previous week _____ 6 _____
24. Remarks:

Figure 12–6. An example of a questionnaire to obtain information about individual staffs' preferences. This provides a data base to use in developing a computerized staffing program. *(From Smith, D.L., & Wiggins, A. A computer-based nursing schedul-ing system. In* Computers and operations research. *Elmsford, N.Y.: Pergamon Press, 1977, p. 195. Reprinted with permission from Pergamon Journals, Ltd.)*

your power and influence in scheduling to punish or reward staff is never appreciated, and is dehumanizing and degrading to the nursing staff.

Being careful about the promises and concessions you make is also part of your image as a competent nursing manager. For example, Douglass states most nursing staff have expected to work every two weekends out of three.[20] Suppose you promise, without prior approval of your immediate supervisor, to give your nursing staff every other weekend off in order to attract or retain staff. The implications of this are that (1) more nurses will be required in order to staff your unit each week, (2) the personnel variable cost in your unit budget will increase, and (3) overtime pay will probably increase because you eventually will need to ask staff or part-time personnel to work extra to cover the unit. Unfortunately, it can be predicted that soon you will be perceived as untrustworthy by all concerned, and you will have generated additional scheduling and budgetary problems for yourself. Everyone will know when you make a mistake as a manager: your staff, supervisor or area coordinator, peers, the vice-president of nursing service and the people in his or her office, and the controller or business manager of the agency.

There will be times when you, as a head nurse, may even need to ask a nurse to work two shifts back to back, as 7 to 3:30 and 3 to 11 shifts, or to take a similar unpleasant assignment. You need to realize this is dangerous, however, not only because of potentially jeopardizing patient safety, but also jeopardizing the nurses' trust of management and staff morale generally. If some of the nurses belong to a union at your agency, then any deviation from the scheduling agreement will probably result in the union steward reporting your actions as a contract violation.

Attending physicians and staff doctors are quick to complain when there is insufficient nursing staff to enable them to do whatever procedures or surgery they need to do. They often have the option of admitting their patients to other hospitals, and may use this as a heavy influence in making changes. Having nurses provide services to their patients is important to their private practice. Physicians try to keep their patients satisfied, particularly those patients who may be prone to file lawsuits.

Patients and their visitors or relatives are quick to note unpleasant attitudes on the part of nursing staff, and patients' evaluations of nursing care received can quickly reflect staffing deficiencies. Generally, for you to have to *occasionally* ask staff to work overtime or extra can be expected, but to do so on a regular basis reveals lack of effective planning, the first task function of leaders, and poor leadership on your part.

Rather than perceiving themselves as one team, staff members too frequently begin to perceive themselves as three groups of nurses according to a particular shift. It is sometimes noted that nurses on the 7 A.M. to 3:30 P.M. (or 3 to 11:30 P.M.) shift will begin blaming and scapegoating the nurses on the 3 to 11:30 P.M. (or 11 P.M. to 7 A.M.) shift for some omission or error, like forgetting to reorder a drug when giving the last dose in the container, or omitting the NPO (nothing by mouth) sign of patients going to X-ray.

Generally it is your responsibility, when you are head nurse, to spend some time on the unit during the evening and night shifts, telling staff directly or indirectly by persuading them about the cooperation and mutual respect you expect of nurses on each shift. Identify individuals by name to personalize, and generate feelings of inclusion by using the word "we" often. You may need to confront individual staff members who are slow to get your message; blaming, scapegoating, and sabotage are not acceptable behaviors. If necessary, write up unacceptable behavior in an interim evaluation report. You need to try to handle these situations at your unit level as much as possible in such a manner that your staff will trust you rather than go over your (organizational) head to your supervisor or area coordinator.

Full-time nursing staff also occasionally becomes resentful of part-time and temporary nursing staff because these nurses are assigned the shift hours and days they want, while the regular staff remain on the staffing pattern and must make concessions. These temporary nurses as well as independent private duty nurses frequently are rejected by the regular nursing staff. Without their professional support (helping find equipment and linens, phone numbers, medications, etc.), the temporary, private duty, and sometimes even part-time nurses find nursing practice unpleasant and unattractive. Such interpersonal behavior merely compounds an already difficult, even stressful, staffing situation. In addition, it is not conducive to effective nursing care. An obvious answer to this situation is to concentrate on retention of the full-time nursing staff so temporary nurses will not be needed. (See page 214 and 228 for further discussion of staff retention.)

As a general principle, we suggest readers consider these statements:

If sound personnel decisions are to be made, then they need to be made slowly and thoughtfully with the participation and consultation of agency and nursing administrators, of representatives of the nursing staff, of nurse recruiters, and of the director of personnel with the expectation that when exceptions are necessary, appropriate approval, appeal, and grievance processes are to be conducted through appropriate organizational channels.

If you and your nursing staff want to initiate policy changes, then as nurses you will need all of others' perceived credibility and trustworthiness, plus any good will you can stimulate in order to have others favorably view the position proposed.

It is best to work within the organizational system if you hope to have an impact and change policies.

EVALUATING

On a regular basis, you need to set up a system of evaluating the total staffing program. This includes the way staffing needs are assessed, the recruitment and screening methods in selecting new staff, and the established systems of scheduling.

To the same degree that you, when you are a head nurse, know what your total staffing program is accomplishing in relation to the objectives you have established, you will be able to determine when to make necessary interventions in order to redirect and maintain control.

Standardizing

First, staffing programs need to be evaluated according to national and local standards. Voluntary national standards include those identified by the American Nurses' Association (see Appendix A) and the Joint Commission on Accreditation of Hospitals (see Fig. 3–1). In addition, Public Law 92-603 established the Professional Standards Review Organization (PSRO) with the charge to stop increasing health care costs and improve the quality of health care, particularly in relation to patients receiving benefits from Medicare, Medicaid, and Maternal and Child Health programs. Gillies reports groups of nurses in several states have developed practice standards based on nursing theories, nursing functions, and nursing care problems.[21] Local standards are the philosophy and objectives of the agency's nursing service department and of the agency itself. Once they have been selected, it is best not to change the standards or criteria so that comparisons can be made from one semiannual or annual report to another to identify trends.

Analyzing

In order to analyze the total program, specific aspects of the program need to be identified as categories and the data available within each category needs to be assembled into summary statements.[22] The categories might be suggested by the criteria or standards you have decided to use.

Look at all of your data and the way they are analyzed, as well as the numerical results of analyses. Ask yourself about each aspect. Look at the work assignment control system being used and the patient forecasting process. How much variance has there been in the budget over the past year or two years or five years? Are the job descriptions effective, or have you had problems with staff because of overlapping areas of responsibility or duplication of tasks? Do the salary scales seem appropriate for the matching job descriptions? How many nurses have been attracted to your agency or unit, and which recruitment method seems most successful? Has there been a complaint regarding discrimination in the screening procedures used? What is the tardiness, absentee, and turnover rate on your unit, service, and agency? How have the new nurses rated the orientation or internship program? Have any of the new nurses quit? What have the exit interviews revealed? Depending on how carefully exit interviews are planned and handled, these can be a source of important information—the "real" reasons why nurses leave. These may be handled by the director or vice-president of nursing, the nurse-recruiter, or a qualified member of the personnel department. See Figure 12–7 for a structured format for exit interviews. Periodic surveys of the nursing staff regarding scheduling can provide important feedback, which might serve as the basis of improvements. If the nursing staff are union members, how have things been going in the relationship between the union and management? Has anyone complained? Summarize each of the categories you have identified, noting in summary form data, both positive and negative.

Appraising

Appraising is concerned, once all things are considered, with how well the staffing program is measuring up to those individual criteria or standards you have established. You may set up a grading system to better indicate areas that need improving and areas of success.

Reporting

This, of course, refers to the formal reports you will need to send through the organizational communication channels, probably both upward and downward. You will need to develop some judgment about what is to be reported, when, and to whom.

Certainly your budget will be the focus of many of your reports. You will need to respond to internal and external audits, the periodic examination of all financial records in the agency. If your nursing unit consumes an extensive amount of supplies, you can expect to be involved with periodic inventory reports, too.

Reports about patients are also necessary. Certainly the actual daily census, acuity levels, and similar information will be necessary to serve as a historical basis for forecasting the number of nurses needed in staffing. In addition, any unique or unusual circumstances will also need to be reported, such as patients' injuries, medication or treatment errors, lost dentures

Nursing Services Department

Please complete this questionnaire and return it within a week in the stamped envelope provided. Be assured that your responses will be treated, without reference to your identity, solely as statistical data for purposes of analysis.

1. Registered Nurse Level at the time of leaving:
   Level 1 _____   Level II _____   Level III _____

2. (a) Please rate the following items on a scale of 1 (least satisfactory) to 3 (most satisfactory) as they reflect your experiences during the period of employment with the Medical Center.
   (b) If any of the following items contributed to your leaving the Medical Center, please check the box at the right opposite the appropriate item(s).

   (a)   (b)
                                                                    Check here if the
                                                                     item contributed
   Rating   to your leaving
   1 2 3
   __ __ __
   __ __ __ Satisfaction with pay and/or fringe benefits   _____
   __ __ __ Extent of responsibility/workload   _____
   __ __ __ Extent of authority given to you   _____
   __ __ __ Communication with superiors   _____
   __ __ __ Communication with colleagues   _____
   __ __ __ Centralization of authority in superiors   _____
   __ __ __ Type and amount of supervision provided   _____
   __ __ __ Orientation and training provided   _____
   __ __ __ Clarity of work instructions   _____
   __ __ __ Effectiveness in dealing with your suggestions,   _____
              opinions or complaints
   __ __ __ Opportunities for advancement   _____
   __ __ __ Work schedule   _____

3. What is/are the reason(s) for your leaving. (Please check more than one item, if applicable.)

   ____ Better position elsewhere.
   ____ Desire to move to another city.
   ____ Spouse moving to another city.
   ____ Retirement.
   ____ Leaving nursing due to: (Check all items which apply).
         ____ Marriage   ____ Other domestic reasons
         ____ Health   ____ Disenchantment with nursing
         ____ Child Care
   ____ Work-related conditions (Please check this item if any of the items listed under question 2 contrib-
         uted to your leaving.)

4. Please use the space below to make other comments about the working conditions at the Medical Center:

Figure 12–7. A questionnaire to obtain preliminary information for use during exit interview. (From Neidermeyer, E., & Neidermeyer, P. A. Journal of Nursing Administration,
1987, 17 (7,8), 8.)

and other articles, and so on. Although you may not be required to keep an account of some of these items, it will be helpful to you to know the incidence of preventable complications, such as urinary tract infection, decubitus ulcers, or pneumonia. Knowing the incidence of these problems, which are known to result from poor nursing care, will provide some vital information about the quality of nursing care being delivered by your nursing staff. Both positive and negative feedback on performance is important to your staff, and you need to collect the information so that you can share it with them. Some patients' diseases, such as tuberculosis, AIDS, or hepatitis, are to be reported to the state or local health departments for follow-up of potential contacts. These items are in addition to the daily census reports and the patients' conditions, which your staff helps prepare for the department of nursing office. (For further discussion of quality monitoring, see Chapter 15.)

While bulletin boards and verbal reports are commonly used in nursing, you may wish to consider using memos for communicating important messages to your nursing staff. By providing a copy for each member of your staff, by name, you will be able to validate that the memo was sent, when, and to whom. You will probably want to maintain a notebook in which to place the memos for reference. Memos really need to be used when you are communicating about an individual's duty schedule; retain a copy for your own files to verify your actions. By reviewing past memos, you have a basis for evaluating the effectiveness of the formal organizational communication network from your unit.[23] You will also want to monitor the effectiveness of all nursing care forms used by your nursing staff, such forms as the Kardex or nursing care plan, nursing notes, and other forms for the patient's chart, as well as intake and output forms and other records used at the bedside.[24,25]

SUMMARY

In this chapter the concept of staffing, continuing from Chapter 11, was discussed. The emphasis has been on the issue of scheduling nursing staff in order to have RN coverage of patients on a nursing unit for 24 hours, 7 days a week, around the calendar. The extensive and detailed coverage of this topic is proportional, we believe, to the importance of staffing to the personal as well as professional lives of nurses. It is our view that the best of humanistic management—the people-oriented functions of the leader—needs to be brought to all aspects of a staffing program. The discussion of staffing ends with our suggestion that you, when you are a head nurse, will probably want to evaluate the entire staffing program. While this is not typical of current management practices, when you are a head nurse, we believe you will find this very helpful. In the current shortage of qualified nursing personnel, it seems reasonable that knowledge about what attracts and retains nurses on a unit is valuable knowledge too long overlooked.

REFERENCES

1. Douglass, L.M. *The effective nurse: Leader and manager* (2nd ed.). St. Louis: Mosby, 1984, pp. 83–84.
2. Gillies, D.A. *Nursing management: A systems approach.* Philadelphia: Saunders, 1982), pp. 214–215.
3. Ibid., 215–218.
4. Trought, E.A. Guidelines for the registered nurse in giving, accepting, or rejecting a work assignment. *The Tar Heel Nurse* (Official Publication of the North Carolina Nurses Association), 1986, *48* (2), 16–19.

5. Ibid., 16.

6. Ibid.

7. Ibid., 17.

8. Rowland, H.S., & Rowland, B.L., *Nursing administration handbook* (2nd ed.). Rockville, Md.: Aspen, 1985, p. 181.

9. Gillies, *Nursing management,* p. 457.

10. Ibid., 456.

11. The legalities of collective bargaining. In *Practices: Nurse's Reference Library* Springhouse, Pa.: Springhouse Corporation, *Nursing84 Books*™, 1984, p. 302.

12. Ibid.

13. Gillies, *Nursing Management,* p. 456.

14. N.Y. nurses end brief strike by approving new contract. *The American Nurse,* July–August 1987, 9.

15. Grievances and arbitration. In *Practices: Nurse's Reference Library,* p. 307–308.

16. Sullivan, E.J., & Decker, P.J. *Effective management in nursing.* Reading, Mass.: Addison-Wesley, 1985, p. 224;

17. Adler, J., McClure, M.L., & Hoover, K. When a nursing staff organizes: Management rights and collective bargaining (programmed instruction). *American Journal of Nursing* 1978 *78* (4), 1–12.

18. Spickerman, S., Lee, B., & Eason, F. Use of learning modules to teach nursing leadership concepts. *Journal of Nursing Education* 27(2), 78–82.

19. Ibid.

20. Douglass, *The effective nurse,* p. 87.

21. Gillies, *Nursing management,* p. 100.

22. Duldt, B.W., & Giffin, K. *Theoretical perspectives for nursing.* Boston: Little, Brown, 1985, pp. 143–144.

23. Langford, T.L. *Managing and being managed: Preparation for professional nursing practice.* Englewood Cliffs, N.J.: Prentice-Hall, 1981, pp. 193–200.

24. U.S. Department of Health, Education, and Welfare. *How to study nursing activities.* (Public Health Service, no. 370).

25. Rowland & Rowland, *Nursing administration handbook,* pp. 192–205.

13

DIRECTING, PART I: COMMUNICATING AND INFLUENCING

INTRODUCTION

The fourth task function of leadership is perhaps the most crucial and trying test of your capabilities as a leader; that of *directing* others to produce the expected quantity of goods or, as in the case of nursing, the expected quality of care to our clients. We believe a leader's directing can only be as effective as the preceding functions of planning, organizing, and staffing. In this chapter, the elements of communicating and influencing are dealt with; in Chapter 14, the other two elements of directing are considered, developing and contracting.

After defining this concept and discussing its function and role in leadership, directing is considered according to the communication styles of leadership described in Situational Leadership theory: telling, selling, participating, and delegating. Integrated into the consideration of each leadership style are the leader's sources of influence or power and the attitudes and communication patterns of Humanistic Nursing Communication theory; some in-service educational needs are also discussed in relation to the readiness of the follower. Characteristics of influence or power are discussed, along with the significance of power, its sources, use, and loss.

THE DEFINITION AND SIGNIFICANCE OF DIRECTING

According to the dictionary, *directing* can be defined by a number of phrases that are not specifically relevant to leadership. For example, the leader first needs to "plan the action and effects" or goals of directing in order to direct others' task-related activities. Being "honest and to the point" and "keeping things straight" are phrases that seem to characterize a good leader. Having "nothing or no one between" the leader and the follower involves giving and receiving directions at first hand, and suggests that directing requires face-to-face interpersonal interactions. The word *supervise* is also used in the general definition of directing; it is derived from *supervidere,* meaning to *oversee* and to *view directly.*[1] This suggests a good leader watches the followers as they work. The result of directing is the production of a product or service of economic value. In summary, the following definition of directing as a function of leadership can be derived from the dictionary:

> Directing requires that the leader talks directly with the followers about the plans and expectations of their work, observes them while the task is being done, and inspects the product or service upon completion of the task.

There are a few references to the term, *directing* in the nursing literature. For example, according to Douglass, directing is the connection between organizing and working:

> . . . directing means the issuance of assignments, orders, and instructions that permit the worker to understand what is expected of him or her, and the guidance and overseeing of the worker so that he or she can contribute effectively and efficiently to the attainment of organizational objectives.[2]

Marriner states that the purpose of directing is to get the work done through others.[3]

In our view, the element shared in common by these definitions and the purpose of directing is *communication*. According to Haney, communication is the key element that holds an organization together:

> But just what is an organization? First, it consists of a *number* of people. . . . Second, it involves *interdependence*. . . . Individuals are *interdependent* when the performance of one person affects and is affected by the performance of others. . . . Interdependence calls for *coordination*. . . . And, coordination requires *communication*. Genesis describes how the building of the Tower of Babel was disrupted by the "confounding of tongues." When men no longer had a common language, when they were unable to communicate, they could not work together.[4]

Writing over two decades ago, Haney also noted that organizations are getting larger, more complex, and more demanding in quality and quantity of goods and services, while society is increasingly imposing other requirements upon organizations. Just as true today is Haney's conclusion that contemporary organizations demand leaders be able to communicate at "unprecedented levels of excellence."[5] This is particularly true of organizations devoted to providing health care and of the leaders of nurses within these organizations. We suggest the reader consider the following as a statement of general principle:

> *The nursing leader who is skillful in using effective communication behaviors will tend to be more successful in directing nursing staff than the nursing leader with limited communication skills.*

The next section concerns directing and the application of the specific communication behaviors defined by Situational Leadership and Humanistic Nursing Communication theories. We believe both theories can enhance the probability of being a successful leader if appropriately applied to leadership situations and relationships between leaders and their followers.

COMMUNICATION BEHAVIORS

The words *communication behaviors* are used here to indicate the specific communication behaviors identified in Situational Leadership and in Humanistic Nursing Communication behavior. The leadership styles of Situational Leadership refer to specific communication behaviors: *telling, selling, participating,* and *delegating.* These four behaviors are labeled *leadership styles* and they consist of varying combinations of *task,* or *directive,* and *relationship,* or *supportive* communication behaviors. (See Chapter 1 and Appendix C for the theoretical discussion of these concepts.) In Humanistic Nursing Communication, the communication behaviors are the five skills or *patterns of interaction: communing, asserting, confronting, conflicting,* and *separating. Humanizing* or *dehumanizing attitudes* refer to the dimension of communicating that is one's demeanor, feeling, mood, or predilection toward someone or something. (See Chapter 2 and Appendix D for the theoretical discussion of these patterns of interaction and Chapter 3 and Appendix B for discussion of humanizing and dehumanizing attitudes.) In this section, we integrate the two theories to provide a theoretical basis for developing communication skills that we believe are particularly appropriate to the directing function of leadership. Let us assume your new staff nurse is an atypical new graduate, Sue, a young woman who has a family to support and who switched from a business major to nursing after several years experience in advertising.

Style 1: Telling.

The first leadership style (S1), or "telling," in Situational Leadership, is defined as one-way communication in which the leader defines the followers' roles and tells them what to do, how to do it, when, and where to do various tasks. This behavior is highly *directive* or task-oriented, with minimal relationship or supportive behaviors. It is appropriately used by a nursing leader, such as a head nurse, when talking to followers or nursing staff members who are at the very first level of readiness (R1).

"Telling" is the leadership style particularly applicable to all new graduates just starting in nursing practice. Upon taking a staff nurse's position, Sue, your new graduate is theoretically at the R1 readiness level in that she is probably unable and insecure about most nursing skills. While some may be unwilling, most new graduates are willing, even anxious, to perform those RN functions that they are comfortable doing, such as bathing patients, doing admission health assessments, and administering oral medications to patients. Many, however, will be unwilling to perform advanced RN functions that they have not performed themselves but have seen performed by RNs.

For example, most new graduates probably have observed but not participated in (1) teaching a newly diagnosed diabetic how to self-inject insulin, (2) administering cardiopulmonary resuscitation (CPR) in an emergency situation, or (3) administering medication intravenously by injecting the drug directly into the vein—an "IV push." Graduates have not participated because these experiences may not have occurred or been required during the clinical laboratory periods while they were in the nursing program. The legal implications are also such that nursing deans and faculty frequently agree with nursing service administrators by contract that these experiences are beyond the scope of the nursing student's educational program, which is, as in other professions, in reality just an extensive introduction to nursing practice. Consequently, such experiences and procedures are usually included in the agency's individualized orientation or staff development programs for RN staff. (See "Orienting," Chapter 11.)

While the instructors in staff development or the in-service education department assume responsibility for the general orientation of all new nurses, it is the responsibility of the head nurses to develop an individualized orientation plan for each new nurse assigned to their units. If teaching new diabetics, CPR, and administering medications by IV push are identified by your new graduate, Sue, as the nursing functions which she is not ready to do, then these functions need to become a part of her individualized orientation plan. As her head nurse, then, your diagnosis of her level for these specific nursing functions would be at low readiness (R1), and you have the highest probability of effectively communicating with her and supervising her by using "telling" (S1) to define her role in these activities, telling her what to do, how to do it, when, and where. Once you have diagnosed the new nurse's readiness level, you can draw a vertical line from that point on the readiness continuum up to intersect the curved line in the leadership style area of the Situational Leadership model.[6] See Figure 13–1.

While the leadership style, "telling" (S1) is high in task or directive behavior, it is low in relationship or supportive behavior. This does *not* mean that you stop *all* of your psychologically supportive behaviors, and it does not mean that you behave in an unsupportive way toward Sue. For example, it is unsupportive in such a situation for you to ask a new graduate which school he or she graduated from or comment about how inept new graduates are these days. It simply means that as you talk to her, you concentrate on the details of the task. You wait to be supportive when the new graduate successfully demonstrates her ability to perform part or all of the task. Your job as head nurse is to increase the maturity level of your new nurses. Behavioral modification theory is applicable here. You wait until you see the behavior you want developed; then you show support by complimenting the new graduate to encourage repetition of the successful behavior. You positively reinforce the desired behavior with your approving and affirming communication behaviors.

The primary method of changing the maturity level of followers or nursing staff is through the use of behavior modification theory. It provides a method of getting cooperation and compliance when you need to work through others to accomplish a task. This theory states that

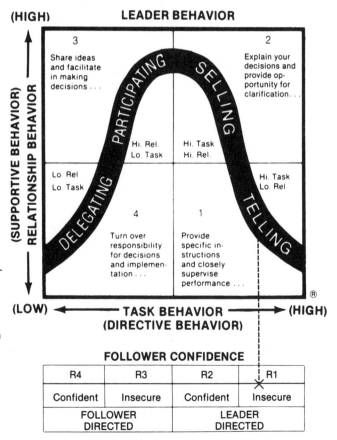

Figure 13–1. To determine the appropriate leader style to use for a follower diagnosed as low (R1) on the readiness continuum, draw a line at right angles from the continuum line to the curved line in the leader behavior styles portion of the model. In this example, using the telling (S1) style has the highest probability of being successful. *(From Hersey, P., Situational leadership: The other 59 minutes. Escondido, Calif.: Warner Books, 1984, p. 69, with permission.)*

one can modify and shape behavior observed in another by use of mutually acceptable goals and interpersonal rewards to develop a desired behavior.

> Its basic premise is that *behavior is controlled by its immediate consequences*. Behavior can be increased, suppressed, or decreased by what happens immediately after it occurs. Because probabilities are difficult to work with, we use observations of the future frequency of the behavior as a measure of the effectiveness of a consequence. Five of the major concepts of reinforcement that help one to make behavioral changes are: positive reinforcement, punishment, negative reinforcement, extinction, and schedule of reinforcement.[7]

To increase the likelihood that a behavior will be repeated, you need to respond positively *immediately* after you observe the least indication of the desired behavior. It is assumed, of course, that both you and your new nurse have the same goal—development of the new nurse's nursing capabilities so that he or she can function to potential in the role of staff nurse.*

It is also assumed that when you, as head nurse, behave in positive, psychologically supportive ways by affirming his or her statements and praising behavior, you will be satisfying the new graduate's need for approval and achievement. Herzberg's work on the concept of job satisfaction supports this idea. In his research, Herzberg found the communication between the employee and the immediate supervisor consistently ranked very high as contributing to the satisfying factors that he defined as motivators.[8] According to Herzberg's theory, having you, as immediate supervisor, recognize a new nurse such as Sue for her good performances and to express appreciation for her accomplishments tends to have a strong positive effect upon her. The effect is an increased feeling of competence and self-confidence. It also contributes to her sense of autonomy, and soon your praise will not be enough; the new graduate will want more responsibility.[9] (See also Chapter 5 on motivating.) Eventually you will want to give the new nurse such as Sue more responsibility, a little at a time, so that it is possible for her to continue to perform well and consistently experience being successful.

Some may critique Herzberg's work by noting that the subjects of his research were a group of accountants (and men); his theory may not be applicable to a group of nurses (predominantly women). To some extent, this question of applicability is justified. There is some evidence that nurses' job satisfaction differs from non-nurses' (and perhaps men's) in that it is more closely related to: "autonomy, supervisory style, interpersonal relationships with superiors and coworkers, organizational climate and self-esteem/recognition."[10] Downs and Hazen investigated one integrative construct, "communication satisfaction," which summarized those aspects of job satisfaction relevant to communication into two variables: information flow variables and relationship or perceptual variables.[11] Factor analyses of 88 communication items resulted in the identification of eight dimensions of this construct, plus the ninth one added later by Pincus.

(1) *Communication climate* (general satisfaction with communication environment)
(2) *Supervisor communication* (immediate supervisor's openness to ideas, guidance in solving job-related problems)

---

*If the new employee does not want the same goal as the manager, then we would be concerned about the ethics involved or the potential of antisocial, manipulative behavior on the part of the manager. This is not the case here, however. We are suggesting managers use behavior modification to help employees become more effective in their jobs, which is a socially desirable goal. Later in this chapter, we also apply behavior modification theory to help managers deal with problem employees and provide constructive discipline. For additional information, see Hersey & Blanchard, *Management of organizational behavior,* pp. 11–15, 234–280.

(3) *Media quality* (written and verbal channels, e.g., meetings, memos, newsletters)

(4) *Horizontal communication* (e.g., grapevine, informal communication with peers)

(5) *Organizational integration* (information relevant to performing job)

(6) *Personal feedback* (information about performance and how performance is judged)

(7) *Organizational perspective* (information about organization as a whole, e.g., policies, procedures, competition)

(8) *Subordinate communication* (refers to supervisors only, e.g., response to downward communication)

(9) *Upper management communication* (top management's direct communication with employees, listening to employees, credibility)[12]

Basing his work on the research of Thiry,[13] and of Downs and Hazen, Pincus investigated the influence of communication upon job satisfaction and job performance. The major finding of this study:

> . . . clearly suggests that a nurse's communication with her/his immediate supervisor is the primary influence on that nurse's job satisfaction *and* job performance . . . This study argues for the need to establish a positive communication atmosphere within the nursing department and the hospital . . . Nurses reported a strong need for frequent, constructive personal feedback on how they are doing their jobs . . . One suggestion . . . for nurse managers . . . [is that] they should receive training in how to administer performance appraisals effectively . . . And, as this study demonstrates, nurses who perceive their communication with other organizational members positively will be more satisfied with their work, co-workers, and supervisors, and perform their jobs more effectively.[14]

Wolf, a nursing administrator, suggests a decentralized organizational structure and participative management styles are appropriate to developing this positive communication atmosphere.[15]

In communicating in "telling" (S1) with the low-readiness (R1) new graduate, you may feel as if you are conveying a dehumanizing attitude. To some extent, this is needed. For example, you will be doing most of the talking, so the communication can be described as monological. You will be giving directives, making judgments, and dealing with categories and parts of the new graduate as a person. To some degree a new graduate such as Sue will be isolated from the rest of the nursing staff as she progresses through the orientation period and she will feel a little helpless and powerless, too, until she becomes familiar with her new environment. You can be humanizing in your attitude, however, by demonstrating a caring, positive regard for her as a person of many dimensions of commitment and responsibility, and showing respect for her as another capable human being and as a new colleague in nursing.

Remember, however, that it is the new graduate, not you, who ultimately decides whether you are "coming across" as humanizing or dehumanizing. As a general principle:

> *To the degree that you are perceived by the recipient of your communication behaviors as being humanizing (or dehumanizing), you are being humanizing (or dehumanizing), whether or not you are intending to be humanizing (or dehumanizing).*

This principle can explain those times you have sincerely intended being humanizing (nice, kind, or sympathetic,) to someone you like or admire, but to your amazement, instead of something approximating a friendly "thank you," you receive a scathing remark in return. Such responses seem to arise from the needs, expectations, or some other internal state of the recipient. If this person is a new graduate or employee, it may be due to anxiety; according to Rothenberg, anger arises from anxiety.[16] This is the way human beings are. In operationalizing humanization as a concept, there are a number of problems in conducting research that Howard has noted.

> How do we judge actions that are defined by recipients as real but are false by other measurements? If a practitioner feels neutral toward a given patient, but the patient feels loved by the practitioner, how do we determine whether the provider's behavior is humanizing or dehumanizing in its consequences?[17]

Basically, it is your perception of human beings that is important, and how you value humanity is reflected in how you treat each individual.[18]

The patterns of interaction of Humanistic Nursing Communication theory are *communing, asserting, confronting, conflicting,* and *separating. Communing* probably is not appropriate or expected when relating in the "telling" (S1) leadership style to a new graduate or new employee who is at R1, or low readiness. With the title of head nurse, you are perceived by the nurse at (R1) low readiness as having *coercive* power; this power is based on fear. You can demote or fire this nurse, so the new staff nurse will follow your directions because it may cost too much to misbehave.[19]

You will need to make *assertive* statements about what is expected of the new graduate like Sue in performance. Errors or misunderstandings need to be *confronted.* A negative, defensive, or angry response can also be confronted, such as the scathing remark mentioned above. You can attempt to influence the individual, *if* you think maintaining the relationship is worth the effort, and for a new graduate and a new employee, you will probably value the individual's potential contribution. In the confrontation of the scathing remark, for example, you might say: "You sound as if you think I am trying to offend or punish you, and I am wondering why you think that of me." If it is important to you and your relationship with this person, then the miscommunication needs to be sorted out for the relationship to be maintained.

You will need to resolve *conflicting* beliefs and behaviors of new graduates or employees as early as possible. By the nature of their role as an orientee, however, they will probably be listening and asking questions for clarification. As head nurse, your position within the agency gives you connection power: you know important people within the agency, and perhaps you also know people outside the agency who are significant to this new nurse. The new graduate or nurse at the (R1) low level of readiness will want you to think and speak well of him or her.[20]

Finally, *separation* may occur in two ways. First, if the graduate such as Sue responds to your directions and to your influence to modify her behavior, then you have the power to reward her appropriate behavior changes through increased relationship behavior, praise, and support, that is, *reward power.* You decrease the amount of direct supervision in relation to that one specific task; you separate yourself from her to allow her a little more independence and room to grow. Second, however, if Sue's performance is very unsatisfactory before the end of the orientation period, then a different separation may be necessary; you may decide to use your coercive power by ending the nurse's association with the agency, that is, fire her. She may feel so uncomfortable that she will resign, initiating the separation herself.[21]

Style 2: Selling

The second leadership style of Situational Leadership, *selling* (S2) is defined as two-way communication in which the leader decreases the amount of task or directing behavior and increases the amount of relationship or supportive behaviors. This leadership style is most appropriate for you, when you are the head nurse, to use for the follower or nurse whom you have diagnosed as being at (R2) low-moderate level of readiness, who is still unable but willing with supervision or unable but confident that he or she can perform. You will need to provide less direction, and you will want to increase your relationship or supportive behavior to reward and reinforce the nurse's willingness and build confidence.[22]

The selling (S2) style is most appropriate for you to use with the new graduate like Sue who has been instructed through the in-service or staff development department, and who is now ready to participate in teaching a new diabetic, administering CPR, or administering a medication by IV push. This nurse, Sue, may still need the supervision of you or one of your staff until she develops the ability and confidence to function independently. The two-way communication occurs, and although she still needs your direction, both you and the new graduate need to participate in a dialogue about the logical, social-psychological, scientific, administrative, or biomedical reasons for performing the nursing function or procedure this or that particular way. You persuade or "sell" her on the way nursing is practiced at your agency. You need to discuss her orientation: "That's not the way we were taught at my school of nursing." You need to convince her this different way of doing is acceptable nursing practice and provide appropriate arguments to support your statements . . . without, we might add, being demeaning in any manner with respect to her school of nursing, faculty, or quality of her education.

Once you have diagnosed the new nurse's (R2) low-moderate readiness level, you can draw a vertical line from that point on the readiness continuum up to the curved line in the leadership style area of the model, as demonstrated in Figure 13–1.

The attitudes of Humanistic Nursing Communication theory that are appropriate for communicating with the (R2) low-moderate readiness nurse follower will continue to seem more dehumanizing than humanizing. In the dialogues with the new graduate nurse employee, however, you will begin showing more humanizing attitudes than previously. For example, by engaging in the dialogue of selling, you will demonstrate more positive regard, caring, and equality, and there will be a decrease in the dehumanizing attitudes, such as tolerance, role-playing, or powerlessness.

The patterns of interaction of Humanistic Nursing Communication theory include *asserting, confronting, conflicting,* and *separating.* As with (R1) low readiness, *communing* is probably not to be expected in communicating with the (R2) low-moderate-readiness staff nurse. The element of trust, however, of each for the other increases somewhat at this level.

In communicating with Sue as the (R2) low-moderate-readiness nurse, you will continue using asserting, confronting, conflicting, and separating in much the same manner as in communicating with the (R1) low-readiness nurse. You will find, however you will be less definite and forceful in your statements. As her head nurse, you are still perceived as being very powerful, but the source of your power base has changed. You are no longer seen by the (R2) low-moderate-readiness level new nurse as coercive, but, in addition to connection power, you are also perceived as possessing *legitimate* power. This means that, because you are authorized to function as a head nurse, you are perceived as having every right to expect compliance and cooperation from her and other nurses, and that you expect even your suggestions to be followed. The new nurse will listen to you and follow your directions because you are the head nurse, a person in an important management position in the organizational structure of the hospital or agency.[23] In selling, the pattern of interaction you will probably be using most is "conflicting" as you resolve conflicting perspectives or differences about how particular aspects of nursing are practiced at this agency. The *separation* pattern of interaction will be used as you continue to separate yourself from her to allow her more independence. Separation in the sense of firing her is becoming less of a probability as her individualized orientation progresses.

Style 3: Participating

The third leadership style of Situational Leadership, *participating* (S3) is also a two-way communication that is high in relationship or supportive behaviors and low in task or directive behaviors. This leadership style is facilitative, and it is appropriate for the follower who is at the high-moderate level of readiness. The new nurse, Sue, at this level is able to do the nursing functions, but still feels insecure without some supervision, or she may be able but unwilling or uncommitted to function on her own. One distinguishing feature of participating is that the directing is now done by the follower, not the leader. As head nurse, you support and encourage Sue to make the decisions and to be self-directive.[24] (See Fig. 13–2.) Once you have diagnosed her new readiness level, the relationship can be charted between this high-moderate level of readiness and the leader behavior curve on the model in a manner similar to that shown in Figure 13–1.

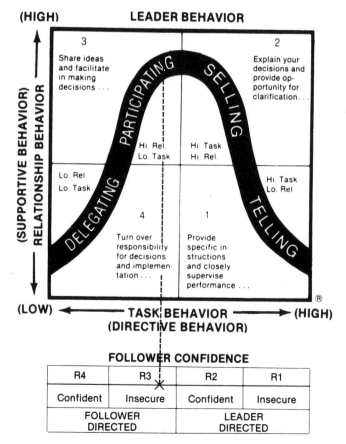

Figure 13–2. For R3 on the readiness continuum, a line is drawn from the readiness continuum line upward to intersect with the Leader Behavior, participating (S3). Note that the task is "follower directed" for both R3 and R4. *(From Hersey, P., Situational leadership: The other 59 minutes. Escondido, Calif.: Warner Books, 1984, p. 69, with permission.)*

At the high-moderate readiness level (R3), the new graduate nurse, Sue, has mastered the knowledge and skills of teaching diabetics, CPR, or "IV pushes," but now needs to develop judgment about the particulars or details of each nursing function. She needs experience in decision making. For example, she will need to think about what time of the day and in what place the diabetic patient would be most receptive to learning about giving insulin to himself or herself. What strategies can she use to quickly get the board under a rather heavy patient before initiating CPR? For the "IV push," medications that are incompatible with certain fluids must be injected into the IV tubing only after flushing the tubing with a compatible fluid. These medications are also to be given very slowly, in one minute or longer, because the medication can reach the heart and brain within 15 seconds and cause speed shock.[25]*

As her head nurse, you will find yourself engaging in dialogue with the new graduate nurse, sharing your stories of success and failure in relation to these nursing functions. For example, you may tell of the diabetic who was admitted with high blood sugar and a severely infected thigh. The patient explained that he was camping for two weeks, and forgot to pack his alcohol swabs for cleansing his skin before giving himself the injection. He just spat on his leg, wiped it off, and injected the insulin. Then you might *participate* in a discussion about what the available options might be so she can teach the current diabetic patient who likes to go camping.

The high-moderate readiness level (R3) follower or new staff nurse like Sue will continue to perceive you, as her head nurse, as having legitimate power, but two other power bases emerge: *referent* and *information* power. Referent power is simply maintaining a good interpersonal relationship with the new staff nurse.

> With people who are *able but unwilling or insecure,* this power base tends to be an important means of instilling confidence and providing encouragement, recognition, and other supportive behavior. When that occurs, the followers will generally respond in a positive way, permitting the leader to influence them because they like, admire, or identify with the leader.[26]

The information power you have is that of providing information (or feedback) about Sue's performance and how she can improve. This is valuable information for her and her potential success as a staff nurse on your unit. In addition, you, as her head nurse, get information from the upper and lateral levels of the organization or outside the unit. You also provide information about personnel policies that apply specifically to her. In nursing, you also provide information about new drugs, procedures, techniques, and so on, that are relevant to her task of providing nursing care to the clients or patients.[27]

It is at this level that the expressions of humanizing attitudes of Humanistic Nursing Communication theory definitely begin to outnumber the dehumanizing. As the incidence of the seemingly dehumanizing task or *directing* behaviors decrease on your part, the apparently humanizing relationship or supportive behaviors increase.

All of the patterns of interaction are used, even communing occasionally. (See Fig. 5–4.) The level of your trust of the new graduate has increased to the point that you willingly self-disclose information about your own nursing practice, and she responds in a reciprocal manner by revealing what she thinks and understands about her patients and her own practice. The

---

*If the medication reaches the brain or heart in high concentrations, it can result in a headache, tightness in the chest, shock (fainting), or cardiac arrest. When administered slowly, the medication and blood have time to mix and blend so that the oxygen and nutrient supply to the heart and brain is sufficiently maintained for the patient's comfort.

positive feedback you give Sue about her ability to function as a nurse is the key factor that builds her confidence. It is the feedback she gives you, probably covert, that tells you how well you are doing in providing her an individualized and effective orientation to your unit, and how successful she feels.

Style 4: Delegating

The fourth leadership style of Situational Leadership, *delegating* (S4), is defined as a two-way communication in which the leader decreases both the amount of task or directing behaviors and relationship or supportive behaviors. This leadership style is most appropriate for you, as a head nurse, to use for the new nurse like Sue who is at the (R4) level of readiness for a particular task, who is both able and willing, confident and committed. You retain your role of identifying the task or function to be done, and you retain the accountability for the nursing care your staff nurse provides to the clients. When you diagnose your new nurse at a (R4) high level of readiness, you can chart the relationship by drawing a line from the readiness continuum up to the leader behavior curve in a manner similar to that shown in Figure 13–1.

At the (R4) high level of readiness, you will find yourself talking very little to a new graduate nurse like Sue. When a new diabetic needs to be taught, when a cardiac emergency occurs and CPR is needed, or when IV push medications need to be given, you may only point to the order, the Kardex, chart, or medication card and say, "Would you please take care of this?" Sue may only nod and move on to take care of it. You trust her to carry out the assignment without further comment, unless some unforeseen complication occurs that needs to be reported to you. When this occurs or when some difficulty arises, you know she will report to you and perhaps ask for your suggestions. Again, remember your power base as perceived by the (R4) high-readiness-level staff nurse. In addition to the information power base, you are also seen as having *expert* power. "Thus, a leader may gain respect from and influence most readily a person who has both competence and confidence by possessing expertise, skill, and knowledge that this follower recognizes as important."[28]

The one additional characteristic a new graduate nurse like Sue may perceive about you is the wisdom you display, which is based on clinical experience. While opinions vary on this issue, it is our belief that first-level managers acquire this expert power base more readily when they have had some clinical experience in comparison with those nurses who have minimal practice as clinical staff nurses.

In communicating with the (R4) high-readiness-level follower or staff nurse, the characteristic is the humanizing rather than dehumanizing attitude of Humanistic Communication Nursing theory. The mutual high positive regard and respect with which both leader and follower view each other precludes dehumanizing attitudes. All patterns of interaction are used in the (S4) delegating leader behavior style and (R4) high-readiness follower level. The communing and separation patterns become unique in that the elements of trust, feedback, and self-disclosure of communing prevail in the relationship even when you, as the head nurse, seldom see the staff nurse. For example, a new staff nurse like Sue may rotate to evenings or nights, and you may have very little direct association with her. The relationship has been so well established, however, that when you do contact her, you both seem to resume the open communication with ease.

As a result of your staff nursing experiences, especially if you practiced in a team nursing situation, you may feel somewhat uncomfortable about delegating tasks to others. In clinical nursing practice as students and later as RNs, nurses learn to complete their own assignments and to avoid depending upon others to help them.

The "ethic" of team nursing created the expectation among auxiliary staff that registered staff nurses would participate in routine general care of patients "just like everybody else." This teamwork notion failed to take into consideration that many nursing units in American hospitals are staffed with only one or two registered nurses per shift. It seems obvious that in such a situation, registered nurses should not be expected to do routine physical care of patients, care that can safely be delegated to individuals with less training. And yet, registered nurses have been taught that they should routinely carry patient assignments, administer medications, assist physicians, and assume all of the other responsibilities of the charge or team nurse."[29]

Poteet suggests some nurses seem to think that they must provide all of the patient care, which is unrealistic, and, if you count yourself among these nurses, you probably need to expend extra effort to learn delegation skills.[30]

As you become familiar with your role as head nurse, some of your tasks will become routine to you. It is these tasks that you can delegate to one of your staff nurses who is an aspiring head nurse. In so doing, you provide your staff with an important experience, and you provide yourself with a replacement for performing those tasks, freeing you to do other tasks, such as planning. It gives you a chance to identify strengths and weaknesses in your staff nurse, and become aware of additional instruction needed. Poteet suggests that you delegate by providing specific directions, sharing potential problems you have anticipated, and describe the results you expect. It is also helpful to set specific times to submit interim reports and time limits for completing the task.[31] Finally, Poteet also notes: "Nurse administrators who repeatedly take all of the credit for themselves will soon find that their work group has few accomplishments."[32] Why should anyone even accept a special assignment or committee appointment when they know in advance they will not receive recognition?[33]

The most difficult part for some nursing leaders to learn is not to interfere after delegating a task to a follower. This behavior, according to Poteet, is an overt display of distrust of the subordinate's ability. Errors will be made, you can expect that. But Poteet suggests that it is important that you, as the leader or head nurse, behave as if you have confidence in the staff nurse's ability to complete the task successfully.[34] "Constantly looking over the employee's shoulder or hovering in the background creates the impression that the employee cannot do the job; this often becomes a self-fulfilling prophecy!"[35] This statement is not merely an opinion, but is supported by some long-standing, but conflicting, research, which we present in the next section.

Matching Leadership Styles and Follower Readiness

In the 1950s, Likert led a research group at the University of Michigan to determine whether there are differences in the styles of leadership of supervisors of high- versus low-producing groups. His results show that supervisors of high-producing groups concentrated on people-oriented aspects of their task group members. These supervisors were labeled "employee-centered." In contrast, supervisors of the low-producing groups were found to continually press for production standards. These supervisors were labeled "job-centered." Likert's research group found that the supervisor of the high-producing task groups tended to emphasize the task goals and details of what needed to be done, and then gave group members freedom to do the work. Thus general supervision tended to be related to high productivity, not close supervision. See Figure 13–3 for a graphic presentation of the findings. One of the 10 (10 percent) high-producing groups had supervisors who were job-centered, and 8 of the 12 (75 percent) low-producing groups had supervisors who were job-centered. Thus, Likert reported

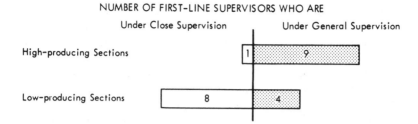

Figure 13–3. A graphic summary of the results of Likert's research. *(From Hersey, P., & Blanchard, K. Management of organizational behavior: Utilizing human resources [5th ed.]. Englewood Cliffs, N.J.: Prentice-Hall, 1988, p. 94. (figure 4–2), with permission.)*

the findings of this study indicated general supervision as desirable, but did not explain the one high-producing group having close supervision and the four low-producing groups having general supervision.[36–38]

Another research project by Halpin and Winer looked at the leadership styles of aircraft commanders and the effectiveness ratings of their crews. They found eight of ten commanders of crews having high effectiveness ratings used leadership styles that were high in "consideration" and "initiating structure"; six of seven commanders of crews having low effectiveness ratings used styles low in these dimensions. As in Likert's report, Halpin and Winer reported the favorable relationship between high "consideration" and "initiating structure" leadership styles and high effectiveness ratings of the crews. They offered no explanation for the data falling in the opposite categories.[39,40]

Hersey replicated Likert's study in Nigeria, a developing country having limited experience in industry and having different traditions, customs, and living standards from those of the United States, the site of the original study. The findings were reversed in comparison with the Likert study. The job-centered supervisors tended to have high-producing groups and the employee-centered supervisors to have low-producing groups. This same distribution of data has been noted in studies conducted in Africa and similar countries in a development phase of industrialization. Hersey explains this conflicting data by proposing that a single leadership style cannot take each situation into consideration. If leadership is a *process* rather than an *intervention*, then multiple leadership styles are necessary. Depending on the situation, then, the leader needs to have the ability to diagnose the follower's readiness and the ability to change the style of communicating to be congruent with the follower's changing level of readiness.[41]

Thus, according to Situational Leadership theory, Poteet's statement is supported by research, depending on the situation. For example, one of your nursing staff may be able to provide excellent nursing care of a patient who is in shock, yet be unable to recognize developing symptoms of shock in patients. Given the opportunity, nursing faculty usually have to point this out to nursing students, and new graduates often need to develop confidence in their ability to recognize the signs of patients going into shock.

Most nurses do learn to recognize shock by the patient's appearance, but some seem to be unable to perceive this easily. It is important to recognize developing shock because the monitors and other technology may not always be available to provide the usual detailed data possible in typical intensive care and other units of hospitals. The patient can progressively become a characteristic ashen gray in skin color and exhibit the classic facial expression of the relaxed jaw, glazed and unseeing eyes staring from half-closed eyelids, arms and legs lying limply about the body, and the torso curved forward slightly as if the chest is collapsing upon the abdomen. Suppose a staff nurse, Jane, repeatedly demonstrates that she is unable to notice the change.

When you tell her or make the diagnosis for her by saying, "This patient is in shock," she is able to provide the care needed. Jane will take and record the vital signs, speed up the intravenous fluids if that is appropriate, notify the physician, actively assist in getting the blood to the room for the blood transfusion if that is appropriate, rush the "crash" (emergency) cart to the room, and anticipate the need for CPR and injection of drugs.

This means that you need to use delegating (S4) when Jane, at (R4) high readiness level, is providing nursing care to a patient who is already in shock. You will need to use participating (S3) or even selling (S2) or telling (S1) when she does not recognize the patient's changing condition and is functioning at (R3) or (R2) moderate or (R1) low readiness levels.

From the above discussion, we can state the following principle:

To the degree you are able to change your leadership style to match the fluctuating readiness level of a nursing staff member as the clinical situation varies and as the nurse's behavior indicates a new readiness level here and now, to that degree you will tend to be an effective leader.

This exemplifies the existential characteristic of Situational Leadership. You need to change leader styles to be congruent with the nursing staff member's current behavior, right now. The faculty of the Center of Leadership Studies state:

> Recognizing a person's level of maturity is critical to the proper use of the Situational Leadership Model. To help this process, the leader should ask two questions about the employee, in terms of the specific task:
> —Is the person able or unable to do the task?
> —Is the person willing or unwilling to do the task?
> The leader who understands how to gauge the maturity (readiness) of followers in relation to specific tasks will find the Situational Leadership Model of immense help in determining the appropriate leadership style to assure success.[42]*

These two questions can be rephrased by asking, "Can you do it?" and "Do you want to do it?"

From a few nurses' participation in Situational Leadership workshops, it has been our experience that nurses may use the participating (S3) leadership behavior more readily than the other styles. This is not surprising, given the strong influence of contemporary efforts in nursing practice to help patients maintain control over their bodies and to practice self-care. To use Participating (S3) most of the time, however, is not effective with all followers. (See Fig. 13–4.) We suggest that what you, as one of many nursing leaders, need to be able to do is use all four of the leadership behaviors. At the Center for Leadership Studies, it has been found that leadership behavior styles tend to differ at various levels of management within an organization. (See Fig. 13–5.) Since head nurses and supervisors usually have registered nurses as their followers, as well as nonregistered aides, orderlies, ward secretaries, and so on, we

---

*Our statement of principle in this paragraph is supported by findings of a survey of managers in a multinational corporation in which Situational Leadership had been in practice for five years.

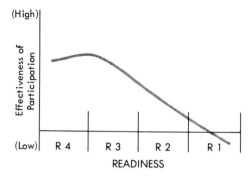

Figure 13–4. The degree of effectiveness of (S3) participating leadership style according to the readiness level of the follower. *(From Hersey, P., & Blanchard, K. Management of organizational behavior: Utilizing human resources [5th ed.]. Englewood Cliffs, N. J.: Prentice-Hall, 1988, p. 196, with permission.)*

would classify them nursing leaders at the middle-management level as shown in Figure 13–5. Thus, we believe there is a need for head nurses and supervisors of nurses to achieve some considerable degree of proficiency with all leadership behavior styles. Depending on how you use your influence or power, you may be able to intensify your degree of proficiency.

POWER

Characteristics of Power

As each of the four Situational Leadership leader styles has been discussed in the sections above, the appropriate power bases of the leader have been introduced also. *Power* in leadership and management is defined as *influence,* and power *bases* refer to the sources or means of influence one possesses. (See earlier discussions of power in Chapters 1, 2, and 4 of this book.) According to Situational Leadership theory, you, as a leader, not only need to know which of the four leader styles to use when communicating to your staff nurse, but you also need to know what power you possess and how to use it.[43]

The amount of power available in any organization is limited. There is only so much legitimate authority available by virtue of your role of head nurse.

Leader power is what is left after subtracting all subordinate power (i.e., collective, legal, economic independence, and expertise), power removed from their grasp by the nature of the

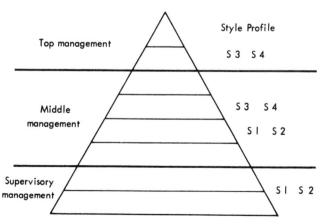

Figure 13–5. The range of styles of leadership behavior that tend to be most effective at various levels of management within an organization. *(From Hersey, P., & Blanchard, K. Management of organizational behavior: Utilizing human resources [5th ed.]. Englewood Cliffs, N. J.: Prentice-Hall, 1988, p. 295, with permission.)*

Figure 13–6. The degree of impact the seven power bases have upon follower behavior increases as the readiness of the follower increases. *(Adapted from Hersey, P., & Blanchard, K. Mangement of organizational behavior: Utilizing human resources [5th ed.]. Englewood Cliffs, N. J.: Prentice-Hall, 1988, p. 208, with permission.)*

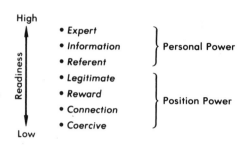

task, i.e., a machine-paced assembly line, lack of proximity, and physical barriers), and that removed by power sources outside their organizational unit (organizational policies, intrusions from their boss, and public sentiment).[44]

This is true of health agencies, particularly in regard to power sources outside the agency: government rules and regulations, insurance companies' policies, and the various private patient care support programs such as the Cancer Society and the Heart Association. As a general principle:

If there is a limited amount of power, then the power you possess as a head nurse will need to be used wisely.

But how?

The Best Power Base

In his review of the research, Natemeyer concluded that (1) a follower's compliance seems to be closely related to expert and legitimate power, and (2) a follower's performance and job satisfaction seem closely related to expert and referent power bases.[45] The results, however, are not entirely clear-cut, so that no one best power base can be identified. Rather, Natemeyer suggests that the appropriate power base is influenced by the situation; it varies. Research supports multiple bases of a leader's power. According to Situational Leadership theory, it is proposed that the variance in the follower's readiness is the decisive factor that dictates which power base is appropriate, and which has the highest probability of success.[46] As discussed earlier in this chapter, the relationship between the follower's readiness level and the power bases can be shown graphically. (See Figs. 13–6 and 13–7.)

There are several sets or categories of power that have been developed. Machiavelli spoke of personal power or love and position power or fear.[47] However, for theoretical analysis, research, and practice, more than two categories are needed. The most commonly accepted set is the five power bases identified by French and Raven, which are the first five listed in Figure 13–8.[48] Later Raven and Kruglanski added the sixth,[49] and Hersey and Goldsmith identified the seventh. *

Which of the power bases you use is determined by your diagnosis of the readiness level of your follower or staff nurse. Generally, you will find the following to be true:

---

*Paul Hersey and Marshall Goldsmith identified the seventh power base, connection power. In addition, some of the original definitions have been modified for use in Situational Leadership theory. (See Fig. 13–8.)

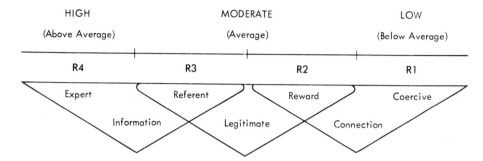

Figure 13–7. The power bases to use to influence followers' behavior at specific levels of readiness. *(Adapted from Hersey, P., & Blanchard, K. Management of organizational behavior: Utilizing human resources [5th ed.]. Englewood Cliffs, N. J.: Prentice-Hall, 1988, p. 216, with permission.)*

People who are dignosed as being at a low readiness level will comply with your directions, those at a moderate readiness will comply and be influenced, and those with high readiness will be influenced.[50]

In order to maximize your effectiveness in influencing others, you not only need to use the appropriate leader behavior style of communicating, but also the appropriate power base according to your diagnosis of your nurse's level of readiness.

---

1. **Coercive Power** is based on fear. A leader high in coercive power is seen as inducing compliance because failure to comply will lead to punishment such as undesirable work assignments, reprimands, or dismissal.

2. **Legitimate Power** is based on the position held by the leader. Normally, the higher the position, the higher the legitimate power tends to be. A leader high in legitimate power induces compliance or influences others because they feel that this person has the right, by virtue of position in the organization, to expect that suggestions will be followed.

3. **Expert Power** is based on the leader's possession of expertise, skill, and knowledge, which, through respect, influence others. A leader high in expert power is seen as possessing the expertise to facilitate the work behavior of others. This respect leads to compliance with the leader's wishes.

4. **Reward Power** is based on the leader's ability to provide rewards for other people who believe that compliance will lead to positive incentives such as pay, promotion, or recognition.

5. **Referent Power** is based on the leader's personal traits. A leader high in referent power is generally liked and admired by others because of personality. This liking for, admiration for, and identification with the leader influences others.

6. **Information Power** is based on the leader's possession of or access to information that is perceived as valuable by others. This power base influences others because they need this information or want to be in on things.

7. **Connection Power** is based on the leader's "connections" with influential or important persons inside or outside the organization. A leader high in connection power induces compliance from others because they aim at gaining the favor or avoiding the disfavor of the powerful connection.

Figure 13–8. The seven bases of power. *(From Hersey, P., & Blanchard, K. Management of organizational behavior: Utilizing human resources [4th ed.]. Englewood Cliffs, N.J.: Prentice-Hall, 1982, p. 178, with permission.)*

While understanding that the various dimensions of power are important to your own success as an influential leader in nursing, you also need to realize that nurses on the average have demonstrated very little wisdom about power.

Power and Nursing

The profession of nursing has a long history of powerlessness. This powerlessness is a covert central theme in Jo Ann Ashley's work, *Hospitals, Paternalism, and the Role of the Nurse,* a documentary of political relationships between and among the hospital administrators, physicians, and nurses.[51] Commenting on the current scene, Kalisch states:

> The critical challenge facing nursing over the next twenty-five years will be to acquire a solid resource and power base upon which to move the profession forward. Ever since the beginning of the profession the absence of such a base has been the most crucially limiting force in nursing's march toward achieving its potential, and economic developments in the years leading up to 2003 will not make it easy to achieve such a base. . . . The 1978 nurse is typically apolitical, largely because her socialization places political involvement outside the purview of professional nursing. The 2003 nurse will recognize the absolute necessity to become considerably involved in the political process.[52]

Contemporary nurses are dissatisfied with the lack of professional autonomy in practice and low economic status in society. "The profession is learning that power and political savvy are essential in assisting professional individuals to accomplish their goals."[53] Power is equivalent to status. Together, power and status give value to an organization's position and the individual holding it. Anything that compromises the power and power bases of this position or individual usually is resisted.[54] Unlike other members of other health care professions, nurses have only occasionally held positions in board rooms or administrative offices of hospitals and health care agencies in the past.

> Most of those other individuals have master's degrees preparation in hospital administration and have had an approved residency in a practice environment before assuming their role as a hospital administrative officer. Not so in nursing. Most nursing administrators with master's degrees are prepared for clinical positions and are not exposed in their graduate programs to significant courses in business, health, or nursing management. . . . Less than 5 percent of all nursing managers have graduate administrative education appropriate to the role of chief nursing officer.[55]

A profession's public image is analogous to its political power; consider, for example, the public image of physicians (since medicare), lawyers, and professional athletes (since drug testing).

> One need only recall how nurses are presented in soap operas, dramas, serials, and other media to get an idea of how they are perceived socially. . . . Viewing a nurse as a competent, knowledgeable, capable professional is difficult for those whose only exposure to nurses prior to hospitalization has left the image of a man-chasing, subservient, obedient, compliant individual with no mind of her own, someone whose most significant decision is which doctor to date.[56]

This public image of nursing need not be reinforced by you and your nursing staff. Thus it becomes exceptionally important that you, as a nurse and particularly when you are a head nurse, know how to accumulate power, how to use it, and how to keep it.

Developing Power

The significance of having power is that it pressures people into following the directions you give as a leader. It enables you to perform the directing function of leadership and management.

The amount of power you have varies according to the position you hold within the health agency, *position power* or, according to you as a person, *personal power*. (See Fig. 13–9.) Position power tends to be related to the followers or nursing staff who are below average in readiness, and personal power is related to those having above-average readiness levels. Position power is usually associated with the follower's *compliance* and the leader's *power over* the followers. Personal power, in contrast, is associated with the leader's *influence over* and *power with* the followers.

> *Position power* is defined as the extent to which you as a leader have rewards, punishments and sanctions which you can bring to bear in reference to your subordinates. This is the authority which has been delegated to you by your superiors. . . .
> *Personal power* is the extent to which you gain the confidence and respect of your people . . . your ability to generate cohesiveness and commitment among the people you are attempting to lead.[57]

Both position and personal power have to be earned every day. As a matter of principle:

> *To the same degree that you, as a head nurse, are able to develop and maintain an interpersonal relationship between you and your immediate superior that is characterized by humanistic communication attitudes, especially trust, you will be able to earn position power.*

Position power is delegated downward in the organization. Just as it is given, it can be taken back. As long as you and your leader (the unit coordinator, supervisor, or the like) are able to maintain an effective, working rapport, you will have your leader's confidence and trust. As

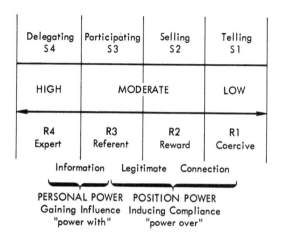

Figure 13–9. This chart shows the relationships among the power bases, the readiness levels, and the leadership styles. *(Adapted from Hersey, P., & Blanchard, K. Management of organizational behavior: Utilizing human resources [5th ed.]. Englewood Cliffs, N. J.: Prentice-Hall, 1988, p. 218, with permission.)*

long as this positive relationship lasts, the upper-level managers will be willing to delegate power to you. Position power, however, is unstable. Upper-level managers will also take the position power, authority, rewards, and sanctions away as soon as you seem to lose personal power or influence over "their" employees.

Personal power comes from the followers and also is earned on a daily basis.

To the same degree that your followers or nursing staff have trust and confidence in your perceived abilities (information power and expert power), you will be able to influence them or earn personal power.

Personal power comes from the followers. It, too, is an unstable power. Its development depends upon the way you treat your nursing staff. You make a few unfavorable, unethical, or unsafe decisions about patient care or staffing schedules, and you can see how few people are willing to support you or follow you. As long as the staff responds to your directing, you have personal power.

Together, power bases, position power, and personal power make up an interaction-influence system. As in systems theory, as one subsystem's changes affect other subsystems, so change in one of the three power subsystems will have an effect on the other two.[58]

Using Power
The power you possess is used when your potential for power is *perceived* by the staff nurses and your superiors. It is not reality but what is perceived by others that is important. For example, suppose a strange man, dressed in a business suit with a stethoscope in his pocket, confidently walks behind the nurses' station, picks up a patient's chart, and begins to read it. Like most nurses, you would probably perceive him to be a private physician and not challenge his presence and behavior. He gives you the impression that he belongs there and has a right to read the patient's chart, a confidential document. In a similar manner, your power base as a head nurse needs to be perceived by others before you can effectively use it.[59] Position and personal power have an interdependent relationship.

> The amount of position power delegated to you by superiors depends to a great extent on *their perception* of how much personal power you have, i.e., the extent to which your people will follow your lead.
> The amount of personal power given to you by your subordinates depends to a great extent on *their perception* of how much position power you have, i.e., the amount of rewards, punishments and sanctions you are able to exercise as a result of management's trust in you.[60]

It is what people perceive that affects their behavior. By implication, then, the way you look, behave, and dress is important.[62-63] If you decide you want to be an autocratic leader, you will need to sustain a high level of position power. If you want to be a democratic and humanistic leader of participative management, then you will need to maintain an ample store of personal power.

Or . . . Losing It!
While some nursing leaders amass a great amount of power, by misusing it, they lose it. For example, the leader with coercive power can gradually lose it by repeatedly making threatening statements but never punishing anyone; the followers decide this leader really does not

have power. The nurse-leader who rewards all his or her followers equally, whether they perform or not, diminishes the value of those rewards; the followers are rewarded for remaining at a low level of readiness. Legitimate power is lost when you fail to make the decisions your nursing staff think you should make or when you make unwise decisions: they will begin to look to your immediate superior for direction. Your referent power is diminished when you give the same psychological "strokes" to those who are being productive and to those who are not meeting standards as well. Your information and expert power needs to be replenished continually by learning new things. If you share too much of your knowledge and information, ultimately you will no longer be needed; everyone knows what you know.

As your power bases, position power, and personal power are eroded, the four styles of leader behavior will no longer be effective. Each of the styles needs the corresponding power base in order for it to be effective. For example, without coercive power, you will be perceived as harmless and unable to deliver the punishment, so your directions will be ignored. In order to be an effective, influential leader, you need to be protective of your power, using it wisely, not misusing it.[64] By definition, principle, and practice:

A LEADER WITHOUT FOLLOWERS IS NOT A LEADER.

Of all the principles we have proposed, this one is probably the most fundamental and, unfortunately, frequently ignored.

In applying Situational Leadership, you need to establish your competence as a head nurse and continuously develop an open, humanistic relationship with the staff nurses. You also need to hand out rewards to those who deserve them and intervene with confidence in problem situations. If you can do these things, you can effectively work through your nursing staff to accomplish the goals of your nursing unit. In the process, you need to develop the readiness level of your nursing staff, the focus of the next chapter.

SUMMARY

In this chapter, two major aspects of directing have been discussed. First, the communication style used by leaders has been drawn from Situational Leadership. The focus has been on the four leadership styles and four levels of followers' readiness. Attitudes and patterns of interactions, drawn from Humanistic Nursing Communication theory, have been incorporated in the discussion also. Second, the concept of influence or power has been defined, and ways in which leaders' power is developed, used, and lost have been considered. The various power bases have been related to follower readiness levels. In the next chapter, consideration of directing continues, focusing on two other elements, *developing* and *contracting*.

REFERENCES

1. Guralnik, D.B. (Ed.). *Webster's new world dictionary* (2nd ed.). New York: Prentice-Hall, 1980.
2. Douglass, L.M. *The effective nurse: Leader and manager.* St. Louis: Mosby, 1984, p. 125.
3. Marriner, A. *Guide to nursing management* (2nd ed.). St. Louis: Mosby, 1984, p. 148.
4. Haney, W.V. *Communication and organizational behavior: Text and cases* (rev. ed.). Homewood, Ill.: Irwin, 1967, pp. 9–10.

5. Ibid., 10–11.
6. Hersey, P., *Situational Leadership: The other 59 minutes*. Escondido, CA: Warner Books, 1984, p. 69.
7. Hersey, P., & Blanchard, K. *Management of organizational behavior: Utilizing human resources* (5th ed.). Englewood Cliffs, N.J.: Prentice-Hall, 1988, p. 245.
8. Herzberg, F. *Work and the nature of man*. New York: World Publishing Co., 1966.
9. Hersey & Blanchard, *Management of organizational behavior*, p. 65.
10. Pincus, J.D. Communication: Key contributor to effectiveness—The research. *Journal of Nursing Administration,* 1986, *16* (9), 19.
11. Downs, C.W., & Hazen, M.D. A factor analytic study of communication satisfaction. *Journal of Business Communication,* 1977, *14* (3), 63–73.
12. Pincus, Communication, 21.
13. Thiry, R.A. Relationship of communication satisfaction to need fulfillment among Kansas nurses. Unpublished doctoral dissertation, University of Kansas, 1977.
14. Pincus, Communication, 24.
15. Wolf, G.A. Communication: Key contributor to effectiveness—A nurse executive responds. *Journal of Nursing Administration,* 1986, *16* (9), 26–28.
16. Rothenberg, A. On anger. *American Journal of Psychiatry,* 1971, *128* (4), 454–460.
17. Howard, J. Humanization and dehumanization of health care: A conceptual view. In J. Howard, & A. Strauss (Eds.). *Humanizing health care*. New York: Wiley, 1975, p. 89.
18. Duldt, B.W., Giffin, K., & Patton, B.R. *Interpersonal communication in nursing*. Philadelphia: Davis, 1984, p. 2.
19. Hersey & Blanchard, *Management of organizational behavior*, p. 214–215.
20. Ibid.
21. Ibid.
22. Ibid., 171.
23. Ibid., 208.
24. Ibid., 171.
25. Pagliaro, A.M., & Pagliaro, L.A. (Eds.). *Pharmacologic aspects of nursing*. St. Louis: Mosby, 1986, p. 64.
26. Hersey & Blanchard, *Management of organizational behavior*, p. 210.
27. Ibid., 179, 183.
28. Ibid., 210–211.
29. Poteet, G.W., Delegation strategies: A must for the nurse executive. *Journal of Nursing Administration,* 1984, *14* (9), 18.
30. Ibid.
31. Ibid., 18–20.
32. Ibid., 20.
33. Ibid., 21.
34. Ibid., 20.
35. Ibid.
36. Likert, R. *New patterns of management*. New York: McGraw-Hill, 1961.
37. Center for Leadership Studies, *The essentials of situational leadership: Participant's manual*. Escondido, Calif.: Leadership Studies Productions, 1980, pp. 61–62.
38. Hersey & Blanchard, *Management of organizational behavior*, p. 94.
39. Halpin, A.W., & Winer, B.J. *The leadership behavior of airplane commanders*. Columbus: The Ohio State University Research Foundation, 1952;
40. Hersey, P. *The essentials of situational leadership: Participant's manual*. Escondido, Calif.: Leadership Studies Productions, 1980, p. 62.
41. The Center for Leadership Studies, *The essentials of situational leadership: Participant's manual*. (Escondido, Calif.: Leadership Studies Productions, 1980, p. 62.
42. Ibid., 66.

43. Hersey & Blanchard, *Management of organizational behavior,* p. 202.
44. Lee, J.A. Leader power and managing change. Unpublished paper, College of Business Administration, Ohio University, Athens.
45. Natemeyer, W.E. An empirical investigation of the relationships between leader behavior, leader power bases, and subordinate performance and satisfaction. Unpublished dissertation, University of Houston, August, 1975.
46. Hersey & Blanchard, *Management of organizational behavior,* p. 211.
47. Machiavelli, N. Of cruelty and clemency, whether it is better to be loved or feared. In *The Prince and the Discourses.* New York: Random House, 1950, Chapter XVII.
48. French, J.R.P., Jr., & Raven, B. H. The bases of social power. In D. Cartwright & A. Zander, (Eds.). *Group dynamics: Research and theory.* New York: Harper & Row, 1968, pp. 259–269.
49. Raven, B.H., & Kruglanski, W. Conflict and power. In P. G. Swingle (Ed.). *The structure of conflict.* New York: Academic Press, 1975, pp. 177–219.
50. Hersey & Blanchard, *Management of organizational behavior,* p. 214.
51. Ashley, J.A. *Hospitals, paternalism, and the role of the nurse.* New York: Teachers College Press, 1979.
52. Kalisch, B.J. The Promise of Power. In E.C. Hein & M.J. Nicholson (Eds.). *Contemporary leadership behavior: Selected readings.* Boston: Little, Brown, 1982, pp. 172–173.
53. Strasen, L. *Key business skills for nurse managers.* Philadelphia: Lippincott, 1987, p..301.
54. Porter-O'Grady, T., & Finnigan, S. *Shared governance for nursing: A creative approach to professional accountability.* Rockville, Md.: Aspen, 1984, pp. 127–128.
55. Ibid., 12.
56. The Center of Leadership Studies, *The essentials of situational leadership,* p. 11.
57. Hersey & Blanchard, *Management of organizational behavior,* p. 217.
58. Ibid., 219.
59. The Center of Leadership Studies, *The essentials of situational leadership,* p. 12.
60. Strasen, L. Power and politics for nurse leaders. In L. Strasen, *Key Business Skills for Nurse Managers.* Philadelphia: Lippincott, 1987, pp. 301–332.
61. Molloy, J.T. *The woman's dress for success book.* New York: Warner Books, 1977.
62. Cho, E., & Grover, L. *Looking terrific.* New York: Ballantine Books, 1978.
63. Hersey & Blanchard, *Management of organizational behavior,* p. 187.
64. The Center of Leadership Studies, *The essentials of situational leadership,* p. 12–13.

14

DIRECTING, PART II.
DEVELOPING AND CONTRACTING

INTRODUCTION

In the previous chapter, directing and its significance was defined, and the communication and influence of the leader were discussed. In this chapter, the directing function of leadership is continued by emphasizing the responsibility of the leader in developing the task skills of nursing staff members and in contracting an agreement with them regarding commitment to performance goals.

In this chapter, the developmental and regressive cycles of Situational Leadership will be discussed, particularly in relation to leader intervention for redirection, discipline, and evaluation. Finally, some of the commonly used combinations of leader styles, *style profiles,* will be presented with comments about the degree of effectiveness typically achieved by each. Examples of directing behaviors of nursing leaders, such as head nurses, will be used throughout to assist you in making applications to your nursing role as a first-line manager of a nursing unit, a head nurse.

DEVELOPING STAFF POTENTIAL

A dynamic aspect of Situational Leadership theory is the development of the readiness level of the followers. As a head nurse, it is not enough for you to be able to appropriately diagnose the readiness level of each member of your nursing staff. You need to devote time to nurture the leadership potential of your nurses, to maximize their expertise in nursing skills, decision making, and problem solving. You need to enhance their self-motivation and cultivate their interpersonal relations skills. Human resources are the most important aspect of all leadership responsibilities and are crucial for the success and reputation of your health care organization for safe, quality care.

> It is vital to emphasize the developmental responsibilities of the Situational Leader. Why? It can be summed up in the saying . . . Give people a fish and they can eat for a day; teach people how to fish and they will eat for a lifetime. It isn't enough to simply provide the appropriate amounts of guidance and support for a given level of readiness. Situational Leaders develop the competence and commitment of their people so they're self-motivated rather than dependent on others for direction and guidance.[1]

A significant aspect of the directing function of your leadership role as head nurse is maximizing the potential of each of your nursing staff members.

That people want to grow and achieve is supported by several theories. (See discussion of theories in Chapter 5.) Maslow's motivation theory stresses growth from one need level to the next higher level. Herzberg's two-factor theory of motivation is based on job-satisfying (motivating versus hygienic or maintenance) factors that emphasize the need for recognition, achievement, challenging work, and increased responsibility as motivating and contributing to job satisfaction. In fact, it has been reported that interpersonal relationships, recognition, and achievement rank very high as job satisfaction for nurses. McClelland's achievement need theory and Mead's role theory also support the idea of an innate drive toward growth and development. We believe you will find most of your nursing staff members interested in having you direct their growth and development, especially if you go about it with an attitude of trust and an expectation that they will perform well.

In discussion of Likert's research (see Chapters 5 and 13), conflicting results are noted. While most of the high producing groups had supervisors who were employee-centered, some high-producing groups had job-centered supervisors. Employee-centered supervisors tend to have high-producing groups. Further investigation revealed that these high-producing followers were primarily responding to their supervisor's trusting attitude and high expectations of them; so their performance was high as they lived up to their boss's expectations of them.[2-3]

> The way managers treat their subordinates is subtly influenced by what they expect of them. If a manager's expectations are high, productivity is likely to be excellent. If his expectations are low, productivity is likely to be poor. It is as though there were a law that caused a subordinate's performance to rise or fall to meet his manager's expectations.[4]

This is *labeling,* a crucial process in mentoring or developing others.

Labeling consists of one or more people associating a symbol with a person. This process covertly carries with it an evaluative and a behavioral dimension.

> The way we use symbols tends to influence the way we perceive and evaluate others. Thus, evaluation is involved when one is labeled smart, dumb, a real neat person, or a "ding bat." Moreover, labeling also serves to identify expected behavior; others know what to expect, for instance, when one is labeled a "ding bat." The person so labeled knows how she may behave; in fact, the person tends to live up to her label.[5]

There is strong research support for the influence of the labeling effect upon performance.[6-9] Rosenthal popularized the concept by moving experiments from the laboratory to the field, demonstrating repeatedly the positive and negative behavioral effects of labeling by teachers upon children's learning.[10,11] Teachers' nonverbal communication is an important factor in the labeling process. This includes increased eye contact, relaxed body, frequent smiling, and being close in proximity. Verbal cues include agreement in attitudes, beliefs, and opinions, as well as providing realistic feedback involving reinforcement of expected behavior or performance. Generally, those children who were able to achieve were the ones who received these positive interpersonal cues from their teachers as well as specific directions for good performance.

In management, when people respond to the high expectations of their manager, an *effective cycle* has occurred (see Fig. 14–1). So the following general principle can be stated:

If your expectations of your nursing staff are high, then their ability to produce will tend to become high.

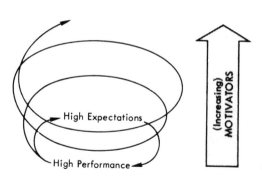

Figure 14–1. The effective cycle: As people perform to live up to the leader's high expectations of them, and the leader continues to reinforce their performance with trust and high expectations, a spiral effect develops. Performance and expectations spiral upward. *(From Hersey, P., & Blanchard, K. Management of organizational behavior: Utilizing human resources [5th ed.]. Englewood Cliffs, N. J.: Prentice-Hall, 1988, p. 232. Reprinted with permission.)*

The opposite tends to be true also. If you tell them what to do with little concern for their feelings or respect for their ideas, then your nursing staff will just do what they *have* to do to meet minimum job standards, and do it with an attitude of resentment, too. With continued communication of distrust and low expectations on your part, an *ineffective cycle* develops (see Fig. 14–2). Once either of these cycles has started between you and your nurses, the interpersonal climate continues to move or spiral; the situation will tend to get better or worse; things usually do not stand still.

> If this downward spiraling continues long enough, the cycle may reach a point where it cannot be turned around in a short period of time because of the large reservoir of negative past experience that has built up in the organization. Much of the focus and energy is directed toward perceived problems in the environment such as interpersonal relations and respect for supervision rather than toward the work itself. Reaction to deteriorating hygiene factors takes such form as hostility, undermining, and slowdown in work performance.[12]

In such a situation, getting a new manager, or in our nursing context, a new head nurse, is probably the best approach. This allows everyone to start off with a clean slate. Behavior indicating trust and high expectations from a new person in the head nurse position tends to be perceived by the nursing staff as intended.

The new person in the head nurse position, however, still has to break the ineffective cycle. It may seem easy; Just fire the personnel who are not performing to expectations and

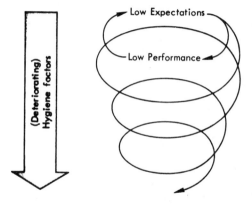

Figure 14–2. The ineffective cycle: As people respond with low performance to the leader's low expectations of them, the leader also reinforces their low performance with distrust and low expectations, so that a spiral or whirlpool effect develops of ever-decreasing performance and expectation. *(From Hersey, P., & Blanchard K., Management of organizational behavior: Utilizing human resources [5th ed.]. Englewood Cliffs, N. J.: Prentice-Hall, 1988, p. 232. Reprinted with permission.)*

hire new people. This often is not available or is not an acceptable option because the nursing staff often have some form of job security (being a union member, civil servant, veteran, and so on) and, given the shortage of nurses, replacements are probably not available. There is an option in which the head nurse can begin by behaving toward staff in a systematic, consistent, and fair way. Situational Leadership theory offers you a way of changing the task-relevant readiness level of your nursing staff by applying the concepts of the *developmental cycle* and the *regressive cycle.*[13]

The Developmental Cycle

The aspect of directing that includes the development of task readiness in nursing staff is an extremely important function of the head nurse. We believe the following principle needs to be considered carefully:

> *The degree to which nursing staff achieve high levels of task readiness corresponds to the degree to which you, as the head nurse, assume responsibility for developing each member of your staff.*

Too often leaders in business and industry avoid accepting responsibility for the performance of their followers, and refer to the Peter Principle: In an organization one will be promoted to his or her level of incompetence. It is easier to say that the job is too much for an employee than it is to help the person grow into the job.

> It has been our experience that when managers have to fire someone or find a place to hide them (this is what Peter called a "lateral arabesque"), or when they are downright worried about someone's performance, these managers should look in the mirror. In most cases the biggest cause of the performance problem is looking back at them. Managers are responsible for making their people "winners," and this is what the developmental cycle is all about.[14]

This is like parents' being responsible for helping their children learn how to behave at the dinner table, how to study and pay attention in school, how to care for a puppy, how to prepare breakfast, or how to drive a car. Children cannot be fired!

One nursing supervisor complained that she had only been in her new position for six months, and she had already fired six people. Then she wondered why one of the authors did not respond favorably to her statements because, after all, she was "cleaning up the place." This is an unfortunate rationalization and excuse this nursing leader used. It is a shame and dishonor to nursing when this type of *colleague abandonment* is used by a nursing manager rather than choosing to help the nurses grow into a broader professional practice. As with any group of skilled and professional employees, your staff nurses are representatives of a select group of above-average people who have been educationally prepared for the job, and they have successfully completed licensure examinations. To hopelessly dismiss such an extensively prepared employee is contrary to social policy and conservation of human resources.

In preparation to initiate the developmental cycle, there are several questions you need to answer. The first question you ask yourself, when you are a head nurse, is: *"What behavior do I want to influence in the staff nurse(s)?"* Is it giving medications on time, following the procedure for disposing of used needles, cleaning and turning patients more often to reduce the number of bedsores, or developing new nursing or management skills?

The next question you ask is: *"How well is (are) the staff nurse(s) doing now?"* Describe the readiness level of the behavior a nurse demonstrates today. How able is the nurse, and how willing? This is not related to educational preparation, nor is it related to how many years or how much experience the nurse has had in nursing at his or her current level of licensure. It means you need to describe how the nurse is behaving or performing today. In order to be accurate, you may ask the nurse: "How well are you doing this (task)?" or "How do you like doing this (task)?" Not all, but most, people are able to respond to these questions. You can verify the nurse's response by observing his or her behavior the next time the task needs to be repeated. This gives you a picture of where the nurse is now; this is your diagnosis of that nurse's readiness level.

The final question is: *"How much farther do you want this nurse's readiness to be developed for each step?"* People learn in small steps, a little bit at a time.

> If a manager wants to influence a staff member in an area in which the person is both unable and unwilling (R1 low readiness level), the manager must begin the developmental cycle by directing, controlling and closely supervising (S1 "telling") the staff member's behavior. If, however, the person is willing (motivated) to do something but not able to do it (R2 low to moderate readiness), the manager must begin the cycle by both directing and supporting (S2 "selling") the desired behavior. If the person is able to do something without direction but is unwilling to do it, or is insecure (R3 moderate to high readiness), the manager is faced with a motivational problem. Individuals reluctant to do what they are able to do are often insecure or lacking in confidence. In this case, the manager should begin the developmental cycle by using a supportive style (S3 "participating") to help the individual become secure enough to do what he or she already knows how to do. Finally, if staff members are both able and willing to direct their own behavior (R4 high readiness), we can merely delegate responsibility to them and know that they will perform well. When that occurs, there is no need for beginning the developmental cycle. The person is already mature in that area.[15]

You are involved in the developmental cycle every time you attempt to teach one of your nurses a new task.

To demonstrate how the developmental cycle works, suppose you hear Mary Jones, one of your nurses, state that she does not know how to apply elastic bandages to the stump of a new patient, Joe Adams, aged 26, who has just had his arm amputated above the elbow. With the prosthesis fitting delayed for about two weeks, until the stitches are removed, you can expect this patient to require daily dressing changes and rewrapping. This will be a daily task, then, which must be completed carefully according to directions or the patient's prosthesis will not fit properly. There will be repeated opportunities for Mary to learn this important task.

First, you decide this is the behavior you want to influence: You want Mary Jones to be able to apply Ace bandages to the amputated arm without direction; you want to be able to delegate this task to her. This is your developmental goal for Mary.

Second, you have diagnosed Mary's ability and willingness to provide this aspect of stump care at (R1) low-level readiness. On the Situational Leadership Model, you can plot a line from R1 up to the appropriate leadership style, S1, or telling, as shown in Figure 13–1 in the previous chapter. This means you will have to tell Mary and show her what to do, when to do it, and how.

The three steps of the developmental cycle are shown in Figure 14–3.

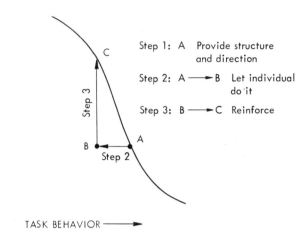

Figure 14–3. The three-step process of the developmental cycle: A, provide structure and direction; B, let the individual perform the task; C, positively reinforce effective performance. *(From Hersey, P., & Blanchard, K. Management of organizational behavior: Utilizing human resources [5th ed.]. Englewood Cliffs, N. J.: Prentice-Hall, 1988, p. 240. Reprinted with permission.)*

Step 1: The first day, at point A on Figure 14–3, you provide the structure and direction; you show and tell Mary how to wrap the patient's stump according to the diagram you provide.[16] In providing telling (S1) high direction and low support, you are not being unfriendly. This just means you are not complimenting Mary before she has earned it. Your communication focus at point A is on the task. (Performing the nursing care, of course, does include talking to the patient and providing information, support, and reassurance as appropriate to Joe's physical condition and feelings. (It is assumed that Mary already knows how to do this, so these psychosociological aspects of nursing care are not included in the discussions here.)

Step 2: On the second day, at point B in Figure 14–3, Mary needs to be encouraged to wrap Joe's stump with you standing next to her, supervising (watching and correcting as needed) her activities.

Step 3: Upon successful completion of the wrapping task, you provide positive reinforcement by complimenting her on those aspects she has performed accurately. Your reinforcement needs to be realistic; acknowledge any errors and quiz Mary on her understanding of what needs to be done in order for the task to be accurate.

As her head nurse, you are making all of the decisions about the accuracy of Mary's performance or the tightness of the bandage. After completing this telling (S1) sequence with her return demonstration, Mary is no longer at R1, but probably into the (R2) level of readiness. Mary has increased in her readiness to perform the task of wrapping the patient's stump.

According to the model shown in Figure 14–3, you need to repeat the developmental process at point C, with the selling (S2) leadership behavior on the third day. This time, you use high relationship or talk to Mary about the logic and reasons why the elastic bandage is applied, attempting to get her to buy into the reasons for performing the task in the manner you have specified. You are still standing beside her as she performs the task, but actually helping her less. You are still primarily responsible for the performance of the task. You are still making the decisions about whether (1) the amount of drainage is within expectations, (2) the elastic bandage is too tight or has wrinkles that may irritate the suture line, restrict circulation, and retard healing, (3) the stump is elevated enough to promote venous return and prevent "dumbbell," or asymmetric edema, and (4) the need for passive range-of-motion exercises to prevent constrictures.[16]

Perhaps you have inaccurately assumed that Mary has handled elastic bandages previously and soon discover she has not. You may find she is unable to comfortably hold the roll of elastic bandage in her right (dominant) hand and unroll it from over the top of the roll, moving it clockwise or to the right around the stump while consistently maintaining a moderate degree of tension on the bandage. If she cannot do this, it means you have overestimated her ability to perform the task. (See Figs. 14–4 and 14–5.) It may be necessary to advance Mary's readiness level in smaller steps. For example, you could show and tell her what to do by demonstrating the complete stump dressing change on Joe's arm. For B' in Figure 14–6 you might demonstrate (show and tell) to Mary the way to handle the roll of elastic bandage. In order to protect and maintain Mary's credibility with Joe, the patient, you will want to do this in the treatment room, away from Joe. Mary may need to practice just this aspect of the procedure until she becomes sufficiently proficient (C'). For B in Figure 14–6, she may assist you (R1 and S1) in doing the dressing one or two times before C, at which point she is able to complete the dressing completely and safely with you standing beside her (R2 and S2).

As you continue to reduce your task behavior and increase relationship behavior to reinforce appropriate behaviors, Mary's level of readiness will advance from (R1) low to (R2) moderate (see Figure 14–7). The next advancement will be for Mary not only to change the dressing herself, but also to make most of the decisions related to specific aspects of the stump care (drainage, bandage tension, and elevation of the stump) after discussing it with you (S3, participating). Topics for discussion might include judging the amount of anticipated edema and the amount of drainage to be expected from the incision or drains. Mary is now able to perform the manual task, but she is not confident about deciding what is normal from what is abnormal and needs to be brought to the doctor's attention. As Mary's readiness level continues to increase, you begin to reduce the amount of both your task behavior and relationship

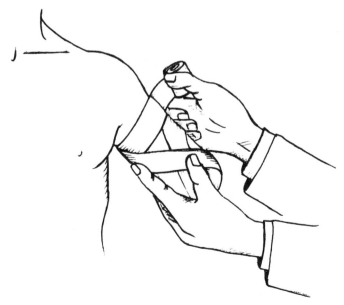

Figure 14–4. The bandage is held as shown at a consistent degree of tension in order to avoid insufficient or excessive compression of the stump tissue. *Graphics by Arch Manning.*

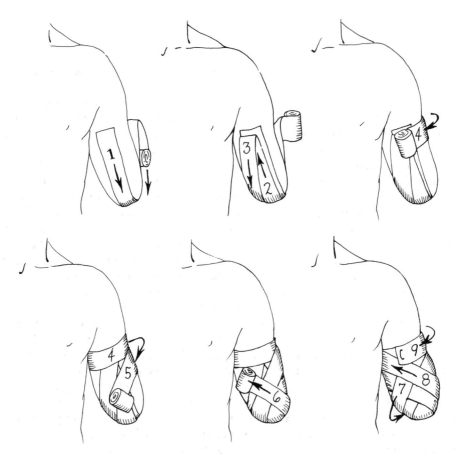

Figure 14–5. The technique for applying elastic bandages is quite specific. *(From Luckmann, J., & Sorensen, K.C. Medical-surgical nursing: A psychophysiological approach [3rd ed.]. Philadelphia: Saunders, 1987, p. 1140, with permission.)*

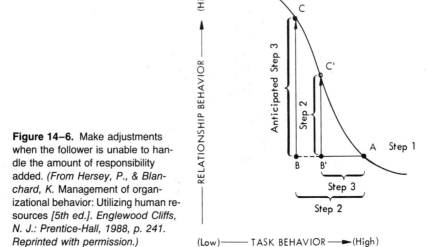

Figure 14–6. Make adjustments when the follower is unable to handle the amount of responsibility added. *(From Hersey, P., & Blanchard, K. Management of organizational behavior: Utilizing human resources [5th ed.]. Englewood Cliffs, N. J.: Prentice-Hall, 1988, p. 241. Reprinted with permission.)*

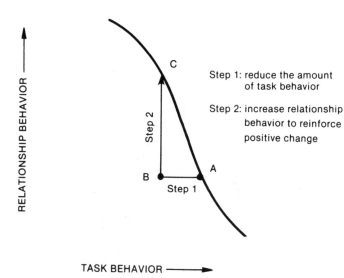

Figure 14–7. Advancing from S1, telling, and R1, low readiness to S2, selling, and R2, low-moderate readiness. *(From Hersey, P.,* Situational Leadership: The other 59 minutes. *Escondido, Calif.: Warner Books, 1984, p. 101, with permission.)*

behaviors. Let Mary begin to make these decisions, reinforcing her when she is correct (see Fig. 14–7).

By the time Mary has reached (R4) a high readiness level, you will find you simply assign the task (S4, delegating) to Mary with no further intervention necessary (see Fig. 14–8). Mary is now able and willing, skillful in applying the bandage, and confident of her own judgments about important aspects of stump care.

In reality, a composite of many developmental cycles are necessary in developing task readiness. Like Mary, people seem to easily learn a little bit at a time. (See Fig. 14–9.) In using the developmental cycle, it is important to reinforce Mary each time she demonstrates behaviors that approximates those behaviors you want her to acquire. People learn a little bit at a

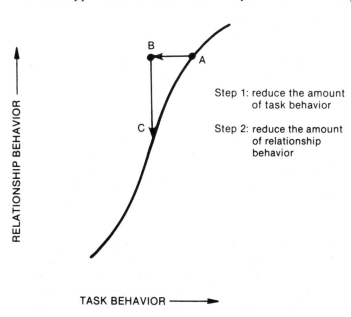

Figure 14–8. Advancing from S3, participating, and R3, high-moderate readiness to S4, delegating, and R4, high readiness. *(From Hersey, P., Situational leadership: The other 59 minutes. Escondido, Calif.: Warner Books, 1984, p. 105, with permission.)*

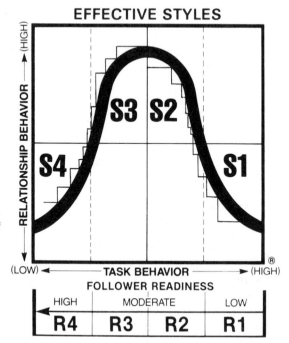

EFFECTIVE STYLES

Figure 14–9. Over time, the developmental cycle for one nursing staff member might look like this. Task readiness increases in small steps. *(From Hersey, P., & Blanchard, K. Management of organizational behavior: Utilizing human resources [5th ed.]. Englewood Cliffs, N. J.: Prentice-Hall, 1988, p. 242. Reprinted with permission.)*

time. When someone is learning something entirely new, it is important to compliment even the slightest progress.[17] This does not necessarily happen in a few days or two weeks, but, from one evaluation period to another, over time you can help your nurses become very skillful and competent nurses. As a head nurse, you can help nurses become successful; you can grow winners!

As your nursing staff increase their readinesss level and demonstrate the upward spiraling effect of the effective cycle, the focus of your own role as head nurse will need to change.

> Through the development of people, Situational Leaders can invest their time in the "high payoff" management functions. These "linking pin" activities enhance the group's performance. When followers can take responsibility for their own tasks on a day-to-day basis, the leader can focus on these activities. These functions include acquiring resources necessary for maximizing the group's productivity, communicating both horizontally and vertically, and coordinating their group's efforts with other departments to improve overall productivity. The leader, instead of getting trapped in tunnel vision, has time for long-range strategic planning and creativity.[18]

As the productivity and quality of care provided by your nursing staff improves, you need to increase your own level of readiness and diversify your own leadership skills. As a head nurse, you may feel one of your staff is competing for your position and threatening your leadership. This can be more than just a feeling, especially when the leader has neglected to arrange for his or her own growth and development. We hope that you will begin to perform some of the "linking-pin" activities (see Fig. 14–10). The focus of your role as head nurse initially will be that of management of the nursing unit, including directing your nursing staff. As your nursing staff's level of readiness develops with the implementation of the developmental cycle, you will find your own trust and confidence in your staff increasing. As the staff develop high-moderate (R3) and high (R4) levels of readiness, your immediate hands-on supervision or directing will decrease. You can begin to focus on your role as representative of your nursing staff in your contacts with other head nurses and with your leader(s). You can be more knowledgeable about what is going on in the nursing service department as well as in other areas of the hospital, and can plan for more effective interface between these areas and your own nursing unit.

In nursing, some examples of the linking-pin activities involve communicating and persuading your leaders, the unit coordinators or the vice-president of nursing—for example, to increase allocations of linens or to consider alternative sources of supply outside the agency. This may be very important to your staff in view of Devereaux's observations about the inadequacy of support services to nurses.[19] (See Chapter 11.) You might argue for administrative support of your nursing staff's efforts in providing a special program they may have developed in patient education or primary prevention. With your linking-pin support, the coordination of patient care between your staff and that of the surgical or physical therapy units might be improved, thus improving the quality of services to your patients or clients. In addition to the long-term planning suggested above, you might engage in writing a grant proposal to a local heart or cancer association requesting funding for a pilot study to test a new nursing intervention. Later, you might write a similar proposal to the National Institute of Health, Center for Nursing Research, seeking funding for a research project designed to test on a larger scale the nursing interventions used by your staff. You might contact a private foundation to help in initiating a special program of care for a target group of patients commonly admitted to your unit. If you do not feel comfortable doing this alone, you might collaborate with other nurses or health care providers.

It is our belief that the following statement of principle merits consideration:

To the same degree that you are able to participate in linking-pin activities, there will tend to be an increase in the level and quality of your own professional nursing practice, as well as that of those nursing staff and colleagues with whom you associate.

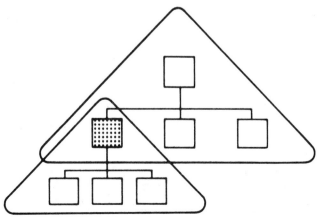

Figure 14–10. The situational leader's role changes from that of supervisor of the group to serving as the group's representative at the next level of the organizational structure. Here, the leader can perform the high-payoff linking-pin functions. *(From Hersey, P., Situational leadership: The other 59 minutes. Escondido, Calif.: Warner Books, 1984, p. 95, with permission.)*

Do not forget to take care of yourself, too. You need to place yourself in the spiraling flow of the effective cycle, as well. As stated earlier, situations tend to get better or worse; things usually do not stand still. You can influence your situation so that it *will* get better.

The Regressive Cycle

There are times when people begin to behave in less mature ways and seem to slip backwards in abilities and willingness or confidence. This phenomenon is labeled the *regressive cycle* in Situational Leadership. It is important to stop this regressive pattern at its earliest point and, as a leader or head nurse, intervene to revert it to a developmental cycle. In order to do this, it is necessary that you identify the regressive behavior and immediately intervene using the leadership style appropriate to this present level of behavior, not that appropriate at the higher level of readiness previously achieved by your staff nurse.[20]

Some regressive cycles are to be expected. For example, you may find the staff nurse, Mary Jones, displaying regressive behaviors by coming back to ask questions about another patient, Harry Smith, who has an immediate prosthesis, because of this patient's return from surgery with a rigid plaster dressing, not elastic bandages.[21] This is the kind of regressive behavior you want to see. As registered nurses, each of us is expected to recognize our own limitations and seek collaborative consultation to protect the patient and provide quality care. Without a conscious diagnosis, you will probably automatically engage in a discussion (S3, participating) with Mary about the comparative unique and similar aspects of nursing care in Harry's specific case versus the delayed-prosthesis method used to treat Joe Adams. Intuitively, you will probably recognize that Mary is not feeling confident (R3, high-moderate readiness) and is seeking your guidance because you have helped her in the past and because she trusts you. After conferring with you, Mary will be able to resume her high level of readiness (R4) and she will be able to provide the appropriate care to the patient having the immediate prosthesis protocol with minimal direction (S4, delegating) on your part.

Undesirable decreases in maturity, however, occur because of high-strength competing responses in the environment. Other things compete for Mary's attention to her work. For example, for the past two years, Mary may have performed at high-moderate (R3) and high (R4) levels of readiness in most areas of her clinical performance areas. Recently, however, you have noticed she has regressed in that she has become forgetful of a variety of details in her assignments. Something in her environment probably has a higher strength in demanding her attention than her nursing practice. It may be an illness in her family, involvement in planning for a family, church, or community event, or the attention demanded by studying for a course she is taking. It may be that you will never know what has distracted her, and as her boss, it may fall beyond your scope of influence (that is, it may be none of your business!). What is within your scope of influence is her level of readiness.[22]

As with the developmental cycle, the regressive cycle needs to be taken one small step at a time. When you notice Mary slipping back from high to high-moderate levels of readiness in regard to several nursing functions, it is important that you intervene using the leadership style appropriate to the behavior displayed. As her performance continues to decline, you need to change your style of communicating with her from (S4), delegating to (S3), participating, to (S2), selling, and, if necessary, to (S1), telling.

> Problem solving needs to be done in a timely manner. The sooner the intervention, the better the chance of stopping the performance slippage. The longer a manager waits, the more directive the intervention will have to be. Therefore, a manager may risk a follower's becoming

anxious, frustrated, or resentful. Even if the directive intervention is appropriate, this may lead to attempts to get out from under the manager or get the manager out.[23]

The longer you wait to intervene, the higher the probability that you will ultimately have to use (S1), telling, as an intervention.

The emotional level you use when making an intervention in a regressive cycle needs to be different than it is for developing people. You need to modulate your voice and control your emotions. Do not yell and scream. Situational leaders can do a lot of (S1) telling when, where, and how to do the task in a respectful, composed, and responsible manner.

> When developing people, you are attempting to expand the present ability of the follower. Therefore, it helps to keep the emotional content of a development intervention at a low level. People often misinterpret Situational Leadership because they think a "telling" style is raising your voice, hollering, or blowing your cool. Actually, a style 1 can be a very soft and caring approach by providing the needed demonstration of how to do things with some hands-on guidance. It would be inappropriate to shout at or raise the emotional level with people who are developing. It could tend to make them insecure about taking risks and continuing to learn in the future.[24]

Even in situations in which you need to discipline a member of your nursing staff, you need to keep your emotional tone at a moderate level of anger to communicate the seriousness of the situation and that you care, but not so much that your credibility is tarnished.

> However, when followers choose not to use their present ability and constructive discipline is appropriate, you can raise the emotional content to a moderate level. This helps to get people's attention and lets them know that you are aware of the performance problem and that you care. It also helps to unfreeze the inappropriate behavior so that change can take place.[25]

Guidelines for Disciplinary Interventions

As a head nurse, you will probably receive some advice from the personnel director about how to handle disciplinary problems with your nursing personnel. This advice, as well as any agency policies or union contract requirements, will probably provide a legalistic perspective. We suggest this extreme perspective need not be used so long as you are able to maintain effective, open communication with your nursing staff. We would propose this general principle for consideration:

> *To the extent that you can effectively communicate with those whom you direct, matching the leadership communication style having the highest probability of success with the appropriate level of readiness of individual nursing staff members, you will be able to maintain open, dialogical communication with individual staff members and decrease proportionately the need for extreme disciplinary action.*

For those times when you decide a disciplinary intervention is necessary, however, you will find the following eight guidelines provided by Hersey and Blanchard helpful:[26-29]

1. *Don't blow your cool.* If at all possible, you need to be quiet and calm, and speak slowly, distinctly, and carefully with an air of seriousness. Behave sternly enough so that you are assured of having the nurse's attention. Make it understood that a prob-

lem exists and that you expect the nurse to do something about it. Avoid becoming angry because this merely betrays your anxiety, diminishes your own credibility, and alienates the person to whom you are speaking.

2. *Don't attack personalities.* Focus on the behavior and performance of the individual, not the person. When disciplining an individual, you need to continually respect the other's worth as a human being and to acknowledge the other's power of choice. It is because you have a high regard for the individual that you are interested in providing authentic feedback so that this individual can choose to change and adjust. In a humanizing approach, try to picture yourself standing beside the individual as, together, you look at his or her behavior and performance problem presenting itself before both of you. This is in opposition to the typical dehumanizing approach of standing in front of the individual and looking at him or her as if the person were the problem.

3. *Be specific.* General feedback is seldom helpful because it is difficult to believe or understand. For example, to say, "Your work is getting sort of neglected lately" is so ambiguous it could be perceived as teasing or joking. Your message and intentions are clear when you identify specifically what the person has or has not done. Do your homework and give specific details. "You neglected to chart the medications you gave at 10 A.M., and the new patient is still waiting for you to give him an admission physical assessment. How has it happened that you are so slow getting these things done?" This identifies specifically what you are noticing, and it also asks for information so that you can further assess the appropriateness of disciplinary action. It enables both of you to develop a solution.

4. *Be timely.* In order to influence future behavior, you need to apply disciplinary action immediately after the poor performance. The timing of your interventions are very important. Avoid being a "gunnysack" discipliner. Some head nurses take note of each incident of poor performance or inappropriate behavior of their nursing staff and store each incident in a file. Then, when the file is stuffed full, they dump everything on the staff member all at once; the annual evaluation conference is usually the time and place the head nurse chooses to do this. The staff nurse usually becomes angry, defensive, and argumentative, and the head nurse becomes defensive and insistent that her perspective prevail: Neither one hears the other. This approach is moving directly from (S1) telling to (S4) delegating, with no provision for development of the staff nurse. By intervening with discipline early, there is a higher probability that you and the staff nurse can calmly and dialogically discuss each behavior or incident at a time, with each of you tending to listen to the other.

5. *Be consistent.* As a head nurse, you need to be consistent in disciplining your nursing staff. The same intervention needs to be applied for the same performance behavior. Your nursing staff will become confused if one person receives a disciplinary intervention for a particular poor performance and others who do the same thing at another time receive no reaction from you. You also need to respond to the performance behavior, not the person doing it. Positive reinforcement also needs to be consistently given for excellent performance. Inconsistency on your part will probably be perceived as picking on one staff member while showing favoritism to another.

6. *Don't threaten.* Some head nurses attempt to intimidate a staff member by saying that if a certain behavior occurs again, they will write up the incident and place it in the staff members' permanent personal file. They never follow through; nothing comes of it. If

your nurses realize you are bluffing, eventually they will ignore your threats. In turn, you seek to regain your loss of power by demonstrating your power through excessive use of some control you have over the staff, like making an example of one staff member by inappropriately assigning him or her to a month of night duty. You need to say what you mean and mean what you say without playing games.

7. *Be fair.* Some head nurses seem to devise a punishment or reward that is grossly out of proportion. Little things are made to count too much, and vice versa. You need to choose punishments and rewards that are commensurate with the deed. Nursing staff resent unfair treatment and will seek justification (and perhaps revenge, such as sand in your gas tank!). When appeals procedures are used by staff, then more people than you would likely become aware of your staff's complaints, and your public reputation is tarnished.

8. *Avoid reinforcing poor performance.* Some staff behave as if they believe "some negative attention is better than no attention at all." You need to avoid being pulled into a reciprocal lock-step response to repeated poor performance by one or two staff members. A leader's attention is important to followers, and if it is important enough, followers may even seek disciplinary interventions. At least they have the leader's attention for a little while. Rather, you need to focus on goal setting and developing performance, making sure the individual knows what to do, when, where, and how.

It is important that you, as head nurse, use these guidelines to intervene and correct your staff nurses who have slipped into a regressive cycle. As a general principle:

To the same degree that you, as a head nurse and first-level manager, are able to intervene effectively and handle personnel problems at your level of authority, you will tend to be perceived by your own leader as being effective in directing your nursing staff.

It is comparatively easy to move people through the developmental cycle, but a true test, an indication of outstanding leadership, is breaking someone's regressive cycle and growing a winner.

CONTRACTING FOR SUCCESS

As a head nurse, you will be involved in evaluating past performance of your nursing staff and in contracting with them about their future performance expectations. By involving each one in his or her own development, your nursing staff members will tend to become committed to their own performance expectations. They voluntarily promise themselves and you to meet these goals.

Management by Objectives

During the 1950s, Peter Drucker introduced Management by Objectives (MBO) as a way of directing followers to reach desirable levels of productivity. This approach became popular, and many organizations have incorporated the MBO process into their management program.[30,31] MBO has not, however, produced the results anticipated. There have been only a few success stories attributed to the process. It is the belief of Hersey and Blanchard that there is a missing link: the leader and follower *do not contract for a leadership style.* While leaders and followers develop agreements on performance goals in the MBO process, there also needs to be a contract between the leader and follower about *how* the leader is going to help the follower achieve the objectives as agreed.[32,33]

According to Hersey, Blanchard, and Hambleton, the MBO process is implemented in the following manner:

> As practiced in most organizations, *Management by Objectives* begins with an agreement among top management on the common goals for the entire organization. At that time, any changes needed in the organization's structure—for example, changes in title, duties, or span of control—are made. Next, each manager and subordinate independently propose time-oriented goals for the subordinate's job and the methods to be used to evaluate on-the-job performance. The two sets of goals are discussed by the manager and the subordinate and a set of mutually agreed upon goals and methods are produced. Also, checkpoints are established. There are times when a manager and a subordinate can compare the expected performance goals with what actually has been accomplished; necessary adjustments can be made and inappropriate goals discarded. At the end of the time period, a final mutual review of performance goals and outcomes takes place. If there is a discrepancy between the two, an effort is made to determine reasons for the discrepancy. With the reasons in hand, steps can be taken by a manager to try and improve performance during the next time period. This sets the stage for a determination of goals or objectives for the next time period.[34]

See Figure 14–11 for a graphic representation of the MBO cycle.

Contracting for Leadership Styles

In using Situational Leadership, the first four steps of MBO need to be completed. The leader and follower can agree upon goals and objectives for the follower, and they identify ways the goals are to be measured. They also come to an agreement about the appropriate leadership style that the leader will use in helping the follower achieve his or her goals.

> It has been found that participation in the formulation of objectives tends to make subordinates feel more personal responsibility for their attainment and is thus more effective than having objectives imposed by an authority figure in the organization. The problem with MBO—and the reason for why few effective implementations occur—is that the role of the manager in helping subordinates accomplish objectives is not usually specified.[35]

Independent Assessment

Instruments, the "Manager's Rating Form" and the "Self-Rating Form," are designed according to Situational Leadership theory and are used for both the leader and follower to independently rate the follower's level of readiness* (see Fig. 14–12). Designed for broad application, these instruments are readily applicable to the head nurse and nursing staff situation. The leader and follower, or you as the head nurse and your staff member, Mary, can compare each other's responses to the instrument, item by item, and come to an agreement about the

---

*The two instruments, the Manager's Rating Form and the Self-Rating Form, were developed by Ronald K. Hambleton, Kenneth H. Blanchard, and Paul Hersey through a grant from Xerox Corporation. The Xerox Corporation not only provided financial support for the instrument development project, but also allowed the authors to involve many of their managers and employees in the development and validation work. Assisting in the development of these instruments were Audian Durham, Warren Rothman, and Ray Gumpert. The instruments are available from University Associates, Inc. 8517 Production Avenue, San Diego, CA 92121.

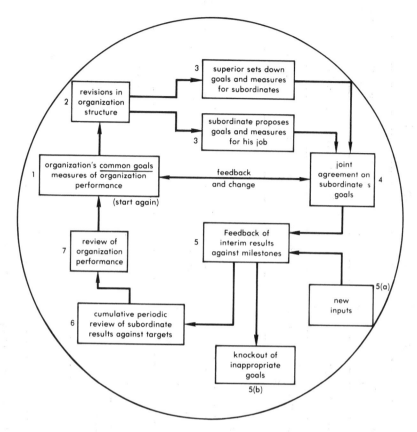

Figure 14–11. The cycle of Management by Objectives. *(From Hersey, P., Blanchard, K. H., & Hambleton, R.K.* Contracting for leadership style: A process and instrumentation for building effective work relationships. *Escondido, Calif.: Center for Leadership Studies, 1977, p. 2, with permission.)*

leadership style to be used with each of the identified goals. This process involves open communication between you and Mary, your staff nurse, since both of you will be stating why each scale was chosen—a cycle of increasing trust, feedback, and self-disclosure (communing) will tend to be established. As a rule, this information is seldom shared between leaders and followers.[36]

Joint Agreement
The leader and follower may disagree about the readiness level of the follower, even after sharing explanations and perspectives. If this seems difficult to resolve, it is advised that the leader accept the follower's perspective. This avoids a situation in which the leader's way is always the one used. The follower quickly decides it is better to keep his or her own thoughts to herself and just try to figure out what the leader wants.[37]

Ultimately, you can expect to contract for a variety of leadership styles that are congruent with the objectives. For example, if you, as head nurse, are discussing goals with Mary, your staff nurse, you both might agree that you need to use (S2) selling, in the event Mary finds another nursing procedure for which she needs skill development. (S4), delegating, might,

ABILITY SCALES

This person •• in performing this objective

Scales	High R4		R3		Moderate R2			Low R1	
	8	7	6	5	4	3		2	1
1. Past Job Experience	Has experience relevant to job					Does not have relevant experience			
	8	7	6	5	4	3		2	1
2. Job Knowledge	Possesses necessary job knowledge					Does not have necessary job knowledge			
	8	7	6	5	4	3		2	1
3. Understanding of Job Requirements	Thoroughly understands what needs to be done				Has little understanding of what needs to be done				
	8	7	6	5	4	3		2	1

WILLINGNESS SCALES

This person •• in performing this objective

Scales	High R4		R3		Moderate R2			Low R1	
	8	7	6	5	4	3		2	1
1. Willingness to Take Responsibility	Is very eager						Is very reluctant		
	8	7	6	5	4	3		2	1
2. Achievement Motivation	Has a high desire to achieve					Has little desire to achieve			
	8	7	6	5	4	3		2	1
3. Commitment	Is very dedicated						Is uncaring		
	8	7	6	5	4	3		2	1

Figure 14–12. A portion of the Manager's Rating Form. (*Developed by P. Hersey & K. H. Blanchard; the LEAD Instruments are available from the Center for Leadership Studies, Escondido, California, 92025. Used with permission.*)

however, be appropriate for Mary's goal of maintaining her current effective interpersonal relationships with her patients. It seems to us highly unlikely that staff nurses like our fictitious Mary would be (R1) unwilling and unable and require (S1), telling, in relation to her performance review goals to cover a three- or six-month period. In dealing with registered nurses, you probably will not be contracting for this leadership style often.[38] The unwillingness of Situational Leadership theory can appropriately be interpreted to mean an ethical concern a nurse might express, as in "unwilling to take the risk of injuring the patient when I think I am unable to perform the task." For example, Mary may be very capable of starting an intravenous (specifically, inserting the needle into the vein), but, because this one patient has very poor veins or the veins are constricted due to cardiovascular shock, Mary may defer or refer the task to someone known to be skilled at hitting collapsed veins. The (S1) or telling style also seems appropriate for very specific tasks, such as bandaging an amputated arm, or for emergency tasks, such as giving the commands during CPR (cardiopulmonary resuscitation).

Decide What Behaviors Exemplify Contracted Style

Once you and Mary, your staff member, have agreed upon a leadership style you are to use, both of you need to explore and describe what this behavior will be. Your staff nurses, such as Mary, need to recognize what you, as the head nurse, are doing when you use a particular style. In addition, this may require meeting daily with the staff nurse who requires an (S1), telling, style when learning a new nursing skill, weekly with the nurse requiring (S2), selling, style when developing judgment, or once every three weeks for one who requires an (S3), participating, style when concentrating on decision-making skills. The staff nurse who requires (S4), delegating, may have sufficient guidance from you by letting you know when she wants or needs to meet with you. As the fifth step (see Fig. 14–11) it is helpful if both you and our hypothetical staff nurse, Mary, make specific appointments before the conference ends, so that Mary's goals will have a specific time frame in which to be accomplished.[39] These appointments provide time for interim feedback, so that steps 6 and 7 (see figure 14–11), cumulative reviews, will tend to show successful performance goal attainment.

The following general principle can be stated about the contract for leadership style:

If the follower achieves the established goals, then the contract for leadership style can be considered open in the sense that it can be renegotiated for achieving higher levels of readiness goals.[40]

Implied Shared Responsibility

Inherent in the contractual agreement for a leadership style is the factor of shared responsibility. If you, as head nurse, contract with Mary for the (S2), selling, leadership style, then you cannot ignore your responsibility to Mary to provide the kind of supervision agreed upon.

Because of the contractual, shared responsibility, if the follower is unable to achieve the stated goals, the leader is considered partially responsible.

Although you may be very busy with other concerns, you need to give a high priority to the contract you have made with your nursing staff members.[41]

Exceptions

Developing contracts between the leader and follower, such as between you and Mary, may not always be appropriate. For example, the follower who is functioning at a low level of readiness, (R1), may view responsibility for a contract as punishment.

> Involvement and participation in goal-setting and contracting for leadership style with people who are "trading time on the job to satisfy needs elsewhere" or who are uncommitted to organizational goals (R1), might lead to less than desirable results. . . . At the other end of the readiness continuum, with people who are "confused about the difference between work and play" and are very competent, self-motivated and committed to organizational goals, mutual goal-setting and contracting for leadership style might be considered a "waste of time." Such people know exactly what needs to be done and how to do it and goal-setting with them might best be done by asking them to send a memo to their boss outlining their job objectives and an evaluation plan. A mutual goal-setting meeting may be unnecessary; a manager needs to merely get out of their way (S4).[42]

Successful application of Situational Leadership to nursing management is reported by Hersey, Blanchard and LaMonica[43] and by Salmond.[44]

Contracting for Your Own Leadership Development
In the process of using the rating forms and developing contracts, you can expect to receive feedback, often covertly, about how you are coming across as a leader. The same instruments that have been suggested can also be used by you, as the follower, and your area director or supervisor, as the leader, to discuss items and identify performance goals for you. In some health care agencies and hospitals, nursing staff members also have the opportunity to evaluate all of the nursing leaders. When such a reciprocal evaluation process is in place, it heightens everyone's sensitivity to the degree to which interrelatedness and interdependence exist among all personnel associated with the institution.

Peer Review
In addition to the performance review or evaluation of individual staff members, there has been some interest in developing peer review of the performance or quality of nursing provided by groups of nurses within a clinical unit or service. A peer review process described by Anderson and Davis consisted of a committee of registered nurses who looked at the way in which the nursing process was conducted within the health care agency.[45]

> A random sampling process was used to decrease the likelihood of a biased patient selection. That is, all wards were given equal chance to be chosen monthly for process review. Then, from each ward chosen, patient names were randomly selected from the ward census that month and listed in numerical order of selection. The reviewers were encouraged to review the first patient on the list. If the patient was unavailable, however, then the reviewer proceeded to the next randomly selected patient. No reviewer was assigned to a patient from the area which the reviewer represented.
>   After receiving the patient list, the reviewer called the head nurse or charge nurse to schedule an appointment to meet with the patient, review pertinent records, and discuss the results of the process review with the nursing staff.[46]

Use of peer review increases the awareness of accountability and enables the nursing staff, individually and collectively, to establish workable standards and goals of nursing care. Used together, the processes of performance review of individuals and peer review of group performance can provide an excellent basis for the leadership function of directing.

SUMMARY

The second half of four major elements of directing have been presented: developing and contracting. The first two elements, communicating and influencing, were presented in the preceding chapter. Applying Situational Leadership theory, the developmental and regressive cycles have been discussed as the basis of advancing your nursing staff through the levels of readiness in order to increase their capabilities. The staff members who demonstrate less effective performance than previously are described as being in a regressive cycle, and approaches are suggested for you, as a head nurse or leader, to intervene. Contracting involves detailed performance review of each staff member's nursing practice and setting goals for the future performance of each. In a similar mode, peer review of a nursing staff's delivery of nursing care is suggested. Taken together, individual performance review and peer review of patient care can serve as a total process of effective directing, the fourth function of leadership.

REFERENCES

1. Hersey, P. *The situational leader: The other 59 minutes.* Escondido, CA: Warner Books, 1984, p. 91.
2. Likert, R. *New patterns of management.* New York: McGraw-Hill, 1961, p. 7.
3. Hersey, P., & Blanchard, K. *Management of organizational behavior: Utilizing human resources* (5th ed.). Englewood Cliffs, N. J.: Prentice-Hall, 1988, p. 231.
4. Livingston, J.S. Pygmalion in management. *Harvard Business Review,* July–August 1969, 81–82.
5. Duldt, B.W. Helping nurses to cope with the anger-dismay syndrome. *Nursing Outlook,* 1982, *30* (3), 171.
6. Storms, M. D., & Nibsett, R. E. Insomnia and the attribution process. *Journal of Personal and Social Psychology,* 1970, *16,* 319–328.
7. Schachter, S. The interaction of cognitive and psychological determinants of emotional state. In L. Berkowitz (Ed.). *Advances in experimental social psychology, Volume I.* New York: Oxford University Press, 1943.
8. Wolf, S.G., & Wolf, H.G. *Human gastric function.* New York: Oxford University Press, 1943.
9. Kiessler, S. Emotion in groups. *Journal of Human Psychology,* 1973, *17,* 19–31.
10. Rosenthal, R., & Jacobson, L. F. Teacher expectations for the disadvantaged. *Scientific American.* 1968, *218,* 19.
11. Rosenthal, R. The Pygmalion effect lives. *Psychology Today,* 1973, 7, 56–62.
12. Hersey & Blanchard, *Management of organizational behavior,* p. 233.
13. Ibid.
14. Ibid., 234.
15. Ibid., 236.
16. Luckmann, J., & Sorensen, K.C. *Medical-surgical nursing: A psychophysiologic approach* (3rd ed.). Philadelphia: Saunders, 1987, pp. 1139–1141.
17. Hersey & Blanchard, *Management of organizational behavior,* p. 243.
18. Hersey, P. *The situational leader,* p. 93.
19. Devereaux, P. McN. Essential elements of nurse–physician collaboration. *The Journal of Nursing Administration,* 1981, *11* (5), 20.
20. Hersey, *The situational leader,* p. 115.
21. Luckmann & Sorensen, *Medical-surgical nursing,* p. 1139.
22. Hersey & Blanchard, *Management of organizational behavior,* p. 250.
23. Ibid., 254.
24. Ibid., 255.
25. Ibid., 256.

26. Hersey & Blanchard, *Management of organizational behavior,* 4th ed., 1982, p. 219; 5th ed., 1988, p. 256.
27. Beletz, E.E. Discipline: Establishing just cause for correction. *Nursing Management,* 1986, *17* (8), 63–67.
28. Marriner, A. Problem employees . . . Poor job performance, tardiness, absenteeism and substance abuse pose knotty problems for nurse managers. *Nursing Management,* 1986, *17* (6), 58,60.
29. News you can use: Coping with pain-in-the-neck employees: (an interview with management consultant Clayton Sherman), *U. S. News and World Report,* 1987, *103,* (24), 74.
30. Odiorne, G.S. *Management by objectives: A system of managerial leadership.* New York: Pitman, 1965.
31. Reddin, W.J. *Effective management by objectives: The 3-D of MBO.* New York: McGraw-Hill, 1971.
32. Hersey, P., & Blanchard, K.H. What's missing in MBO? *Management Review,* October 1974, 25–32.
33. Hersey, P., Blanchard, K.H., & Hambleton, R.K. *Contracting for leadership style: A process and instrumentation for building effective work relationships.* Escondido, Calif.: Center for Leadership Studies, 1977.
34. Hersey, Blanchard, & Hambleton, *Contracting for leadership style,* p. 2.
35. Ibid.
36. Ibid., p. 8.
37. Ibid.
38. Ibid.
39. Ibid., 9.
40. Ibid., 10.
41. Ibid.
42. Ibid.
43. Hersey, P., Blanchard, K., and LaMonica, E. A Situational approach to supervision. *Supervisor Nurse,* 1976 , *7* (5), 42–46.
44. Salmond, S.W. Supporting staff through decentralization. *Nursing Economics, 3* (September–October, 1985), 295–300.
45. Anderson, P.A., & Davis, S.E. Nursing peer review: A developmental process. *Nursing Management,* 1987, *18* (1), 46–48.
46. Ibid., 47–48.

15

CONTROLLING

INTRODUCTION

The fifth and last task function of the leadership process is *controlling.* It is the litmus test, distinguishing fact from fantasy and revealing the degree of effectiveness of leadership. In this chapter, controlling and its significance as applicable to effective leadership is defined, and controlling is approached using the following set of elements: *standardizing, reviewing, rating, reporting,* and *intervening.*

A DEFINITION OF CONTROLLING

This management or leadership function is generally defined as the process of checking or verifying some accomplishment by comparison with a standard. It also refers to regulating, curbing, and restraining organizational activities, and it involves the use of influencing and power to impose regulations. The term is derived from the Old French word *cont(r)eroller,* meaning "to check by a counter roll or duplicate register." Noun synonyms of controlling include authority, jurisdiction, mastery, power and clout; verb synonyms are command, pilot, dominate, reign, govern, adjust, guide, restrain, curb, check, and bridle.[1] (See previous discussion of influencing and power in Chapter 13.)

Control Systems

The three basic types of control systems used in most organizations vary according to the amount of control upper management delegates to employees. See the discussion of these systems in Chapter 6 and Figure 6–1. The reader may also want to refer to Chapter 11 for the definitions and application of these control systems to the delivery of nursing care; case, functional, team, and primary nursing. Graphic descriptions of these are presented in Figures 11–1 to 11–4. Appendix E presents a chart decribing each approach to nursing care delivery according to key factors, enabling the reader to easily make comparisons. These systems vary in the amount of control management has over the role definition and autonomous functioning of the Registered Nurse. The following principle can be stated:

> *The degree to which you, when you are a head nurse or manager, control the practice of nursing is directly related to the degree of freedom your registered nurse staff have to control (autonomy and accountability) their own nursing practice.*

Thus the functional and team methods of organizing delivery of nursing care is designed in such a way that management maintains considerably more control over nursing practice.

Primary nursing, on the other hand, is characterized by autonomous practice and is congruent with limited control by management.

Significance

The significance of controlling as a leadership and management function is that this process assures consistent and continuous performance and quality of an organization's service or product. It is comparable to a thermostat on an air conditioner or heater in that it prevents excessive variances beyond a predetermined range within an organization. As Marriner states:

> In management, controlling involves selecting standards, measuring performance against these standards, reporting results, and taking corrective actions. Controls should be designed for specific situations and should report potential or actual deviations promptly enough for corrective action to be effective. . . . Controls must be determinable, verifiable, and flexible. Alternative flexible plans help achieve flexible controls. Controls must be understandable, economical, and must lead to corrective action. Adequate control systems disclose deviations, identify who is responsible, and recommend corrections.[2]

Although Marriner refers to "control systems," or methods such as peer reviews, audits, and quality assurance programs, we believe controlling is not vested in some administrative process or procedure, but rather lies in each individual manager or leader who personifies, performs, and monitors the function of controlling within a health care agency. It is the manager or leader such as a head nurse who must *understand* and be able to *use* whatever controlling systems and methods are in place in order to have clout and be able to make effective interventions. We can state the following principle:

> *To the same degree that you, as a nursing manager or leader, are able to identify relevant data, understand the control systems, and plot outcomes over time, you will be able to maintain control and tend to make timely interventions when appropriate.*

While there are some differences between managers and leaders, in this aspect of controlling they are identical.

Distinguishing Between Leadership and Management

Leadership and management have many characteristics in common. Both are involved in the same processes, such as planning, organizing, directing, and controlling. Both are concerned with meeting an organization's goals. Management, by definition, achieves these goals by working through and with one or more people within the organization. Leadership, however, in contrast with management, includes attempts to influence the behavior *beyond* the organizational goals.

> Leadership occurs at any time one attempts to influence the behavior of an individual or group, regardless of the reason. It may be for one's own goals or those of others, and they may or may not be congruent with organizational goals.[3]

In considering the degree of effectiveness of a nursing manager, then, one would review and rate those outcomes relevant to the health care agency's organizational goals. In evaluating the effectiveness of a nursing leader, however, one would not only look at achievement of organizational goals, but also at the interpersonal influence upon followers or nursing staff.[4]

For example, a nursing manager may not encourage one of the nursing staff to go for a

BSN or study for a certification test because this would make staffing more difficult; this staff member would need extra considerations, such as specific days off duty. In the short term, then, this would be viewed as contrary to organizational goals. On the other hand, a nursing leader should be personally encouraging and administratively supportive of the efforts of any member of the nursing staff who tries to achieve additional or higher nursing credentials. The leader would have a positive attitude toward such personal development efforts and view this as ultimately contributing to the quality of nursing care provided in the unit. Thus the manager looks primarily at the organizational product or service, while the leader also looks beyond. (See a brief discussion of this distinction in Chapter 3.)

The Effectiveness Dimension of Situational Leadership®

Effectiveness of a leader depends upon how the leadership style of Situational Leadership matches the situation or environment in which the leader and followers interact in their particular context. The *environment,* then, is really the third dimension of the Situational Leadership Model (see Fig. 15–1). However, it is here labeled "effectiveness" instead. According to Hersey and Blanchard:

> It is the interaction of the leadership style with the environment which results in the degree of effectiveness or ineffectiveness. We call the third dimension *effectiveness* because in most organizational settings various performance criteria are used to measure the degree of effectiveness or ineffectiveness of a manager or leader. . . . the third dimension is the environment in which the leader is operating. One might think of the leader's basic style as a particular stimulus, and it is the response to this stimulus that can be considered effective or ineffective. . . . those taking a situational approach to leadership are evaluating the response or the results rather than the stimulus.[5]

The degree of effectiveness of a leader is represented in Figure 15–2. Conceptualized as a continuum, the degree of effectiveness of any one leadership style can fall anywhere along this continuum, and that slice of the continuum is then assigned the four quadrants of the Situational Leadership Model. Descriptions of effective and ineffective leadership styles according to the four basic styles are presented in Table 15–1.

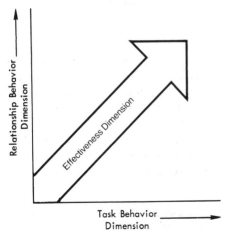

Figure 15–1. The Situational Leadership Model with the effectiveness dimension added. *(From Hersey, P., & Blanchard, K. Management of organizational behavior: Utilizing human resources. [5th ed.]. (Englewood Cliffs, N.J.: Prentice-Hall, 1988, p. 118. Reprinted with permission.)*

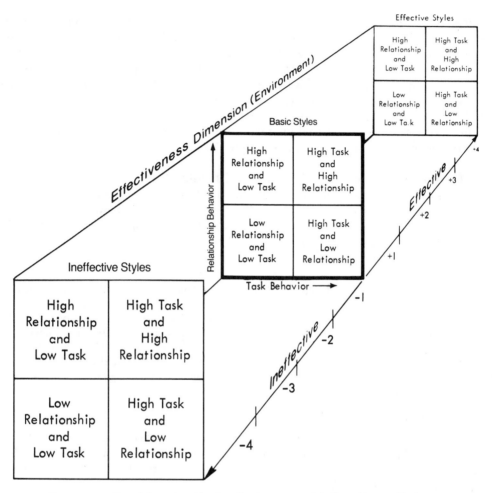

Figure 15–2. The tridimensional leader effectiveness model. *(From Hersey, P., & Blanchard, K. Management of organizational behavior: Utilizing human resources [5th ed.]. Englewood Cliffs, N.J.: Prentice-Hall, 1988, p. 119. Reprinted with permission.)*

Diagnosing and Developing Leadership Effectiveness

Instruments have been developed to yield data about effectiveness of leader behavior. You can use these for self-evaluation, for leadership skill development, or for research. The instruments consist of twelve situations in which you and your follower(s) select one of twelve options that most closely describes your behavior as perceived by you on the Lead-Self and by one or more members of your nursing staff on the Lead-Other.*

These instruments are generic and applicable to any leadership context, whether in industry, business, or health care. You, as either a potential or practicing nursing leader, can use these instruments to diagnose your own strengths and weaknesses as a leader. Repeated use of

---

*For those interested in assessing leadership effectiveness, the Lead instruments are available from the Center for Leadership Studies, P.O. Box 1536, 230 West 3rd Avenue, Escondido, CA 92025-0312.

TABLE 15–1. THE FOLLOWING CHART SHOWS HOW THE BASIC LEADER BEHAVIOR STYLES MAY BE SEEN BY OTHERS WHEN THEY ARE EFFECTIVE OR INEFFECTIVE.

Basic Styles	Effective	Ineffective
High Task and Low Relationship Behavior	Seen as having well-defined methods for accomplishing goals that are helpful to the followers.	Seen as imposing methods on others; sometimes seen as unpleasant and interested only in short-run output.
High Task and High Relationship Behavior	Seen as satisfying the needs of the group for setting goals and organizing work, but also providing high levels of socioemotional support.	Seen as initiating more structure than is needed by the group and often appears not to be genuine in interpersonal relationships.
High Relationship and Low Task Behavior	Seen as having implicit trust in people and as being primarily concerned with facilitating their goal accomplishment.	Seen as primarily interested in harmony; sometimes seen as unwilling to accomplish a task if it risks disrupting a relationship or losing "good person" image.
Low Relationship and Low Task Behavior	Seen as appropriately delegating to subordinates decisions about how the work should be done and providing little socioemotional support where little is needed by the group.	Seen as providing little structure or socioemotional support when needed by members of the group.

From Hersey, P., & Blanchard, K. Management of organizational behavior: Utilizing human resources (4th ed.). Englewood Cliffs, N.J.: Prentice-Hall, 1982, p. 99.

the instruments after a period of training or experience provides feedback on your progress. Generally, we can state the following principle:

When the leader style you use is appropriate to the situation, then your leadership tends to be effective in meeting goals.[6]

(See a discussion of organizational versus personal goals in Chapter 9; see Chapter 8 for the discussion of integrating organizational and personal goals. See Chapter 1 for the theoretical definition of leadership.)

Research on Leadership Effectiveness in Nursing

There has been a limited amount of research on leadership in nursing per se, and Situational Leadership has rarely been mentioned. In the instances in which the theory has been noted, however, Situational Leadership theory and the Lead-Self, Lead-Other instruments have been praised. For example, in their review of 58 published research reports on leadership in nursing, McCloskey and Molen found that none of the researchers had used the Situational Leadership instruments; however, they included these instruments in their survey "because they are of recent origin and are some of the best tools currently available."[7] Their work represents the formal style of reporting research.

On a more informal level, some studies have been presented orally or in poster sessions at local, state, or regional research conferences sponsored by nursing associations or schools. Hundreds of reports are given annually in this manner. Two such oral presentations known to us reported use of the Situational Leadership instruments.

Berhang-Doggett used the Lead-Self and Lead-Other instruments in a study of 127 RN staff in a 450-bed acute care teaching hospital. She found staff nurses who perceive their head nurse as "high consideration (humanistic and supportive)" have greater job satisfaction in comparison with staff nurses who perceive their head nurse as "low consideration (nonsupportive)" ($p < .01$).[8]

Wittenauer reported using the Lead-Self for a descriptive study of 204 graduates of a master's degree program. The dominant leadership styles were Style 2, or selling (60 ss.), Style 3, or participating (22 ss.), and a combination of both Styles 2 and 3 (9 ss.) The graduates' Graduate Record Exam (GRE) scores were found to be significantly correlated with leadership styles: Total GRE correlated with the dominant style range ($p < .05$) and dominant style adaptability ($p < .01$); verbal GRE scores correlated with the effectiveness score ($p < .05$) and the dominant style range ($p < .02$). A similar relationship was found between leadership style and perceived level of the graduates' present position in a health agency ($p < .01$). In addition, the graduates' grade point average (GPA) and leadership effectiveness score also correlated significantly ($p < .01$). Wittenauer makes the following recommendations: ". . . there is a need to develop testing and counseling programs for prospective and enrolled students which take into account their leadership style and aspirations for specific job positions."[9] She also suggests that graduate faculty may wish to consider using the tests for diagnosing leadership styles upon entering the program. Throughout the program, faculty would be able to individualize guidance of their graduate students in shaping and developing leadership styles. Thus the students could increase their probabilities of becoming effective leaders after graduation.[10]

Often such presentations at research conferences may not be published, and consequently have a limited life. There may be other relevant nursing research studies using Situational Leadership theory and instruments. Certainly, the studies cited have important implications for nursing leadership education and practice, and tend to support the application of Situational Leadership to the nursing context.

In a related study, Dolan et al. studied the congruency of people versus task orientations in the leader–follower relationship. Since the effectiveness of the leader is so closely related to the leader's sensitivity to the follower's perceptions of goals and needs, it would seem that the more similar the leader and follower in people versus task orientation, the more effective the leadership. Using RNs in the area of rehabilitation nursing, Dolan et al. had 28 pairs of subjects, a nurse-leader and nurse-follower, respond to a Task-People Questionnaire developed by Sergiovanni, et al. No statistically significant relationship was found between people versus task perceptions of leader and follower. In fact, there was a wide distribution of both the task and people scores for both leaders and followers. The task scores were lower than the people scores, however, indicating the rehabilitation nurses in the study were primarily people-oriented. While replication with a larger sample is indicated, this study suggests a variety rather than a similarity of task versus people perceptions can be expected in leader and follower relationships in nursing.[11]

Controlling has now been defined as a concept and as a function of leadership, and its significance discussed in establishing the effectiveness of the leader and manager role. The next issue is the elements of controlling: *standardizing, reviewing, rating, reporting,* and *intervening*.

Standardizing
Standardizing refers to the establishment of criterion, goals, and expectations that serve as a guide for practice or the activities used to operationalize organizational goals and plans. It is through setting standards that the expected level of excellence is established.

Quality Assurance Program and Peer Review Committees

In 1972, the Social Security Act was amended by Public Health Law 92-603, which requires that health care agencies establish professional standards review organizations to review the quality of care provided to clients or patients on federal health care programs, such as Medicare and Medicaid. This law requires the establishment of peer review committees to set standards and determine the degree to which the services provided by an agency meet these standards concurrently and retrospectively. The review committees' membership consists of representatives of all health care professions and disciplines in the agency. Consequently, the quality of the review process itself has become a dynamic and significant aspect of nursing leadership roles.[12]

In nursing and health care, there are numerous sets of standards that have been established on national and state levels, particularly since the enactment of the 1972 Social Security Act. At the national level, the Joint Commission for the Accreditation of Hospitals has established criteria for reviewing and rating hospitals. (See Chapter 3, Table 3–1.) In addition, the American Nurses' Association has published standards for nursing services. (See Appendix A.) At the state level, most state boards of nursing have developed and accepted statements that serve as standards. A statement developed by the North Carolina Nurses' Association about appropriate and inappropriate nursing care assignments has been previously discussed. (See Chapter 12.) Often the state boards of nursing and the nursing associations work together and support one another's statements, and together they provide direction and guidance to the RNs in their state. Although a struggle, congruency is usually achieved in statements of standards of the medical, dental, pharmacist, and other associations of health care professionals. Ultimately, the health care laws of the states and the nation as a whole have evolved through collaboration between associations of health care professionals and citizens.

At the agency levels, standards are reflected in many documents. The philosophy of a health care agency such as a hospital provides general statements of direction. Policies and procedures provide more specific instruction about what one must do to satisfy requirements. Job descriptions state expectations of behavior necessary to meet standards. Audits, budgets, and inventory control systems are, by their very nature, statements of standards. In the nursing division or department, the nursing administrators and staff have statements that serve as standards of nursing care, and are responsible for maintaining a quality assurance program. Nursing rounds, peer reviews, in-house educational programs, nursing care plans, and career ladders are reflections of the formal criterion statements used regularly in practice.

Informal criteria are also established as you go about practicing nursing. For example, the standard of comfort provided patients on bedrest is reflected in what you do. It makes a remarkable difference whether the bedfast patient is bathed with only one basin of water or with numerous basins of fresh water; the flannel sheet is used rather than a towel to cover the patient during the bath; the top sheet is moved to the bottom and a clean top sheet is put on each day or two clean, fresh sheets are put on daily; or whether you offer water that has been in the pitcher overnight or offer fresh, iced water when giving oral medications. . . . remarkable because too many former patients *do* make remarks about their care. The nursing care plan serves as a formal channel of communication among nurses so that each agency develops customary or implicit standards of care. Similar unwritten criteria exist not only for nursing care practices but probably for all aspects of services provided by hospitals and health care agencies.

Clarifying and Translating Standards

It is the responsibility of upper management, usually the vice-president or director of nursing and his or her administrative team, to interpret and spell out what the standards mean. Translating the national standards and agency's philosophy into the nursing context and understanding the implications for nursing practices is important and cannot be sidestepped. According to Marriner:

> Top management clarifies policies, goals, and objectives, and these are further developed by each succeeding lower level. For example, top management sets the overall budget, but each department then works with its own budget. Specifying goals and objects directs personnel and determines priorities and the use of resources. Management by objectives promotes this.[13]

As the clarifying and translating process moves to the lower levels of the organizational structure of the hospital, you, as a head nurse, will become very familiar with additional facets included in the review process.

For example, peer reviews as suggested by Anderson and Davis are an important part of an agency's quality assurance program.[14] A review of feedback from patient questionnaires provides the patients' perspective of the kind of care provided, and it often reflects the community's view of how your unit is coming across—your local reputation. Your own nursing rounds are a source of important information about the quality of care being provided. Many head nurses we have known seem to quickly look in on each of their patients immediately after receiving report. As a head nurse, you will probably do this, too. Notation is made of any needs, whether related directly to the patient's care and nursing procedures, or indirectly, such as repair or replacement of equipment, orderliness of the room and general housekeeping, and so on. This is a very fundamental review process; practiced daily, it is the basis for translating ambiguous standards to specific situations and for developing and maintaining the quality of care expected.

Reviewing

Reviewing refers to the assessment of all decisions, behaviors, activities, achievements, productivity, and other data relevant to meeting standards. It is analogous to adding up all of a student's test scores to obtain an average score representative of learning over a semester or school year. In management, this involves an array of review processes involving the budget, performance, inventory control, audits, and program evaluations. The significance of reviewing is that it provides a summary perspective of how well nursing on each unit has met standards for a specified period of time. Many of your research skills are applicable because the information gathered for review purposes is typically obtained by using questionnaires, surveys, and statistics. This is applied research, or what Polit and Hungler refer to as "evaluation research," and your goal is to decide how well the organization is functioning.[15]

The Budget Review

Second only to the human relations skills or the communication style of leaders is the ability to control through the budget. Money is power in any organization. Herein lies a problem for nursing leaders.

> . . . the legacy of nursing education at the undergraduate and at the graduate levels has produced almost three decades of nurses with little or no theoretical basis for sound financial

management. Part of the blame for this deficiency in the curricula may rest with the health care industry's tendency to discourage the involvement of nurses in the financial arena. Many experienced nurse managers have encountered a long line of fiscal officers who communicated that nurses need not worry about these matters.[16]

To exclude nurses, who as a group are primarily women, from fiscal matters may be due in part to sexual discrimination, and this exclusion may have limited the development of nurses' degree of readiness for management and leadership. This is also in opposition to the generally accepted definitions of management and leadership functions, and the controlling function specifically. All of these terms include the financial dimension by definition. The budget is the primary basis of determining funds available to provide the necessary human and material resources in order to deliver the quality of nursing care desired. That financial management has been omitted from nursing educational programs is attested to by the following statement by educators identifying essential content for baccalaureate nursing education: "socialization, values and professional behavior, knowledge and nursing practice, provider of care, coordinator of care, and professional membership."[17] No reference is made to management and financial information.

On a more positive note, Poteet and Goddard list three reasons for nursing leaders' being involved in the fiscal life of a health agency:

1. Other nurses depend upon the nursing administrators to control fiscal resources.
2. Nursing administrators speak for the needs of patients and nurses during the bargaining and negotiating process of fiscal management of any health agency.
3. Participation enables nursing administrators to be accountable and responsible for the fiscal dimension of management and leadership roles.[18]

In addition, criteria for the accreditation of baccalaureate and higher degree programs in nursing state financial matters are expected to be included in the curriculum.[19]

Since upper and middle nursing managers make rounds in the clinical areas daily, it is the nursing leaders who have personal knowledge of patients' or clients' needs, while other health agency administrators and managers seldom have such direct contact with the health care customer.[20] This reminds us of Peters and Waterman's recommendation for success: Stay close to the customer.[21] We can state another principle:

As a nurse-manager, you have important information about health care needs, which, when made available to decision-making groups, has potential for being a source of power and influence.

(See also the discussion of influence and power in Chapter 10 and in Chapter 13.)

Another aspect of fiscal management that many nursing leaders are actively investigating is identifying actual costs of nursing services. Historically, costs of nursing services, along with housekeeping and maintenance, has been included in the catch-all category of "room charges," and nursing has been viewed as an expense rather than a source of revenue. As cost efficiency has forced in-depth exploration of fiscal affairs, it has been revealed that nursing is a significant source of revenue. This has changed others' perception of nursing and nurses' own self-image as well. According to Porter-O'Grady:

One of the hottest topics in nursing management is cost accounting for nursing services—providing a basis for determining their value so that they can be evaluated and, in the final analysis, directed to generating revenue. It is hoped that the issue becomes a long-term practice reality. One of the important components of developing the viability of nursing is to determine its value and contribution to the delivery of health care services.[22]

As a general principle, we propose the following statement:

The degree of access and influence you, as a nursing leader, have in regard to your unit's budget as well as your agency's budget, tends to be closely associated with your power to control resource distributions and effect desirable outcomes for nursing.

In our estimation, cost accounting for nursing services needs to be given high priority by nurse-leaders.

Performance Reviews
Usually, once or twice each year, performance review or evaluation of your nursing staff will demand a great deal of attention on your part as a head nurse or nursing leader. Just as the development of job descriptions and standards are to reflect the philosophy and objectives of the health agency generally, the evaluation of effectiveness in job performance needs to reflect the job description and standards. Jernigan and Young have published a set of general standards, job descriptions, and performance evaluations that seem congruent in this respect. These might be used as a guide in evaluating or revising similar statements in your agency.[23]

Performance Review of Nursing Staff
If Management by Objectives (MBO) has been used in the performance review and evaluation process, then the individual nurse's objectives become a part of the standard for evaluation. Commendations and incident reports, which usually mean something is amiss and a serious error has been made, found in a personnel folder need to be summarized and prepared for administrative decisions. The personnel decisions usually involve the following: giving a warning, placing the individual on probation, demoting, dismissing, promoting, giving merit raises, and perhaps reassigning some personnel.

Verification of Licensure
It is also the nursing administrator's responsibility to verify the licensure of all RNs. This is particularly true in states having mandatory licensure laws. In most states, the RN license renewal occurs on an annual or biannual basis, so that one check on a similar basis will identify those practicing without a license. This is a serious offense, and in some cases, the nursing administrator's own licensure is in jeopardy if any of the nursing staff are found to be violating this law. It is easy to understand the forgetfulness of a busy person who lets a renewal date slip by, but the number of people who try to impersonate a nurse is astounding. The nursing administrators, including the head nurse, are primarily responsible for verifying the qualifications of nursing staff members, so it is wise to set up a schedule for checking licenses if there is not an established, department-wide mechanism already in process.

Performance Review of the Administrative Team
The vice-president or director of nursing is primarily responsible for reviewing the leadership performance of the area directors or supervisors and head nurses, as well as other line and staff

personnel functioning in her administrative team. The peer review process as described by Anderson and Davis is being implemented by some executive nursing leaders.[24] In other words, the middle-management nursing leaders also become involved in self-evaluation and peer evaluation in relation to the agency or hospital goals and objectives. In such cases, the Situational Leadership instruments, Lead-Self and Lead-Other, have potential application. (See Chapter 14 and Fig. 14–12.) While it is important for middle managers to be loyal to the executive officer of the nursing unit, it is important that the administrative team members at all levels are able to work effectively together as well as with nursing staff in achieving administrative goals.

Inclusion of the nursing staff in the evaluation and performance review of their immediate administrator, such as the head nurse, tends to strengthen leader–follower relationships. If the Lead-Self and Lead-Other instruments are used, the openness that occurs in discussing the individual items promotes a humanistic relationship. This process also heightens the middle managers' sensitivity to the need to respect individual nursing staff as individuals and as a group holding considerable power. Weaknesses in the relationships or in the leader's ability to function effectively tend to surface early. The process is time-consuming, however. Nursing staff also may be so dissatisfied with administrative policies or responses to their requests that they use the head nurse as a scapegoat.[25] (See discussion in Chapter 4.) While there is some risk, the major advantage is that any member of the administrative team who is an ineffective leader can be identified relatively early and redirected or eliminated before extensive disruption of the organization has occurred. The nursing executive officer can help members of the management team deal with scapegoating. Kelly states the viable alternative to scapegoating is "individual responsibility."[26] A performance review of individual nursing staff may serve to adjust perspectives and attitudes.

As a general principle, we suggest the following statement:

If systematic peer evaluation of all personnel, both followers and leaders, is conducted at regular intervals, then repeated refocusing on goals and objectives tends to reinforce appropriate behaviors of all personnel so that there is a higher probability of working interpersonal relations, effective performance and, ultimately, attainment of organizational goals.

It is the responsibility of the executive officer of the nursing unit, the vice-president or director of nursing, to validate the appropriate qualifications and performance of all personnel under his or her direction. This executive officer is accountable to the agency administrator and the governing board for maintaining adequate, qualified, and effective nursing personnel.

Staffing

The entire administrative team in a nursing unit, from the executive officer to the head nurses, reviews staffing policies and procedures on a regular basis. This includes assessing, selecting, scheduling, and evaluating. Since staffing has been presented in considerable detail in Chapters 11 and 12, our discussion here is brief. In relation to the controlling function of leadership, you, when you are a head nurse, will need to study the staffing history of your unit and plot the effects of any interventions you have initiated. On an agency-wide basis, you may become involved in an assessment of staffing from a broad perspective. Data concerning the comments of patients or clients, visitors, physicians, and even the community at large will probably be included. Such broad spectrum reviews may generate recommendations for charting new directions and solving long-standing problems.

The challenge of burnout and job dissatisfaction, along with concerns about high turnover among nurses, have become examples of long-standing problems. In recent years, the focus of interest and research has turned from the overt causes, such as salary and scheduling, to covert influences, particularly interpersonal relations. For example, Prescott and Bowen found that nurses who left for work-related reasons cited lack of flexible scheduling and head nurse characteristics and behavior (unfair, unresponsive to staff nurses' needs, poor orientation, and poor supervision). Factors that seem to be important in retaining nurses were found to be child care facilities, salary, and promotion opportunities. Respect by administrators and physicians was also frequently cited by both groups.[27]

> These concerns are complicated by the effects of Diagnostic Related Groups (DRG's) and cost containment. As computer facilities and expertise increase, comparisons of patient-specific nursing care costs have become possible between a national data base and hospitals-specific data base.[28]

Wiser decisions can be made when nursing leaders in administration have information available to them. Overtime costs tend to increase with the increasing number of vacant staff nursing positions, yet spending too much on overtime merely results in having to make cuts elsewhere in the nursing budget. Head nurses need to keep overtime at a minimum.[29] Staffing of RNs will be a major concern for you when you, as a head nurse, look at these issues of burnout, job satisfaction, morale, and so on among your own staff. If interpersonal relationships are a part of the problem, you will probably have more guidance available to you than head nurses have had in the past.

Inventory

Staff nurses, are all too familiar with the careful counting or inventory of narcotics and other prescription-only drugs. If the count is off, the RNs responsible for the narcotic box stay on duty until an accurate count can be verified. They are also familiar with the practice of hiding linens, surgical gloves, and whatever other items are difficult to obtain within the hospital. This is probably about the extent to which most new graduates and many experienced RNs think about inventories.

When you are a head nurse, however, it becomes your responsibility to maintain an adequate inventory of equipment, office supplies, record forms, medications, and many other items in order to meet the needs of your nursing unit. According to Marriner:

> The manager needs to determine the most economical level of inventory, as supplies represent a significant cost factor. The purchasing, order, carrying and long and short stock costs must all be considered to determine the most economical level of inventory. . . . A high inventory turnover is desirable.[30]

It costs money to purchase and order; *ordering costs* include the time and materials involved for an employee to order, receive, and place goods in storage. *Carrying costs* include storage space (refrigeration or special conditions may be required), the costs of maintaining records, and losses incurred due to spoilage or contamination. *Stock out* costs means running out of stock. Lack of supplies may cost patients extra days in the hospital or require the patient to be transferred to another agency that can provide the materials needed. *Reorder point* is the quantity of stock maintained over and above normal usage in order to avoid stock out.[31]

Long stock costs are due to supplies becoming outdated and unusable, such as sterile supplies, intravenous fluids, and some medications. *Short stock* costs refers to expenses incurred when a company runs out of an item. What if your hospital surgical supply ran out of Swan-Ganz catheters? This catheter allows continuous direct monitoring of the pulmonary artery pressure and is used in intensive care for patients suffering from cardiogenic shock. The effects of short stock may require that the patient be taken to another hospital, resulting in a loss of revenue for your hospital, or it may mean, worse, that the patient dies.[32]

Major challenges in the appropriate management of inventories in health care revolve around the unpredictable nature of the demand for health care services, as well as the life-and-death nature of some health care services. In managing inventories, it is important not to tie up excess capital in stock or inventory. On the other hand, if inventory of a particular item is used up, the institution's supply may run out. Supplies such as temporary pacemakers and endotracheal tubes may be infrequently used items, yet capable of determining life and death in certain circumstances. Because of these factors, nurses have traditionally stock-piled supplies (maintained excessive inventories) to ensure that they "never run out." This is an important area for nurse administrators to focus on in a cost-conscious operating environment.[33]

There are several approaches to the inventory process, to which you will need an orientation when you become a head nurse. As a general principle, we suggest the following statement:

To the same degree that you, as a head nurse, are able to correlate retrospective data about inventory on your nursing unit, the future plans the physicians have for their practice (new surgical techniques, drugs, skills or certifications), and the annual budget for your unit, to that degree your predictions and judgments will probably tend to be reasonable.

While we have mentioned three important factors that have an influence on deciding what and how much inventory to maintain, we also acknowledge that many other factors are involved. Whether the patient's care is financed by a federally funded health care program or by a private insurance, for example, is merely one other factor. Certainly biomedical ethics and the human factor need to be included in your decision. Unfortunately, you also have to consider the problem of pilferage by hospital employees. In one case, hospital employees (including the professional members of the staff) were searched, including spot searches of their cars, at irregular intervals as they left the building. Hundreds of sheets and towels were retrieved as a result of one spot check alone. In accord with the usual organization policy, the employees involved were fired immediately. As you become involved in making judgments about inventory, you need to maintain a sensitivity to the many factors involved in this controlling function.

Program or Project Evaluation

Some of the aspects of the nursing service department within a health care facility may be uniquely classified as programs or projects. Typical examples include the educational programs for personnel designed to orient, update, and maintain knowledge and skills of the RN staff, and those designed to train ward clerks, secretaries, nurse aides, and orderlies. Programs may be established in order to initiate a change; a special orientation may be established to increase retention of graduates embarking upon new careers or of nurses returning to practice after years of inactivity. In addition, there may be clinically oriented programs conducted by the nursing staff that are designed to educate particular high-risk groups of patients or clients, such as self-care programs for those having diabetes, cardiovascular and hypertensive heart diseases, as well as prenatal care and parenting programs. Other programs may include a range of primary prevention programs such as smoking cessation, osteoporosis, and cancer detection classes.

The purpose of these programs is to improve the organizational operation or the services provided.

> But evaluation can also be used for such secondary purposes as defense against attack, justification for expansion, support for status quo, boosting of morale, personnel appraisal and promotion, and institutional reorganization.[34]

The evaluation process involves collecting data, often using tools or instruments that probably have been introduced in a nursing research course.[35] The focus is on how much the participants learned, how consistently their behavior has changed (improved work habits for employees or compliance to self-care instructions for clients), and how the program affected the organizational operation or services. You would seek answers to such questions as whether or not more nurses stay than before initiation of the program, or whether there are fewer readmissions of patients or clients who received instruction in self-care.[36,37]

Projects usually include long-range grants originating at the community or state level to develop health resources. The goal might be to construct a building, increase bed capacity of a hospital, or provide a new health care service. Federal, state, and private funding is usually involved; criteria for review and evaluation are usually written into the grant proposal. As a nurse-leader, you may become involved in a variety of ways, such as a grant writer, board member, consultant, reviewer, or employee. Such long-term projects are typically influenced by political, socioeconomic, and government personalities and events.[38]

Rating

Rating refers to the process of establishing and applying a ranking or grading to measure all aspects assessed in the reviewing process. Actual achievements are compared to the established standards or goals, and a total grade or score is assigned to indicate the degree to which the standards or goals have been achieved or met. These ratings serve as the basis of periodic reports to a wide range of audiences within and outside a health care agency.

Recognition of Clinical Excellence

Another "hot issue," as Porter-O'Grady would label it, is retention of nursing staff in clinical nursing and keeping highly qualified nurses at the patients' bedside. While nurses easily recognize excellence in clinical practice and know when they are performing very well, the overt and public rewards for nurses have been nonexistent. People working in sales and manufacturing receive bonuses, cruises, or shares of company stock. Nurses in administration can be promoted through the ranks of a health care agency or hospital, and in academic settings, nurses can move from assistant instructor to associate to full professor; promotions are typically accompanied by salary increases and public recognition of their advancement. There has been nothing comparable for clinical nurses to receive. Historically, this lack of overt recognition of excellence in clinical practice has been a concern in nursing because nurses have had little motivation to improve.[39]

Mobility in clinical nursing has meant moving from one place to another, not moving up in one's career. The only way good clinical nurses have been able to get promotions, advancement, and salary increases has been to move into nursing administration or faculty positions—and away from the bedside. The number of vacant positions is increasing, there is a declining number of people entering nursing education programs, and there is an increasing diversity of career options available other than nursing to young women. The shortage of RNs looms before hospital and nursing administrators, and they are considering potential incentives for the job of staff nursing.

One such incentive is the career ladder or clinical ladder. This provides the nursing administrator with a management tool to identify through a peer review those nurses who demonstrate clinical excellence, meeting and sometimes exceeding stated standards. The clinical ladder developed by the nursing staff of Mount Vernon Hospital is provided to serve as an example. (See Appendix F for the Nursing Clinical Ladder of Mount Vernon Hospital, Alexandria, Virginia.) In this ladder, two tracks are identified, administration and clinical, with four levels of practice, which seems to be a common approach. Kneedler et al. also report four levels based on competencies in three major areas: job knowledge, judgment, and responsibility. The levels identified by Kneedler et al. are:

I. New employee, no experience.
II. New employee with experience.
III. Teaching, management, and practice review process.
IV. Meets higher education requirements and practice with autonomy, leadership and clinical competency.[41]

Furthermore, they report using a five-point rating scale that extends from "needs to improve" (1) to "exceeds standard" (5).[42] These progressive levels of performance can easily be associated with the four levels of follower "readiness" of Situational Leadership. A variety of categories have been identified for evaluation of performance. For example, Tower et al. identified the following categories: skills, communication, nursing process, medications, and professional responsibility.[43] Roedel and Nystrom state: "Ideally, each level on a clinical ladder ought to offer greater job enrichment in addition to pay improvement."[44] They also note, however, that nurses do not necessarily experience more job satisfaction at higher levels.[45] According to Hesterly and Sebilia, career ladders may not be *the* answer for many nursing personnel problems.

> Theoretically clinical ladder systems, in which the bedside nurse could ascend to higher levels of salary based on clinical performance, would improve the quality of patient care, motivate employees to develop their skills, increase retention rates, and reward the skilled practitioner economically. How successful clinical leaders have been in achieving these goals is unclear. Anecdotal reports from institutions where clinical ladders are in place demonstrate varying results. The issues of quality patient care, motivation, and retention are so complex that it is difficult, if not impossible, to isolate the impact of a clinical ladder on any of these areas. The issue is further clouded by the impact of current economic constraints on quality of care, motivation, and retention.[46]

Most of the authors cited above go on to describe how the clinical ladder concept was implemented in their agency, indicative of the variety of ways clinical ladders can be developed. While the results and effects are variable, this would seem to be a step in the appropriate direction of recognizing clinical expertise and enabling advancement while the nurse remains beside the patient or client.

Reporting

Managers or leaders are required to submit a verbal or written account of task or goal achievement in the assigned area of responsibility. When you are a head nurse, you will also be presenting or writing reports at regular intervals.

Official Reports

Some of the information you report is used in the health agency and beyond. Langford notes that "in hospitals, there will be census reports and summaries of patient conditions prepared for each shift."[47] This must be accurate because these data are the basis for inventory, staffing, budgetary and many other management decisions within the nursing department. They are also the basis of similar decisions in other departments throughout the hospital or health agency, and they provide information necessary for accreditation and licensure surveys.[48] Some reporting is required by law.

> All states have health statutes that require the reporting of certain public health information to specified government officials. Generally, the individual making reports required by statute is immune from suit under the doctrine of the public's right to know.[49]

Typically, reportable information includes the following: child abuse, ophthalmia neonatorum, infant phenylketonuria, communicable diseases, births out of wedlock, gunshot wounds, suicide, rape, and use of unprescribed narcotics.[50]

Computerized Nursing Information Systems

In some agencies or hospitals, a computerized nursing information system has been developed.

> Computerized nursing data typically deal with staffing and scheduling and with patient classification, which is often correlated with patient census and nursing staffing data. Many nursing divisions already have their quality control systems included in the nursing information package. Some nursing divisions are now exploring adding nursing diagnoses and nursing regimens to the data bank.[51]

If such a system has yet to be installed, then the nursing administrative team will probably want to start planning for the information needs of nursing and requesting computer space. Once an agency's system is in place, it is difficult to incorporate nursing needs. It is wise to have nursing representation on computer services planning committees in order to be included in the process.[52]

In those agencies in which a computerized information system has already been installed, you will find your work as a nursing manager or leader greatly facilitated in comparison with the old-style papershuffling. More information can be stored in less space, reviewed and analyzed rapidly, and statistical reports generated quickly. The system, however, must be designed to meet the specific administrative, business, and practice needs of the agency; a poorly designed system can be equally as frustrating. The computerized information systems can provide excellent support to the administrative decision-making process, particularly in regard to staffing, duty schedules, inventories, and patient classification. The business office is usually the first department to be computerized, facilitating the recording of charges, billing, payrolls, and financial statements. Information from medical records can be analyzed, reorganized, and compared to provide a depth and scope of information otherwise not accessible manually. Medical and nursing notations about patient care can be made directly into the computer, eliminating the problem of being unable to read handwriting, a common source of aggravation and error. Maintenance of standards of care is facilitated as nursing care protocols develop as "screens" that provide options in patient care planning and facilitates complete recording of care given. Most people are already aware of the many uses of computers in monitoring vital signs of patients in intensive care units. In the area of in-service education, computers assist in maintaining schedules for recertifying staff members on such important skills as cardiopulmonary resuscitation (CPR), as well as record and report on the number of correct responses to computer-assisted instructional (CPI) programs.[53] This is only a sample of the applications of the computer to information systems within a health agency. You will need to consult the latest texts and journals throughout your career in order to keep up with this rapidly advancing technology.

Controlling What Is Reported

Less regimented, but highly controlling information systems exist in the verbal reporting that occurs between the nurse-leader and followers, between you as a head nurse and your nursing staff. Your nursing staff will be particularly attentive to any cues from you about what is important to report, and in this sense, reporting becomes a means of controlling.

> The superior controls the perceptions of subordinates by controlling the flow of input to others and by controlling the form of response from others. March and Simon note that the organization's vocabulary screens out some parts of reality while magnifying others. This mode of control also applies to the selection of vocabulary and subject matter addressed by the nurse executive. Her vocabulary is attention-directing and cue-establishing since it predisposes the employee to a certain mind-set by supplying the accepted categories and classifications of thought. Attention-directing and cue-establishing communications are unobtrusive but effective means for control.[54]

Stevens suggests that the questions a nursing leader asks provide more cues about what is important for nursing staff members than one's statement of philosophy and goals. For example, rather than asking a vague question, such as "How are things going?", according to Stevens, it is more appropriate to ask questions that provide direction and information about the staff members' role and function; for example: "What are you doing about the discharge planning needs of the Korean patients who do not speak English?" The nursing leader can design report forms to promote the desired perspective and thinking processes of nursing staff. For example, a report form based on problems identification and solution will differ in the perspective developed from one based on Management by Objectives.[55]

The Annual Report

Once a year, the director or vice-president of nursing writes an annual report summarizing all accomplishments of nursing within that agency. This report is typically not only available to the nurses, but also to upper administrative officers and governing boards of a hospital. Reports to accrediting agencies require some of the same information typically found in annual reports. This document is an important management tool and offers a rare opportunity to reach a variety of audiences beyond the health care agency itself. It is common for many of the head nurses and other middle-management nursing leaders to participate in the development of this document.

As a head nurse, you will want to read the annual reports and similar documents for the previous one or two years in order to get information and a view of your agency's progress and direction. As a general principle, we suggest the following statement about reporting:

If you, as a head nurse, are aware of the recent organizational history of the health agency or hospital in which you practice, then you will be able to identify what is important to include in your own administrative reports.

"Whistle Blowing"

"Whistle blowing" is a corporate phenomenon that frequently occurs when an employee, typically a scientist or engineer, reports that something is amiss to his immediate supervisor. This report, however, is perceived as negative by the supervisor, who does nothing. Historically, the most famous is Judas Iscariot, and Martin Luther is probably one of the only whistle blowers to achieve tremendous influence with the public.[56]

Whistle-blowing can be categorized with betrayal, subversion, and treason. According to Ralph Nader, whistle blowing is:

. . . the act of a man or woman who, believing that the public interest overrides the interest of the organization he serves, publicly "blows the whistle" if the organization is involved in corrupt, illegal, fraudulent, or harmful activity.[57]

James M. Roche, chairman of General Motors, however, suggests a different definition:

Some of the enemies of business now encourage an employee to be disloyal to the enterprise. They want to create suspicion and disharmony and pry into the proprietary interests of the business. However this is labeled—industrial espionage, whistle blowing, or professional responsibility—it is another tactic for spreading disunity and creating conflict.[58]

Generally, it is an indication that management processes within an organization designed to handle dissent are not working, and the employee places humanistic values and public duty above his own commitment to the organization. The employee feels management is unresponsive to his expressed concerns and reports directly to the public. While all Americans do have the constitutional right of free speech, Stewart identifies fear of being fired as a factor that usually stops employees from speaking out. American society does expect that professional experts have sufficient honor and veracity to be trusted; professionals are supposed to assure society that organizational decisions will not inflict harm.[59] American society expects this of health care providers, too.

In his analysis of 51 incidents, Stewart identifies the following sequence of events characteristic of whistle blowing:

1. The employee observes a service/product/policy that seems unethical, immoral or illegal, and harmful to the public.
2. The employee reports these observations to the supervisor, but understands that the supervisor is not going to do anything about it.
3. The employee (a) resigns voluntarily, with or without publicity, or (b) is fired or forced to resign.

4. The employee reports the observations to (a) the regulatory body (commission, licensing board, or the courts), or (b) to the public press.[60]

According to Stewart, the employee's rationale is as follows:

> Potential whistle blowers often consider their information to be favorable because they feel they have discovered an organization problem which needs to be remedied; thus their concern shows that they are conscientious employees. Their information is unlikely to be passed up the organizational hierarchy by their superiors, however, because this information, by definition, is unfavorable to their superiors.[61]

Stewart proposes the primary causes arise from communication overload occurring between the leader and follower, and he offers two correctives. First, he suggests the "exception" principle as a corrective: employees reporting only significant deviations from standards, policies, and so on to their immediate supervisor. Second, Stewart suggests the use of an ombudsman to facilitate upward communication within the organizational structure. This would be someone within an organization who could listen to the employee, investigate, decide whether or not the dissenting view is worth further inquiry, and offer to help or to explain reasons for management's views and behavior.[62]

As a head nurse or similar nursing manager and leader, you can expect to encounter a whistle blowing incident among your nursing staff, given the variety of biomedical-ethical-legal alternatives possible, the clients' preferences, and the court decisions that have been made recently. For an extreme example, brain-dead accident victims have been kept alive and acephalic, newborn infants have been sacrificed in order to "harvest" human organs for transplants. These issues are scary, and because of the need for confidentiality, you would not always have full disclosure of facts. There may be times you feel as if you, too, want to be or are being a whistle blower.

Bearing in mind the two correctives offered by Stewart, we offer another perspective. In the nature of nursing, medicine, and related health care disciplines and professions, all are inherently whistle blowers. Nurses and physicians are continually communicating facts or bad news to people, talking to them about illnesses, restrictions, and pain.[63] This expected or necessary whistle-blowing behavior as a nurse may inadvertently predispose you to behave in a similar manner in relation to organizational matters and consequently reflect negatively on your career. We believe that by establishing this awareness and sensitivity in you, by reading this section on whistle blowing, you will be able to maintain a more comfortable balance between your values and your view of management decisions.

Finally, whistle blowing does not have to happen. As a head nurse dealing with your nursing staff, you can be sensitive to the beliefs and values of your followers and keep them informed about the actions you take based on their reports. By maintaining open communication and developing integrative behaviors within the group, you have an opportunity to resolve the concerns at your level of the organizational structure. We suggest the following statement of principle for your consideration.

> *Reporting involves truth, trust, and human values, and what is ethical to report, when and to whom is not always clear.*

Reporting provides you an opportunity to show a leader characteristic we have indirectly discussed—wisdom.

Intervening

An *intervention,* according to the dictionary, is any interference into the current state of affairs.[64] In the management or leadership process of planning, organizing, staffing, and directing, *intervening* is the element of controlling which links up with planning, so that the process is recycled continuously over time. Depending upon the reports or feedback of what has been achieved, the leader may decide an intervention is indicated in order to maintain congruency between activities, standards, and the original plan.[65] Just as a thermostat is sensitive and controls temperatures within a certain range, so a leader or manager maintains conformity between plans and activities. Thus, the basic control system is *feedback.*[66]

Examples of task-oriented interventions that can be made include budget revisions, changing standards, decreasing or increasing inventories, or continuing programs or projects. There are a number of people-oriented examples of positive interventions you might make as a head nurse. These may include a promotion, increase in salary, and praise. Your intervening may be negative, such as disciplining, punishing, or terminating a member of the nursing staff; or the intervention may be relatively neutral, such as transferring nursing staff from one service to another. You cannot always anticipate how people will respond to your interventions, however, because some may become very upset. (See the discussion of legal responsibilities in scheduling in Chapter 12.) It is important in maintaining managerial control that you be able to distinguish between a normal "griping" level and insubordination.

Insubordination

In accepting employment in an organization or health care facility, you make a contract in which you agree to spend time and to perform certain assigned duties or roles as stipulated in your job description. As payment, the agency or hospital agrees to give you money, health insurance and other benefits, and conveniences (a locker or parking space). In this contract, the agency, through its managers, reserves the right to tell you what to do, when and how to do it. As long as these assigned duties fall within your job description, you give up the right to refuse to do the assigned tasks.[67] According to Barbara Stevens:

> Refusal constitutes a breaking of the contract between the two parties. Thus insubordination, the refusal to carry out a legitimate assignment, is a case of self-firing. The employee breaks the contract and has no right to expect further benefit from the employing agency.[68]

Stevens also states that refusing reassignment to another nursing unit is the most common basis of insubordination among nursing staff. To be sure the nursing staff member understands the implications of refusal, you, as a head nurse, need to provide this information. The Labor Management Relations Act is interpreted as follows: "An employer has a fundamental right to assign employees to positions which he deems, in the exercise of his managerial discretion, to be most expedient."[69,70] As head nurse, your decisions regarding placement of personnel are to be defined by patient needs, not personnel preferences. In addition, a reassigned nursing staff member is expected to continue performing to standards. "Employees have a right to strike, but they have no right to continue working on their own terms while rejecting standards desired by their employer."[71,72] Stevens also points out the following: "Thus there is legal support for the supervisor's position in maintaining control of assignments and in determining that standards be met."[73] While it would be unfair to manipulate or push a follower into being insubordinate, it is a fair question for you to ask when a follower is apparently unwilling to accept your direction, but you know the individual is able. Just ask, "Are you saying that you are declaring yourself insubordinate and are refusing to perform this assignment?" If the individual says, "Yes," then you need to take the appropriate actions to immediately reassign his or her duties to another nurse. More than likely, however, the nurse will immediately change the direction and attitude of his or her comments and conform to expectations. "The nurse manager's legal responsibility for quality control of nursing services imposes upon her the duty to observe, report, and correct the incompetence of individual patient care personnel within her unit."[74] As long as you carry the title of head nurse, you are the authorized representative of management, and you are to maintain control of all organizational activities within your scope of authority and responsibility. As a general principle, we suggest the following:

> *The degree of control you maintain is related to the degree to which you consider feedback in your intervention decisions.*

The primary basis of knowing when and how to intervene are the control systems of *feedback* and *feedforward*.

Feedback Control Systems

Very little is written these days about feedback control systems, but this process seems to be a rather elementary theory or understanding of management. We include it here because it connects controlling and planning, providing a cyclical model of the process elements of leadership or management. There are two aspects: *feedback* and *feedforward*.

Feedback

Similar to feedback in the communication model presented earlier (see Chapter 4), feedback in the control system provides information about organizational activities that have occurred (see Fig. 15–3). It reports errors that have occurred and are occurring in the planned activities to meet organizational goals. This information, measurements of samples of activities, is compared with planned standards or criteria set by management. As long as the measurements are consistent with the criteria, no intervention is necessary. When an error or deviation from the standard occurs, then intervention is indicated, and the plan is revised accordingly.[75]

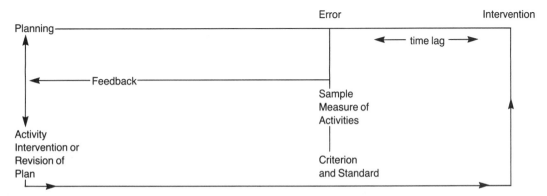

Figure 15–3. A model of the feedback control. *(From a similar model in Filley, A. C., House, R. J., & Kerr, S. Managerial process and organizational behavior. Glenview, Ill.: Scott, Foresman, 1976, p. 441.)*

An example of this feedback system is the orientation and training program for nurses aides and orderlies. The program is planned and implemented to prepare individuals to perform in these jobs. After the individuals complete the program and begin to work in the units, the nursing managers and staff take note of the errors the aides and orderlies make. The intervention is to change the course of instruction in such a way that the next group will have a higher probability of avoiding these errors.

The weakness of this process, however, is that it must rely on *error*. Something has to go wrong before the system works. In addition, the time lag between the deviation from the standard, the correction, and corrected activity allow for a potentially wide variance in the performance of the activity. Thus, the manager has the problem of trying to reduce the time lag as well as correct the error.[76]

Feedforward

Unlike feedback, *feedforward* control systems rely on indicators of anticipated deviations of activities from standards (see Fig. 15–4). Looking forward into the future, an estimate is made of how well the organizational activities will maintain the standard or criteria. This estimate is based on related activities; if these happen, then the organizational activity will be influenced. "The controlling activity, which we shall call the 'related activity,' is ahead of the primary activity and 'feeds forward' information to it."[77] Based on information about the related activities, control is maintained through revision of plans or adjustment of activities to meet the same or revised standards.

For example, a new hospital wing is being added, and it is decided that the standard of 50 additional nurses will be needed to appropriately staff the new units when opened in one year. Future-related activities that indicate the number of RNs to be available then would be the current enrollment of nursing programs in the region and the number of unemployed RNs living in the surrounding counties. This feedforward control system is often used in adjusting inventories, purchasing, and productivity. Whether or not certain business ventures are developed often depends upon feedforward information about emerging population demographics,

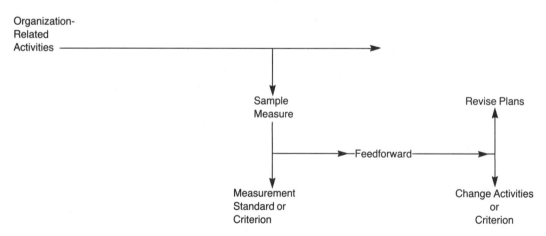

Figure 15–4. A model of the feedforward control. *(From a similar model in Filley, A. C., House, R. J., & Kerr, S. Managerial process and organizational behavior. Glenview, Ill.: Scott, Foresman, 1976, p. 443.)*

such as the so-called "baby boomers" and "gray power" population changes, advocates, and whether a market exists for the proposed product.

This system also has limitations, according to McGuire. "First, it requires an accurate determination of the relationship between two or more processes or activities. Second, the system cannot deal with unusual circumstances."[78] It seems wise to consider using data from both feedback and feedforward in making controlling decisions.

Controlling and Planning

The degree to which you, as a nursing manager or leader, can depend upon feedback and feedforward control systems, however, is open for discussion. While it is important to know what errors have occurred and try to prevent recurrence, in health care, there may be litigation rather than a second chance to correct performance. Patients or clients may be so harmed or inconvenienced that legal settlements seem to be the only recourse. Examples of this are found in the prescribing of new medications that, after a while, are found to be harmful in some unanticipated manner.

While feedforward control is used to anticipate patient acuity and, from that, staffing needs, the demands on health care services are very difficult to predict. One freeway pileup or a chemical spill can quickly disrupt organizational plans and control systems in nearby health care facilities. The AIDS epidemic is a nationwide example of how the urgency of illness can overtax the health care system and frustrate planning and control efforts at many levels. Illness and accidents simply are not planned, and elective care has its limitations.

Theoretically and practically, authorities present differing views on the relative balance between planning and controlling. Green suggests that, on the whole, planning tends to be poorly done, so control is a cover (or coverup) for poor planning.[79] As a general principle, Green states: "The less confidence the manager has in his plans, the more time he should devote to control and vice versa."[80] Hughes, however, proposes that controls compensate for ineffective planning in some situations by reducing the impact of uncertain situations.[81] He proposes as a general rule that: "In essence, effective control requires effective planning."[82]

Controlling is difficult to research because, as anticipated events or activities do or do not occur, managers intervene to change plans, standards, or activities. Consequently, controlling, as a function of management and leadership, remains hypothetical and theoretical in nature. As a matter of practice, control needs to be incorporated in planning: As you plan, you ask yourself, "How do I control the plan?" and "How do I build control into the plan?" Some visualize the whole management process—planning, organizing, staffing, directing, and controlling—as being a circular process (see Fig. 15–5). In practice, however, the process involves a reciprocal relationship between planning and controlling if you are to reach your goal (see Fig. 15–6). Just as you need to repeatedly look at a map as you drive on a long trip in order to verify that you are following the right road signs, so you need to look at the control data to verify that you are on the right track for reaching your goal. In maintaining your personal checking account, you can record all of the checks, waiting until the end of the month to determine whether or not you have exceeded the amount deposited, that is use a little budget planning and no controls. You can also record each check and calculate the amount of money remaining in the account, planning and controlling as you proceed through the weeks until your next check.[83]

As a nurse-leader or manager, we believe you do need to be aware of the close relationship between controlling and planning and the influence of this relationship upon the other elements in the process, organizing, staffing, and directing. This management process is analo-

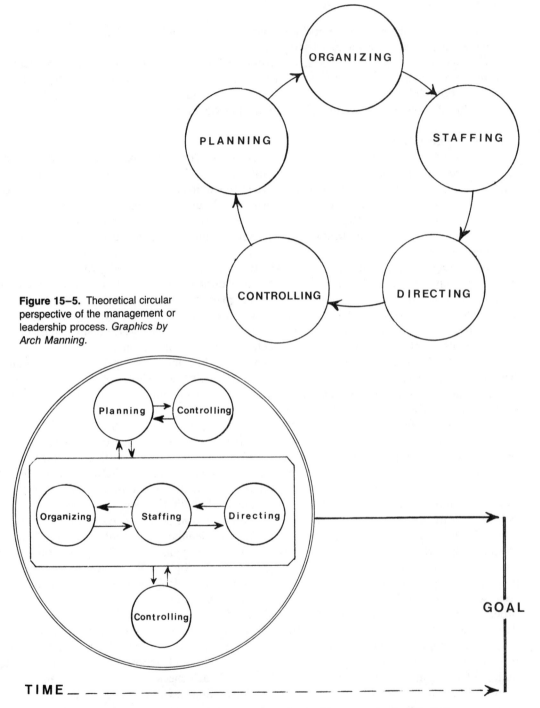

Figure 15–5. Theoretical circular perspective of the management or leadership process. *Graphics by Arch Manning.*

Figure 15–6. Perspective of the management or leadership process in practice, demonstrating the dynamic reciprocal relationship among all elements of the management or leadership process. *Graphics by Arch Manning.*

gous to the nursing process; assessing, planning, implementing, and evaluating.[84] As a practical matter, evaluating is the equivalent of controlling. You continually evaluate or control assessing, planning, and intervening in relation to your goal, which is improvement of the client's health status. Just as the nursing process is applicable to all patients to insure quality care,[85] so the management process is applicable to all types of organizations and levels of management.[86]

SUMMARY

The discussion of controlling has been divided into a set of five elements: standardizing, reviewing, rating, reporting, and intervening. The differentiation between management and leadership has been considered. In addition, the focus has been on effectiveness as a dimension of a leader or manager, and ways in which effectiveness can be assessed, evaluated and, more importantly, developed have been suggested. Of contemporary interest, certain issues associated with controlling were noted, such as the need for incentive programs that allow nurses to remain at the bedside yet achieve career advances, ethics in reporting versus whistle blowing, and intervening to control without violating employees' rights.

REFERENCES

1. Guralnik, D.B. (Ed.). *Webster's new world dictionary* (2nd ed.). New York: Prentice-Hall, 1980; *American heritage dictionary: Word finder* (computerized synonym dictionary). San Rafael, Calif.: MicroPro International Corporation.
2. Marriner, A. *Guide to nursing management* (2nd ed.). St. Louis: Mosby, 1984, p. 238.
3. Hersey, P., & Blanchard, K. *Management of organizational behavior: Utilizing human resources* (5th ed.). Englewood Cliffs, N.J.: Prentice-Hall, 1988 , p. 5.
4. Hersey & Blanchard, *Management of organizational behavior,* p. 127.
5. Ibid., 118.
6. Hersey & Blanchard, *Management of organizational behavior,* p. 96.
7. McCloskey, J.C., & Molen, M.T. Leadership in nursing. In J.J. Fitzpatrick & R. L. Taunton (Eds.). *Annual Review of Nursing Research,* Vol. 5. New York: Springer, 1987, p. 193.
8. Berhang-Doggett, J. Head nurse leadership style and staff nurse job satisfaction. Paper presented at RESEARCH: 85, sponsored by the College of Nursing, University of South Carolina, Columbia, S.C. May 16, 1985.
9. Wittenauer, M.A. Leadership style of master's graduates as related to present position and selected educational variables. Paper presented at RESEARCH: 85, sponsored by the College of Nursing, University of South Carolina, Columbia, S.C. May 16, 1985.
10. Ibid.
11. Dolan, P.R., Mendius, R.K., Anspaugh, D., & Enck, G. A Study of leadership styles of rehabilitation nurse leaders. Submitted for publication, December 1987.
12. Marriner, *Guide to nursing management,* p. 282–284.
13. Ibid., 74.
14. Anderson, P.A., & Davis, S.E. Nursing peer review: A developmental process. *Nursing Management,* 1987, *18* (1), 46–48.
15. Polit, D.F., & Hungler, B.P. *Nursing research: Principles and methods* (3rd ed.). Philadelphia: Lippincott, 1987, pp. 158–162.

16. Poteet, G.W., & Goddard, N.L. Issues in financial management. In B. Henry et al., (Eds.). *Dimensions and issues in nursing administration.* Boston: Blackwell Scientific Publications, in press.

17. Essentials of collegiate and university education for professional nurses: Report to the membership of AACN—October, 1986. *Journal of Professional Nursing,* 1987, *3(1)*, 54.

18. Poteet & Goddard

19. *Criteria for the evaluation of baccalaureate and higher degree programs in nursing* (5th ed.). New York: National League for Nursing, 1983, p. 7 (Pub. No. 15-1251).

20. Essentials of collegiate and university education for professional nurses: Report to the membership of AACN—October, 1986. *Journal of Professional Nursing,* 1987, *3(1)*, 54–69.

21. Peters, T.J., & Waterman, R.H., Jr. *In search of excellence: Lessons from America's best-run companies.* New York: Warner Books, 1982, pp. 156–157.

22. Porter-O'Grady, T. *Creative nursing administration: Participative management into the 21st century.* Rockville, Md.: Aspen, 1986, pp. 207–208.

23. Jernigan, D.K., & Young, A.P. *Standards, job descriptions, and performance evaluations for nursing practice.* Norwalk, Conn.: Appleton-Century-Crofts, 1983.

24. Anderson & Davis, Nursing peer review, 46–48.

25. Johnson-Soderbert, S. Theory and practice of scapegoating. *Perspectives in Psychiatric Care,* 1977, *15* (4), 153–159.

26. Kelly, L.Y. Endpaper: Escape by scapegoat. *Nursing Outlook,* 1979, *27* (11), 752.

27. Prescott, P.A., & Bowen, S.A. Controlling nursing turnover. *Nursing Management,* 1987, *18*(6), 60–66.

28. Marquess, R., & Petit, B.J. An analysis of the effect of percent of R.N. staff on nursing costs by DRG: A national costing study produces intriguing—though mixed—results. *Nursing Management,* 1987, *18*(5), 33–34.

29. Myslenski, J.V. Controlling overtime costs: Strong administrative direction yields genuine reductions. *Nursing Management,* 1987, *18*(1), 51–54.

30. Marriner, *Guide to nursing management,* p. 290.

31. Strasen, L. *Key business skills for nurse managers.* Philadelphia: Lippincott, 1987, pp. 244–246.

32. Ibid., 70.

33. Ibid., 69.

34. Knowles, M.S. *Modern practice of adult education.* New York: Association Press, 1973, p. 223.

35. Polit & Hungler, *Nursing research,* p. 158–163.

36. Kirkpatrick, D.L. Evaluating training programs: Evidence vs. proof. *Training and Development Journal,* 1977, *32* (11);

37. Parker, B.K. *Health care education: A Guide to staff development.* Norwalk, Conn.: Appleton-Century-Crofts, 1986, p. 50.

38. Penbreth-Valentine, M. *Health planning for nurse managers: Strategies for success.* Rockville, Md.: Aspen, 1984.

39. Merker, L.R., Mariak, K.A., & Dwinnells, D.W. *The clinical career ladder: Planning and implementation.* New York: Springer, 1985, pp. 1–16.

40. Ibid.

41. Kneedler, J., et al. Competency-based career ladders. *Nurse Managers,* 1987, *18*(7), 77–78.

42. Ibid.

43. Tower, B.L., et al. Behaviorally based clinical evaluation. *Journal of Nursing Education,* 1987, *26*(3), 120–123.

44. Roedel, R.R., & Nystrom, P.C. Clinical ladders and job enrichment. *Hospital Topics,* 1987, *65*(2), 22.

45. Ibid., 24.

46. Hesterly, S., & Sebilia, A.J. Recognizing clinical excellence. *Journal of Nursing Administration,* 1986, *16*(2), 34.

47. Langford, T.L. *Managing and being managed: Preparation for professional nursing practice.* Englewood Cliffs, N.J.: Prentice-Hall, 1981, p. 199.
48. Ibid.
49. Gillies, D.A. *Nursing management: A systems approach.* Philadelphia: Saunders, 1982, p. 451.
50. Ibid.
51. Stevens, B.J. *The nurse as executive.* Wakefield, Mass.: Nursing Resources, 1980, p. 353.
52. Ibid.
53. Tomey, A.M. *Guide to nursing management* (3rd ed.). St. Louis: Mosby, 1988, pp 16–17.
54. Stevens, *The nurse as executive,* p. 353.
55. Ibid., 354.
56. Stewart, L.P., "Whistle blowing": Implications for organizational communication. *Journal of Communication,* Autumn 1980, 90.
57. Nader, R., Petkas, P.J., & Blackwell, K. (Eds.). *Whistle blowing: The report of the conference on professional responsibility.* New York: Grossman, 1972, p. vii.
58. Flint, J.M. G.M.'s chief scores critics of business. *New York Times,* March 26, 1971, p. 52.
59. Stewart, "Whistle blowing," p. 95–96.
60. Ibid.
61. Ibid.
62. Ibid.
63. Duldt, B.W. Anger: An alienating communication hazard for nurses. *Nursing Outlook,* 1981, *29*(11), 643.
64. Guralnik, *Webster's,* p. 738.
65. Filley, A. C., House, R. J., & Kerr, S. *Managerial process and organizational behavior.* Glenview, Ill.: Scott, Foresman, 1976, p. 440.
66. Ibid., 464.
67. Stevens, *The nurse as executive,* p. 308.
68. Ibid.
69. Ibid.
70. *American Jurisprudence,* vol. 48, section 606, (2nd ed.), 1970, p. 421.
71. Stevens, *The nurse as executive,* p. 308.
72. *American Jurisprudence,* vol. 48, section 624, (2nd ed.), 1970, p. 431.
73. Stevens, *The nurse as executive,* p. 308.
74. Regan, W. Nursing service problem: Incompetent personnel. In *The Regan report on nursing law,* August 1974.
75. Filley et al. *Managerial process and organizational behavior,* p. 440–441.
76. Ibid., 441.
77. Ibid.
78. Ibid., 143–144.
79. Green, T.B. Control: The cover for poor planning. *Managerial Planning,* 1976, *24*(5), 42–43.
80. Ibid.
81. Hughes, R. E. Planning: The essence of control. *Managerial Planning,* 1978, *26*(6), p. 1–3, 10.
82. Ibid., 3.
83. Interviews with R. Eugene Hughes, Professor and Chairman, Department of Business Management, East Carolina University, Greenville, North Carolina, January 4 and February 7, 1988.
84. Yura, H., & Walsh, M.B. *The nursing process* (4th Ed.). Norwalk, Conn.: Appleton-Century-Crofts, 1983.
85. Ibid., 307.
86. Hersey & Blanchard, *Management of organizational behavior,* p. 5.

Appendix A: STANDARDS FOR ORGANIZED NURSING SERVICES

Standard I

THE DIVISION OF NURSING HAS A PHILOSOPHY AND STRUCTURE THAT ASSURE THE DELIVERY OF HIGH QUALITY NURSING CARE AND PROVIDE MEANS FOR RESOLVING NURSING PRACTICE ISSUES THROUGHOUT THE HEALTH CARE ORGANIZATION.

Criteria

1. The Division of Nursing has a philosophy and objectives compatible with ANA standards, the *Code for Nurses,* and the mission of the health care organization.
2. The philosophy of the Division of Nursing provides for individual authority and accountability on the part of nurses and for their participation in the management of the division.
3. The organizational plan for the Division of Nursing specifies lines of authority, accountability, and responsibility for all nurses employed within the health care organization, including the nursing management team.
4. The organizational plan specifies the nurse executive as a member of corporate administration.
5. The Division of Nursing is represented with voting privileges on policy-making boards and committees of the health care organization.
6. The Division of Nursing encourages representation and particpation by its members in professional organizations and in community and governmental activities related to health care.
7. Data are systematically collected for use in planning, budgeting, and evaluating the Division of Nursing.

Standard II

THE DIVISION OF NURSING IS ADMINISTERED BY A QUALIFIED NURSE EXECUTIVE WHO IS A MEMBER OF CORPORATE ADMINISTRATION.

Criteria

1. The nurse executive is a qualified licensed registered nurse who is knowledgeable in nursing practice and administration.
2. The nurse executive is prepared at the graduate level in a program that includes administrative concepts or is qualified through years of experience and ANA certification in nursing administration.
3. The nurse executive is knowledgeable about current advances in technology and trends that affect health care delivery.
4. The nurse executive collaborates with the nursing staff in the development and implementation of objectives and program strategies and in the joint evaluation of progress within the Division of Nursing through the process of participative management.
5. The nurse executive establishes and maintains formal and informal relationships within the organization to accomplish the goals of the Division of Nursing.
6. As part of corporate administration, the nurse executive participates in the planning and evaluation of organization effectiveness.
7. The nurse executive participates in fiscal management decisions to assure resources to provide consistently effective nursing care.
8. The nurse executive provides leadership for innovation and research in nursing.

Standard III

POLICIES AND PRACTICES OF THE DIVISION OF NURSING PROVIDE FOR EQUALITY AND CONTINUITY OF NURSING SERVICES THAT RECOGNIZE CULTURAL, ECONOMIC, AND SOCIAL DIFFERENCES AMONG PATIENTS OF THE HEALTH CARE ORGANIZATION.

Criteria

1. The policies and practices of the Division of Nursing incorporate or take into account the

health values and traditions of various cultures related to health maintenance and the care of illness.
2. The Division of Nursing provides means to meet the needs of persons who are unable to speak for themselves or lack sufficient knowledge to obtain necessary services.
3. Planning and delivery of nursing care reflect diverse patient preferences, needs, and capacities for self-care.

Standard IV

THE DIVISION OF NURSING ENSURES THAT THE NURSING PROCESS IS USED TO DESIGN AND PROVIDE NURSING CARE TO MEET THE INDIVIDUAL NEEDS OF PATIENTS/CLIENTS IN THE CONTEXT OF THEIR FAMILIES.

Criteria

1. Nursing practice policies and standards of practice encourage collaborative planning with patients and their families to meet their needs and to establish priorities of care.
2. Policies and standards for practice recognize the role of patients' families in the delivery of care prior to and after discharge.
3. Policies and standards of practice encourage attention to the unique needs of families.
4. There is a mechanism for collaborative practice by nurses with nurses, with physicians, and with others.
5. Nursing staffing patterns and assignments are made by use of a system that determines patients' requirements and priorities for care, and matches those requirements with the knowledge and skills of nursing staff.

Standard V

THE DIVISION OF NURSING PROVIDES AN ENVIRONMENT THAT ENSURES THE EFFECTIVENESS OF NURSING PRACTICE

Criteria

1. The Division of Nursing has specific policies that provide for advancement in clinical practice.
2. Policies of the Division of Nursing provide for the granting of clinical nursing privileges to recognize nurses qualified in clinical specialties.
3. The Division of Nursing has a quality assurance program that evaluates the effectiveness of the division as well as the performance of the individual staff member.
4. The Division of Nursing rewards the performance of the nurse, as well as her educational preparation and experience, by its recognition and compensation policies.
5. Adequate support services are available, enabling nurses to give primary attention to clinical practice.

Standard VI

THE DIVISION OF NURSING ASSURES THE DEVELOPMENT OF EDUCATIONAL PROGRAMS TO SUPPORT THE DELIVERY OF HIGH QUALITY NURSING CARE.

Criteria

1. Each employee of the Division of Nursing receives an orientation that introduces her to the philosophy, objectives, and practices of the health care environment and assesses the employee's level of knowledge and skill.
2. Planned, ongoing learning experiences are developed to assist nursing staff to meet their learning needs, as documented in patient care studies and in nursing staff evaluation, and as indicated by changes in the characteristics of the patients served.
3. The Division of Nursing provides resources for the participation in educational programs designed to meet the continuing learning needs of the nurse for growth and advancement.

4. Learning experiences are selected with consideration for the preferences of the individual nurse as well as the needs of the overall nursing service and patients.
5. The Division of Nursing collaborates with educational institutions to provide clinical learning experiences for nursing students and other health care providers.

Standard VII

THE DIVISION OF NURSING INITIATES, UTILIZES, AND PARTICIPATES IN RESEARCH STUDIES OR PROJECTS FOR THE IMPROVEMENT OF PATIENT CARE.

Criteria

1. The Division of Nursing provides a mechanism to analyze nursing practice problems so that scientific knowledge and methods can be used in formulating solutions.
2. Nurses are encouraged to analyze published research findings and to implement them in practice.
3. Nurses are provided the resources to test ideas about patient care, thereby improving the quality of care as well as their own professional satisfaction.
4. Nurses are encouraged to initiate studies and to publish their own research findings.
5. Collaborative relationships with other health care providers are used in pursuing research to study patient care practices.
6. The Division of Nursing reviews clinical study proposals for considerations necessary to protect the human rights of patients and nurses and others in concert with organizational protocols.
7. The Division of Nursing participates actively in reviewing, evaluating, and recommending approval of all clinical studies that involve or affect nursing practice.

Components of a Professional Nursing System

ACKNOWLEDGMENT: These components, under the title, "Characteristics of a Professional Climate in a Nursing Department," were initially developed by the Task Force on a Nursing Practice Climate—A Professional Model. The list below is the result of ongoing development of these characteristics by the Commission on Nursing Services and the Task Force on Standards for Nursing Services.

This checklist may be used for self-assessment by a division of nursing.

Where the Standards for Organized Nursing Services established by the ANA Commission on Nursing Services are being met, the nursing division will have the following characteristics:

1. The Division of Nursing communicates directly with the Board of Trustees and has mechanisms for shared governance, including contracted agreements, nursing staff bylaws approved by the Board of Trustees, and/or rules and regulations which provide for clinical privileges and for accountability to the governing body and to the patient.
2. The Division of Nursing has sufficient autonomy and budgetary control to be able to assume accountability for the quality of nursing practice and the outcomes of nursing care.
3. A nursing management information system and other resources are used to develop and manage divisional planning, budgeting, and monitoring the quality of nursing care.
4. Nursing administration participates fully, by title and action, in top-level administrative decision making and with the governing body.
5. Nurses who are appointed to managerial and administrative positions have preparation and practice backgrounds consistent with the roles, responsibilities, and qualifications for nursing administrators identified by the ANA Commission on Nursing Services.
6. A professional practice committee promotes collegial relationships between and among nurses, physicians, and other professionals.
7. Nurses receive administrative support in their role of patient advocate.
8. Effective around-the-clock services are available to support the practice of nurses.
9. Planning and budgeting recognize staffing patterns based upon patients' requirements and priorities for care that are matched with the knowledge and skills of nursing staff.
10. Nursing policies and practices are congruent with the ANA *Code for Nurses,* the ANA *Standards for*

Organized Nursing Services, the ANA *Standards of Nursing Practice,* the state nursing practice act, the standards of the voluntary accrediting body appropriate to the agency, and the requirements of the regulatory body appropriate to the agency.

11. A plan is in operation to maintain and enhance the competence of nurses through promotion strategies, scholarship resources, and continuing education programming in order to meet the increasingly complex needs of patients and the requirements of high technologies.

12. The compensation system for nurses recognizes educational preparation, prior professional experience, and level of clinical competence, as well as length of service.

13. Nurses effectively recommend decisions on admission, placement, and discharge of patients.

14. Practicing nurses have individual accountability for the care of each patient/client.

15. Provision is made for nurse-to-nurse consultation within the facility and between agencies or institutions.

16. Institutional policies administered by the Division of Nursing assure shared responsibility between the institution and the individual nurse for the development and maintenance of the competence of practitioners.

17. The Division of Nursing investigates staff utilization methods that have likelihood of improving the quality of care and of containing costs.

18. An evaluation program assesses practitioner performance and administrative effectiveness, as well as patient outcomes.

19. Staff and administrative support are provided for nursing studies and research.

From Standards for nursing service. *American Nurses' Association. (Publication No. #NS–1) Kansas City Missouri. 1982.*

Appendix B: HUMANIZING INTERPERSONAL COMMUNICATION.
B. W. Duldt.

These statements of nurse–client relationships versus statements of nurse-leader–follower relationships have been drawn from humanistic and holistic philosophical perspectives of nursing and from the theory that describes behavior, that is, Situational Leadership, and the theory that describes attitudes, that is, Humanistic Nursing Communication. These statements are designed to serve as a basis of discussion, however, rather than be viewed as facts to be accepted without question. We believe these statements uniquely capture the best available: (a) research and knowledge about how people communicate interpersonally, and (b) the essence of sound leadership theory, research, and practice as applicable to leader–follower relationships and roles in all areas of nursing practice. The sets of attitudes of Humanistic Nursing Communication theory are used as the organizing genre or categories.

For Nurse–Client Relationships	*For Nurse Leader–Follower Relationships*
1. Dialogue versus Monologue	*1. Dialogue versus Monologue*
Dialogical communication requires the nurse and client to genuinely listen to each other to say something new about one's own unique, here-and-now life situation.	Dialogical communication requires the leader and follower to genuinely listen to each other to say something new about his or her own unique, lived, here-and-now experience.
Communication in dialogue is a humanizing, two-way interaction in which each person participates by sharing with another information about oneself as well as being open and responding to similar information shared by the other. Each is aware of the other's presence—of "being there" and "being with." It is an encounter that involves the interpersonal concepts of trust, self-disclosure, feedback, assertiveness, confronting, conflicting, and separation. The nurse is involved on two levels: (1) as a unique human being with a warm, genuine person; and (2) as a responsible, accountable professional person making one's special knowledge and skills available to the client. The client is also involved on two levels: (1) as a unique human being and person experiencing some degree of experiential distress and struggling to cope in a critical life situation; and (2) as a client needing and, intentionally or unintentionally, seeking the special knowledge provided by the nurse.	Dialogical communication is a two-way interaction in which each person participates by sharing with another information about one's self that is relevant to the task as well as being open to the other and responding to similar information shared by the other. It is an encounter that involves the interpersonal concepts of trust, self-disclosure, feedback, assertiveness, confronting, conflicting, and separation. The leader is involved on two levels: (1) as a unique human being and a warm, genuine person; and (2) as a responsible, accountable professional person making his or her special knowledge and skills as a leader available to the follower. The follower is also involved on two levels: (1) as a unique human being and a genuine, warm person, and (2) as a follower making his or her special knowledge and skills available to the leader, intentionally or unintentionally seeking the special knowledge and skills provided by the leader. Both are assumed to be committed to a reasonable degree to achieving task goals of the employing health agency. Both may be experiencing some degree of experiential distress and struggling to cope and achieve task goals. By working together and maintaining dialogue, each assists the other not only in avoiding a critical job (life) situation, but also in attaining the highest level of functioning possible through one's professional practice.
The polar opposite is monologue or a one-way interaction in which the nurse informs, directs, and instructs the client with minimal consideration of the client as an individual. A monologue encounter tends to involve distrust, lack of self-disclosure and feedback, submissiveness, and lack of confrontation. Personal involvement is minimal. The nurse is perceived as a closed, cold, role-playing individual; this tends to reduce for the client the general availability of the nurse's	The polar opposite is monologue; usually

special knowledge and skills. The client tends to be viewed by the nurse as a problem or a disease entity requiring the nurse's professional attention. In the more technical clinical settings, the client is ignored as the nurse cares for the equipment attached to the client.

this takes the form of policies, orders, and standard operating procedures. The follower may seek a special request or offer a suggestion about the task. This "upward communication" is ignored by the leader. The follower's suggestions are filed away, and nothing is done. The follower is expected to take directives without question.

2. Individuality versus Category

Individuality requires the nurse to be aware of the client as a unique, irreplaceable human being.

2. Individuality versus Category

Individuality requires the leader to be aware of the follower as a unique, irreplaceable human being, separate and distinct from categories and classifications commonly used in occupational settings.

Individuality is the recognition of another as a person and choosing to enter into a meaningful interpersonal relationship. Treating a person as an individual involves the deliberate use of humanizing communication attitudes and patterns of communication. The nurse remembers seemingly minor details of care or preferences in routines—details which, when attended to without prompting, assure the client's self-perception as a person. In this way, the nurse validates the client as someone special.

    The opposite is to categorize the client as one of a set to whom nursing care, treatments, or procedures are applied with minimal variation in routine.

Individuality is the recognition of another as a person and choosing to enter a meaningful interpersonal relationship with her or him. It involves the deliberate use of communication as a tool to establish recognition of the total character of the follower as a person rather than one of a set of objects to which a category of supervision, productivity, or personnel policies are applied.

    The opposite is for the leader to classify followers as aides, staff nurses, or other job categories. Categories do provide a useful "shorthand" for discussion about task, employee issues among leaders, or both. However, to be called, "Hey, Nurse!" rather than by one's own name by one's leader is interpersonally alienating and dehumanizing.

3. Holistic versus Parts

The element of holism requires the nurse to perceive the client as a complex totality of coherent characteristics (or systems) functioning together as one undiminished entity constituting the full of a person.

3. Holistic versus Parts

Holistic requires the leader to perceive the follower as a complex totality of coherent systems functioning together as one undiminished entity constituting the full of a person.

Holistic is a way of perceiving the client on two levels "all at once," as a total system of the whole and as a part that is a subsystem of the total. In providing care, the nurse necessarily focuses professional attention on a particular part(s) or subsystem(s) that is maladaptive. Simultaneously, the nurse also focuses both professional and personal attention on the organized set of parts or subsystems comprising the total human being, that is, a holistic view of one seeking to maintain a harmonious relationship with the environment.

    The opposite of "holistic" is fragmentation of the person by focusing only on the malfunctioning

Holistic is a way of perceiving the follower on two levels "all at once," a total system of the whole and subsystem as a part of the total. For example, in controlling, the nurse-leader necessarily focuses attention on a particular subsystem of a task that is maladaptive. Humanistic nursing leadership requires the nurse-leader to also focus both professional and personal attention on the organized set of subsystems comprising the human being who, as follower, is performing the task. While many organizational policies give appropriate attention to the biological, social, and mental factors of employees, the "spiritual," a

part. For example, an intensive care nurse may concentrate so intently on the tasks and procedures of caring for the client's body that she may experience some degree of surprise when the very ill client speaks, turns over, or initiates some independent action.

vital dimension of holism, often is recognized to some lesser degree. The spiritual includes temperament, attitude, state of mind, motivation, and mood. The humanistic nursing leader, then, seeks to develop and maintain positive attitudes and temperaments, and to develop sensitivity to the follower's state of mind and moods. Reward systems are developed to affirm the follower's motivation. The humanistic leader has a sensitivity to the follower's perceptions of his or her own situation and a commitment to fairness.

The fragmentation of the follower is achieved by requiring a set level of productivity with no exceptions; all preoperative medications given by a certain time, all patients' dinner trays returned by 12:30 P.M., and all bed baths completed by 11 A.M. Development of a supportive relationship with patients or clients is frustrated by changing the nurses' patient care assignments every other day. "A nurse is a nurse is a nurse" seems to be the view of the dehumanizing leader. So the maternal-child nurse is reassigned to the psychiatric or orthopedic unit with little concern for the nurse's career goals, not to mention patient or client safety.

4. Choice versus Directive	*4. Choice versus Directive*
Choice requires the nurse and the client to have freedom to consider alternatives and make decisions about issues encountered in the existential "here and now."	Choice requires the leader and the follower freedom to consider alternatives and make decisions about issues encountered in the existential "here and now."

Choice is a privilege and a responsibility for all human beings and is a key concept in existential philosophy. To be able to choose allows a human being to be more than merely a "reactor" to stimuli, but to be an "actor," producing novelty and change in human behavior. Having thus initiated change, the human being is then accountable for the outcomes and consequences of decisions. In humanistic nursing, both the nurse and client as persons have choice in regard to whether or not to communicate, with whom, regarding what, and in what manner. The nurse as a knowledgeable professional has choice regarding decisions about care offered and provided for the client. The client has choice, to the extent of capabilities, regarding whether or not to accept the care offered and provided. And the nurse needs to validate that the client has knowledge of alternatives and consequences of choices and to respect and honor the client's choices.

The opposite of choice is directive. The

Choice is a privilege and a responsibility for all human beings and is a key concept in existential philosophy. To be able to choose allows one to be more than merely a "reactor" to stimuli, but to be an "actor," producing novelty and change in human behavior, and controlling outcomes to some degree. Having once initiated change, one is then accountable for the outcomes and consequences of decisions. In humanistic nursing leadership, both the leader and follower as individuals have choice in regard to whether or not to communicate, with whom, regarding what, and in what manner. The leader as a knowledgeable professional has choice about options offered and provided for the follower. The follower has choice, to the extent capable, regarding whether or not to accept options offered and provided. The leader needs to validate that the follower has knowledge of alternatives and consequences of his or her options, and needs to respect and honor the follower's decisions. Just as the client or patient has

nurse may dehumanize the client by issuing orders and expecting compliance, often without questioning the appropriateness or validity of the order. Some professional colleagues and perhaps the total health care system may dehumanize the nurse and the client by issuing directives and policies that unnecessarily limit professional and personal choices of the nurse and the options of health care for the client.

the right to choose whether or not to accept care offered, so the follower has a right to choose whether or not to follow a leader. The client has the option to reject care; the follower has the option to reject a directive. And such choice, as any other, carries responsibility and risk.

The opposite of choice is directive. The dehumanizing, patronizing, paternalistic leader assumes the follower is incapable of choice and will make the "wrong" choice in relation to organizational goals (or the leader's personal goals). To neglect to inform followers of options available for job advancement, educational opportunities, new policies, and so on, is typical of the leader who makes all the decisions.

5. Equality versus Degradation

5. Equality versus Degradation

Equality requires the nurse to approach the client with an awareness that both are human beings sharing all characteristics of existential human beings and living in an inescapable "here and now."

Equality requires the leader to approach the follower with an awareness that both are persons sharing all characteristics of existential human beings and living in an inescapable "here and now."

Equality involves being aware that, beneath all of the roles, status symbols, positions, and classifications people use in presenting themselves to one another, all are united in being human. People share the struggles of essence or being that involve ambiguity, anxiety, pain, joy, grief, and loneliness. The nurse is privileged to "be there" in critical life situations that involve very human struggles with inescapable "here-and-now" threats to health, well-being, and life itself. Equality means to perceive oneself as one person, a nurse, standing beside another person, a client, and together looking at a health-related problem, concern, or burden owned by the client, but shared; together, nurse and client seek ways to solve the problem, alleviate the concern, or lift the burden—and endure the ambiguity.

The opposite of equality is degradation, a dehumanizing process of depriving another of due rank, honor, and status. Degradation means to perceive oneself as a nurse, standing before a client, and to perceive the client as a problem, concern, or burden—not as another person. The nurse seems to be above having such a problem. Thus, the nurse keeps a safe distance, physically as well as interpersonally, as if to avoid being contaminated by the client.

Equality involves being aware that, beneath all of the roles, status symbols, positions, and classifications we use in presenting ourselves to one another, we are united in being human. We share the struggles of essence or being that involve ambiguity, anxiety, pain, joy, grief, and loneliness. The leader is privileged to "be there" in critical career situations of the follower, such as employment, transfer, promotion, or termination, which involve very human struggles with inescapable "here-and-now," threats to self-image, coping abilities, well-being, and earning capabilities. Equality means to perceive oneself as one person, a leader, standing beside another person, a follower, and together looking at a job-related problem, concern, or burden owned by either the follower or leader, but shared; together leader and follower seek ways to solve the problem, cope with the concern, or achieve the goal—and endure the ambiguity and risk. Although each person may play different roles within the organization, the different roles are of equal importance and value to the organization and the achievement of task goals and productivity. In operationalizing equality, the nurse-leader needs to communicate openly to all followers about job assignments, openings, benefits, privileges, and rewards. Everyone is to have the opportunity to receive recognition and opportunity for advancement in order to choose whether or not to accept challenges.

The opposite, degradation, is to deny followers due advancement, recognition, and status. The dehumanizing leader degrades followers by viewing them as tools to achieve productivity goals and mere means to an end. Any difficulties or concerns of the follower are reflected back on the follower so that he or she is seen as a complainer, goldbricker, or incompetent. The leader withholds self from the relationship, remaining impersonal, aloof, and superior. The followers learn to distrust the leader and loose confidence in the leader's ability to fairly apply job evaluation standards, criteria, and expectations. Ultimately, a third-party arbitrator, such as a union or lawyers, becomes a necessity to negotiate basic employment issues.

6. Positive Regard versus Disregard

Positive regard requires the nurse to label the client as potentially being capable of positive growth, of being able to cope, so that the client will tend to live up to this label.

Positive regard involves establishing an interpersonal climate that assumes the client does like one's situation or problem. It also assumes the client is capable of choosing to improve one's life situation. The client is seen as having potential for growth and learning not only in relation to health care and maintenance practices, but also in relation to personal maturity. In such a climate, help can be extended to the client, and the client may move more readily into open communication patterns that include trust, self-disclosure, and feedback. According to Rogers and Truax,

> It involves as much feeling of acceptance for the client's expression of painful, hostile, defensive, or abnormal feelings as for his expression of good, positive, mature feelings. . . . It is non-possessive caring for the client as a separate person. The client is thus freely allowed to have his own feelings and his own experiencing.[1]

Disregard is the dehumanizing opposite of positive regard. To communicate to a client with disregard is to assume the client prefers one's situation or problem and is incapable of improving. To provide more than minimal or routine help is believed relatively pointless; the client is seen as

6. Positive Regard versus Disregard

Positive regard requires the leader to label the follower as being potentially capable of positive growth and able to cope so that the follower will tend to live up to this label.

Positive regard involves establishing an interpersonal climate which assumes the follower does like his or her task and is growing in task competency. The follower is seen as having potential for growth and learning not only in relation to task performance and productivity, but also in relation to personal maturity. It is in such a climate that help can be extended to the follower and he or she may move more readily toward open communication patterns, which include trust, self-disclosure, and feedback. In discussing this approach in relation to clients, Rogers and Truax state the following:

> It involves as much feeling of acceptance for the client's expressions of painful, hostile, defensive, or abnormal feelings as for his expression of good, positive, mature feelings. . . . It is non-possessive caring for the client as a separate person. The client is thus freely allowed to have his own feelings and his own experiencing.[1]

Recognizing that this is not a counseling context, but a work context, it is believed that this attitude is to some considerable degree applicable to the leadership role in the leader–follower relationship. Such positive labeling tends to release the

incapable of using the help. The client is socialized into a submissive, uncomplaining, manipulative "client role" with limited acceptance of expressions of feelings and needs in a closed communication system.

follower to attain greater quality and quantity in job performance than with negative, distrustful climates. However, the leader needs to recognize the distinction between normal and therapeutic relationships. Generally, the role of leader excludes being a therapist, and appropriate personnel policies usually provide some direction when the need for professional counseling is indicated.

The leader who disregards followers, their requests and suggestions, ultimately disregards his or her own source of power and influence. If the follower does not accept the leader, then the leader is unable to influence the follower to change behaviors and participate in meeting goals. It is imperative that the follower accept the influence of the leader in order for leadership to be effective. This acceptance is, to a considerable extent, based upon the follower perceiving the self as being positively regarded by the leader.

---

7. Acceptance versus Judgment

Acceptance requires the nurse to establish a climate of psychological safety and support so that the client perceives the nurse as a trustworthy listener.

Acceptance involves nurses receiving clients as they are, not for what they are, but for their potential.[2] It includes making favorable responses to clients' expressions of feelings, personal meanings, and attempts to change and cope. Clients need to feel free to risk revealing the positive as well as the awkward, unsuccessful, and negative side of themselves, knowing the nurse will acknowledge, agree, and welcome these things without denial, manipulation, or defensiveness. Acceptance is a life situation. The effect of interpersonal acceptance is, for the nurse, recognizing the client as a unique self and, for the client, a releasing of the individual to self-disclose and trust.

Judgment is the dehumanizing opposite of acceptance and requires both the client and nurse to meet certain criteria in order to receive. For the client, one may need to be on Social Security or Medicare in order to qualify for certain types of nursing care. Or the nurse may need to behave in a certain manner in order to be worthy of receiving a particular privilege. Since one is continually aware of the other's role of judge, one is prone to compare what is received with that of

---

7. Acceptance versus Judgment

Acceptance requires the leader to establish a climate of psychological safety and support so that the follower perceives the leader as a trustworthy listener.

Acceptance involves the leader receiving followers as they are, not for what they *are,* but for their *potential,* for what they can *become.*[2] It includes making favorable responses to the followers' expressions of feelings, personal meanings, and attempts to change and cope. Followers need to feel free to risk revealing the positive as well as the awkward, unsuccessful, and negative side of themselves, and trusting the leader to acknowledge, agree, and welcome these things without denial, manipulation, or defensiveness. Acceptance is a pleasant state of being approved, believed, and acknowledged in one's own "lived world." The effect of interpersonal acceptance is for the leader, recognizing the follower as a unique self and, for the follower, a releasing of the individual to self-disclosure and trust, to risk growth and actualization.

The dehumanizing leader who emphasizes judgment stresses meeting criteria and standards. Followers experience concern about negative evaluations when concurrent feedback is not forthcoming from the leader. As the leader makes critical and evaluative comments, the fol-

others to determine one's own ranking in the regimented scheme of things. It makes a difference what or who one is. The threat of rejection is continual.

lower does not feel free to speak up and attempt to correct or influence the perceptions of the leader. The working relationship becomes unpleasant, unstable, and unattractive. The followers cope by taking sick time, seeking transfers, or leaving.

8. Empathy versus Tolerance

8. Empathy versus Tolerance

Empathy requires the nurse to actively listen for significant cues communicated by the client in order to sense the client's view of the world, to anticipate feelings and reactions, and ultimately to assess needs.

Empathy requires the leader to actively listen for significant cues communicated by the follower in order to sense the follower's view of the job world, to anticipate feelings and reactions, and ultimately to assess needs.

Empathy is the nurse's ability to communicate understanding of the client and to demonstrate a sensitivity to the client's current feelings, needs, and concerns. This ability is achieved through selection of language, voice qualities, posture, gesture, and attitude. The nurse does not experience the client's feelings, but has an awareness, an anticipation, and an appreciation of expressed feelings. The nurse is able to understand the association between the client's current health status, the progress in the client's response to therapy, and the impact of the nurse's own subsequent behavioral acts upon the client. As the recipient of empathy, the client is able to cope more easily with his or her life situation and perceive the nurse as communicating "I am with you." The client is subjectively aware of the nurse's "presence."

It is particularly discouraging and disappointing to expect empathy and to receive only tolerance. Here the nurse endures, bears, or puts up with the client. There is a lack of sensitivity to the client's feelings, needs, or fears. When the latter are expressed, the nurse may deny the importance or relevance of each.

Empathy is the leader's ability to communicate understanding of the follower and to demonstrate a sensitivity to current feelings, needs, and concerns. This is achieved through selection of language, voice qualities, posture, gesture, and attitude that are attractive to the follower. The leader does not experience the follower's feelings, but has an awareness, an anticipation, and an appreciation of expressed feelings. The leader is able to understand the association between the follower's current job status, the progress of the follower's response to leadership styles of communication, and the impact of the leader's own subsequent behavioral acts upon the direction of the follower's behavior. As the recipient of empathy, the follower is able to cope and grow more easily with his or her job situation and have a greater tendency to perceive the leader as communicating, "I am with you."

Without some degree of empathy, one merely encounters tolerance. One's work is merely "passable." One's leader seems to endure one's comments, ideas, contributions, and even one's mere presence. The total climate becomes unfavorable for one's very existence as co-workers take up the leader's attitude of tolerance. The negative implications for fair application of personnel policies, salary increases, promotions, and similar issues are inevitable. The attitude of tolerance soon becomes reciprocal, and easily moves to hatred.

9. Authenticity versus Role Playing

9. Authenticity versus Role Playing

Authenticity requires the nurse to be his or her own self, openly and honestly a human being, nothing more or less, in interpersonal relations with others.

Authenticity requires the leader to be his or her own self, openly and honestly a human being, nothing more or less, in interpersonal relations with others.

Authenticity is a personal recognition and acceptance of one's self as a human being, caught up in all the struggles, dilemmas, and contradictions characterizing humanity. It is the recognition and study of one's own struggles with choice, and the dilemmas arising from knowing perfection, yet being trapped in an animalistic, materialistic, time- and-space-bound world of inevitable contradictions of values, feelings, and behaviors. Authenticity excludes pretense and facades. Rather, it involves honesty in personal and professional feedback to self and others, as well as an openness and spontaneity in expressing feelings. It includes a commitment to deliberately communicate interpersonally with responsibility and accountability as a person having unique and singular capabilities, limitations, feelings, values, and perceptions. It is being true to one's self, and it is a call to others to be interpersonally authentic also.

The opposite of authenticity is role playing. In clinical practice, there are times when the nurse is to withhold information for the client's welfare, or at least allow it to be conveyed by another professional. Thus, some role playing is occasionally necessary in certain nurse–client relationships. However, one can role play to the extent that the individual, whether client or nurse, is perceived interpersonally to be an empty shell of a person or hiding behind a facade. The client plays the "sick" role, seemingly for secondary gain. The nurse may act "professional," seemingly to protect the self from becoming involved. One tends to wonder where the "real" person's values, feelings, and intentions truly lie.

Authenticity of the leader is a personal recognition and acceptance of one's self as a human being, caught up in all the struggles, dilemmas, and contradictions characterizing humanity. It is the recognition and study of one's own struggles with choice, and the dilemmas arising from knowing perfection, yet being trapped in an animalistic, materialistic, time- and space-bound world of inevitable contradictions of values, feelings, and behaviors. Authenticity excludes pretense, facades; the opposite is role playing. Rather, it involves honesty in personal and professional feedback to self and others, as well as an openness and spontaneity in expressing feelings. It includes a commitment to deliberately communicate interpersonally with responsibility and accountability as a person having unique and singular capabilities, limitations, feelings, values, and perceptions. It is being true to one's self, and it is a call to others to be interpersonally authentic also.

The opposite of authenticity, role playing, involves inherently manipulative, managerial facades. There are times when leaders are aware of new policies or procedures that are destructive to the followers in some way; an appropriate role is to be maintained until the information is provided by the appropriate management representative. However, the leader who acts angry to motivate followers, who acts cold and uninvolved to maintain a "proper" distance from the followers, is perceived as cold, calculating, and uninvolved. The leader may look human, but in reality is only the company robot programmed to follow standard operating procedures.

10. Caring versus Carelessness	*10. Caring versus Carelessness*
Caring requires the nurse and client to help each other struggle and strive, cope and achieve in the human existential state through confirmation of each other's being and understanding of each other's feelings.	Caring requires the leader and follower to help each other struggle and strive, cope and achieve in the human existential state through confirmation of each other's being and understanding of each other's feelings.
Caring is having a positive regard for another person so that one can accept the other as each grows, unfolds, and blooms in his or her own unique way. It includes validating each other in worth of self, desires, beliefs, perceptions, and feelings through a process of trust, self-disclosure, and feedback. Caring is not feminine in the sense of classical sex-role stereotypes of lover-	Caring in leadership is having a positive regard for one's followers so that one can accept the followers as each grows, unfolds and blooms in his or her own unique way. It includes validating each other in worth of self, desires, beliefs, perceptions, and feelings through a process of trust, self-disclosure, and feedback. Caring is not feminine in the sense of classical sex-role stereotypes

wife-mother behavior. It excludes the classical male sex role stereotype of unemotional stoicism, dominance, and self-serving competitiveness. Rather, it is one person caring for another, regardless of sex, because one has a stake in the other's fate. One becomes involved to *give* out of one's strengths. One gives time, energy, attention, and thought to another's existence.

In humanistic nursing, the nurse gives of personal and professional strengths and resources to help the client struggle and strive to survive illness (or to die, to let go), to heal, and hopefully to achieve wellness of body and of spirit. And this caring is reciprocal. The nurse is able to study each existential relationship with clients, to mature in personal and professional resources, and to be validated in those communication and nursing skills and behaviors that prove most effective in achieving meaningful interpersonal relationships with clients and others. Each caring experience gives promise of another caring in the future for both nurse and client.

The dehumanizing opposite of caring is to be careless. There is a tendency to be ignored and disregarded. For the client, it means carelessness in nursing care. Details of care are left undone: call lights are unanswered; medications are given erroneously, if at all. It means losing personal items of clothing, dentures, or eyeglasses, and it means receiving salt on the low-salt dinner tray.

of lover-wife-mother behavior. It excludes the classical male sex-role stereotype of unemotional stoicism, dominance, and self-serving competitiveness. Rather, it is one person, caring for another, regardless of sex, because each has a stake in the other's fate. One gives of one's self or becomes involved to *give* out of one's strengths. One gives time, energy, attention, and thought to another's existence.

In humanistic nursing leadership, the leader gives of personal and professional strengths and resources to help the follower struggle and strive to succeed (or fail, to leave) and hopefully, to achieve career objectives and perhaps a fullness of life personally and professionally. And this caring is reciprocal. The leader is able to study each existential relationship with followers, to mature in his or her personal and professional resources, and to be validated in those communication and leadership skills and behaviors that prove most effective in achieving meaningful interpersonal relationships within the task group. Each caring experience gives promise of greater caring in the future for both leader and follower.

The leader who is careless about followers' job needs and expectations sets up barriers. For the staff nurse follower, this means not being informed of a change in one's duty hours, not being relieved by another nurse for lunch or bathroom breaks, and having the guards refuse to provide escort service to one's car when leaving the hospital late at night. No one plans for these needs. No one counts the vacation days due, and no one shows concern when too much is inaccurately deducted from a paycheck. No one notices what happens to the nurses on the unit. Management seems to care less about what happens to "me!"

---

11. Irreplaceable versus Expendable

Irreplaceability requires the nurse to recognize one's own life as well as that of clients as having intrinsic value.

Irreplaceability means human life cannot be replaced or substituted as one might replace a light bulb. Each client is to be supported, maintained, and enhanced through respect and enhancement of self-concept, body image, and reality presentation. One's self-concept is the spirit and center of the human being. According to Mead, one's image of one's self, of one's body, and of one's life

11. Irreplaceable versus Expendable

Irreplaceability requires the leader to recognize one's own life as well as that of others as having intrinsic value.

Irreplaceability means human life cannot be replaced or substituted as one might replace a light bulb. Each human being and his or her career is to be supported, maintained, and enhanced through respect and enhancement of self-concept, body image, and reality presentation. One's self-concept is the spirit and center of the human being. According to Mead, one's image of one's self, of situation is heavily influenced by interpersonal relationships.[3]

It is important that the nurse recognize his or her own being as having intrinsic worth and value. The nurse needs to care for his or her own self-concept, body image, and lived world. It is important to treat one's self in a humanistic manner by recognizing one's feelings and needs, learning to express positive as well as negative feelings, and to meet needs, yet not in a self-serving fashion. It is recognizing one's own worth and irreplaceability to limit one's personal and professional commitments, responsibilities, and obligations to that degree at which one can function with optimal ease. In the degree this is accomplished, the nurse will tend to operationalize humanistic nursing.

To assume the human being is expendable is the ultimate in dehumanization. Clients come to be viewed by nurses as machinery on an assembly line in a factory. For a client to die would be the equivalent of relief from a taxing routine of trying to get the machine fixed. The death may hardly be noticed at the charge nurse's change-of-shift report, and the empty bed is quickly filled with another client. There begins to be for the nurse a quality of sameness about the clients. Little progress seems to be made, and the need of making any real effort to value human beings seems pointless. This is particularly true when the clients tend to be socially unattractive, such as the retarded, the mentally ill, the senile, and the chronically ill and disabled—the very people who need the extra dose of all the humanizing elements identified here.

one's body, and of one's "lived world" is heavily influenced by interpersonal relationships.[3]

It is important that the leader recognize his or her own being as having intrinsic worth and value. The leader needs to care for his or her own self-concept, body image, and lived world. It is important to treat one's self in a humanistic manner by recognizing one's feelings and needs, learning to express positive as well as negative feelings, and to meet needs, yet not in a self-serving fashion.

One needs to recognize that leadership roles are vacated and filled with considerable ease. One's role as a leader is analogous to dipping one's hand into a bucket of water: upon removing your hand, the water comes together so that there is minimal indication that the hand was ever there. Leadership is hard to achieve, seldom permanent, and easily lost. This sense of expendability helps maintain attentiveness to task and productivity goals. It is the vitality of being human that has irreplaceable value, not of being a leader or follower.

---

12. Intimacy versus Isolation

Intimacy requires the nurse to be receptive of client's need for disclosure of personal feelings, perceptions, and experiences, especially those disclosures having relevance to health.

12. Intimacy versus Isolation

Intimacy requires the leader to be receptive of follower's need for disclosure of personal feelings, perceptions, and experiences, especially those disclosures having relevance to task accomplishment, job advancement, and career development.

Intimacy is listening to another's self-disclosures and caring about the meaning and implications for the other's well-being.[4] It involves establishing an interpersonal climate of trust so that the risk of self-disclosure might be minimized. In nursing, there is a social "permission" to disclose so that the health care might be based on all rele-

Intimacy is listening to another's self-disclosures and caring about the meaning and implications for the other's well-being.[4] It involves establishing an interpersonal climate of trust so that the risk of self-disclosure might be minimized. In nursing, there is a social "permission" to disclose so that the health care might be based on all relevant health or illness information. Clients often disclose to nurses personal things never before revealed to others. The nurse needs to be committed to receiving clients' disclosures with caring and respect in order to promote the client's interpersonal growth and to support the client's coping and adaptive processes. In nursing, intimacy also includes touching as one administers nursing care. Hall identifies intimate space as being up to 18 inches from one's body. He describes this interaction space as appropriate to lovemaking, comforting, protecting, struggling, and fighting.[5] In the process of "laying on of hands," as nurses we need to recognize the potentially powerful impact of invading clients' intimate space, and nurses need to use this to support the clients' well-being.

The dehumanizing opposite of intimacy is interpersonal isolation, which seems to be too often the experiences of clients needing care and of nurses wanting to give safe, quality nursing care. The client finds himself or herself isolated from familiar faces and places while experiencing strange sensations and behaviors of the body. While many people, nurses and others, may come near to perform certain tasks, too often it seems that no one, even the nurse, is able or willing to provide adequate information or answers to questions posed. And all quickly withdraw to other tasks, busily rushing down halls in opposite directions, hopefully coordinated in some unknown way—the so-called team approach. Very few of these people use one's name, and those who do often merely use it to check the identification bracelet: one becomes a bed or room number or a diagnosis. If one displays the normal symptoms of isolation, the nurses soon stop using the bed or room number and begin using labels such as "difficult," "problem," or "fussy."

vant health or illness information. Followers often disclose to leaders personal things never before revealed to others. While this personal disclosure is not to be encouraged, the leader needs to be committed to receiving follower's disclosures with caring and respect in order to promote the follower's interpersonal growth and career development, and to support the follower's coping and adaptive processes. In nursing, intimacy also includes touching as one administers nursing care. Hall identifies intimate space as being up to 18 inches from one's body. He describes this interaction space as appropriate to lovemaking, comforting, protecting, struggling, and fighting.[5] In the process of "laying on of the hands," as nurses, we need to recognize the potentially powerful impact of invading clients' intimate space; as leaders, we need to respect the privacy and dignity of the follower's personal space and need for territory. In the leader–follower relationship, touching tends to be limited. Leaders and followers need to give each other the "18 inches of personal space," except for a rewarding "pat on the back." Rather, intimacy is most appropriately relabeled "inclusion" in the leader–follower relationship. The humanistic leader includes the follower in the process of achieving task goals through directing, guiding, listening, and developing followers, promoting their efforts, capabilities, and careers.

Isolation is easily achieved for the nurse-follower on solitary assignments such as the nursery, intensive care, and night duty. The sense of being alone is enhanced by limiting the opportunity to meet with other staff nurses informally or formally, and limiting general information about the organization and its goals. Unless the leader makes a special effort to include staff from other shifts or isolated posts, it is easy for these followers to develop hostile attitudes toward the day shift or staff on other units. Isolation is enhanced by the "them and us" perspective. Because contact and responsibility are fragmented in the typical team or functional organization of nursing staffs, individual nurses have limited opportunity to get to know the client, and have limited power over what happens to the client; they feel frustrated professionally and very isolated personally.

13. Coping versus Helplessness

Coping requires the nurse to assess, support, maintain, and augment the client's abilities to

13. Coping versus Helplessness

Coping requires the leader to assess, support,

achieve an optimum level of functioning in one's existential state.

Coping, according to the dictionary, means to encounter problems and difficulties in such a manner that one is "on even terms with" or "is successful"; it is fighting a battle and winning.[6] For the existential person, coping involves being a reflective, subjective, lonely, future-oriented person existing in a time- and space-bound setting characterized by the objectivity, reason, and structure of scientific knowledge. Humans daily encounters problems and difficulties that require continuous striving, choosing, and doing. Coping permeates all areas of human life. The nurse is particularly concerned in determining the client's modes of coping as a biological being, as a cognitive being, and as a subjective being. The goal of the nurse is to assist the client in achieving not only survival, but also the fullest expression of "being" human, even in dying.

Helplessness is the dehumanizing opposite of coping. The client is helpless when without accurate and complete information with which to develop a plan of action. Without individualized guidance and support of the nurse and others, the client tends to feel overwhelmed and may not grasp the total situation and its implications. Panic tends to develop, along with anger and even revenge (I'll sue for this!) for the dehumanizing treatment. Distrust and rejection of all health care professionals becomes common as clients turn to self-help groups who understand or to "quick-cure" commercial shams.

maintain, and augment the follower's existential state in the job setting.

Coping, according to the dictionary, means to encounter problems and difficulties in such a manner that one is "on even terms with" or "is successful"; it is fighting a battle and winning.[6] For the existential person, coping involves being a reflective, subjective, lonely, future-oriented person existing in a time- and space-bound setting characterized by the objectivity, reason, and structure of scientific knowledge. Humans daily encounters problems and difficulties that require continuous striving, choosing, and doing. Coping permeates all areas of human life. The leader is particularly concerned in determining the follower's modes of coping as a biological being, as a cognitive being, and as a subjective being. The goal of the nurse-leader is to assist the follower in achieving not only survival, but also the fullest expression of "being" possible through task accomplishment and job success.

Yet feelings of helplessness are not unknown in nursing leadership and clinical practice. The nurse feels helpless because of the responsibility for, yet inability to control, the nursing care plan of even one patient. Any decision about a client's care that one nurse makes will probably not be respected and followed by nurses on succeeding shifts in the typical hospital setting. Communication between the nurse and the client's physician tends to be very limited, so that the nurse is often unable to coordinate the nursing care plan with the medical plan for care. Consequently one can know the inevitable outcomes and watch them happen. All of the education and knowledge goes for nothing as no one will listen. What is the use of trying?

14. Power versus Powerlessness

Power requires the nurse to be accountable for personal and professional choices in his or her own life and nursing practice, and to recognize the client's fundamental responsibility and freedom as well as accountability for choice, particularly in regard to health-related issues.

Power is not only answering for one's conduct and obligations but also being accountable for one's choices of right and wrong. It implicitly assumes the capability to initiate change and to be a

14. Power versus Powerlessness

Power requires the nurse-leader to be accountable for personal and professional choices in his or her own life and nursing practice, and to recognize the follower's fundamental responsibility and freedom as well as accountability for choice, particularly in regard to job-related issues.

Power is not only answering for one's conduct and obligations but also being accountable for one's choices of right and wrong. It implicitly assumes the capability to initiate change and to be a cause of some event. One is responsible for one's own communicative behavior. In responsible interpersonal relationships, one evaluates feedback from others, becomes congruent with inner feelings, and changes if one chooses to do so. Responsible interpersonal relationships are at the core of humanistic nursing. Communicative acts on the part of the nurse are embodied in the nursing process and are significant factors in the individual client's plan of nursing care. The nurse needs to respect the client's power to choose and to be responsible for his or her own choices. Equally, the nurse needs to respect the client's feelings of dread, anxiety, and anguish, which, inevitably for existentialism, follow choice.

Powerlessness is the dehumanizing opposite of power. The client is rendered powerless by nurses and others who ignore, do not consult, or even talk about him or her in the client's presence as if the client were absent.

cause of some event. In existentialism, the power of choice is man's ontological freedom, and choice is followed by a feeling of dread and sense of responsibility. The coward and hero alike are responsible for their acts. One is responsible for one's own communicative behavior. In responsible interpersonal relationships, one evaluates feedback from others, becomes congruent with inner feelings, and changes if one chooses to do so. Responsible interpersonal relationships are at the core of humanistic nursing. Communicative acts involving power on the part of the leader are embodied in the leadership process and are significant factors in the individual follower's career development. The leader needs to respect the follower's power to choose and to be responsible for his or her own choices. Equally, the leader also needs to respect the follower's feelings of dread, anxiety, and anguish, which, inevitably for existentialism, follow the power of choice.

To be powerless means to be without choice, influence, and accountability, and to merely react to events. It means being charge nurse with all the accountability and responsibility inherent in the role but without the authority of the head nurse or unit supervisor positions. It is being the nurse who is moved from unit to unit to meet emergency staffing needs or who is manipulated (coerced?) into working double shifts by the supervisor. It is being as powerless as a tin soldier in a child's toy battalion.

REFERENCES

1. Rogers, C.R., & Truax, C.B. The therapeutic conditions antecedent to change: A theoretical view. In G. Egan, *Encounter groups: Basic readings.* Belmont, Calif.: Brooks/Cole, 1971, p. 264.
2. Giffin, K., & Patton, B.R. *Personal communication in human relations.* Columbus, Ohio: Merrill, 1974, p. 124.
3. Mead, G.H. *Mind, self and society.* Chicago and London: University of Chicago Press, 1934.
4. Giffin, K., & Patton, B.R. *Interpersonal communication in action.* New York: Harper & Row, 1977, pp. 347–348.
5. Hall, E. T. *The hidden dimension.* Garden City, New York: Doubleday, 1969.
6. Guralnik, D.B. (Ed.). *Webster's New World dictionary* (2nd college ed.). New York: Simon & Schuster, 1980.

Appendix C: SITUATIONAL LEADERSHIP THEORY®
Phenomenon: Leader-Follower-Situational Communication;

Assumptions	Concepts	Relationship Statements	Evaluation
1. A single, ideal type of leader behavior is unrealistic; the leadership process is a function of the leader, follower, and other situational variables (p. 99).	1. *Leadership*: the process of influencing the activities of an individual or a group in efforts toward goal achievement in a given situation (p. 86).	1. If a leader is to be an effective manager of change, then the leader must be able to analyze the demands of the environment; diagnose and adapt leadership style to fit these demands; and develop means to change some or all of the other situational variables.	1. Research support: a. Stinson, J.E., & Johnson, T.W. "The path-goal theory of leadership: A partial test and suggested refinement. *Academy of Management Journal*, 1975, *18*(2), 242–252.
2. The style of leadership needs to be adapted to the situation and to the needs of the followers (p. 106).	2. *Leadership style*: the consistent behavior patterns used when leaders are working with and through other people as perceived by those people (p. 146).	2. The appropriate leadership style (communicating by telling, selling, participating, or delegating) for given levels of follower readiness is in a curvilinear functional relation to the task and relationship behaviors.	b. Gumpert, R.A., & Hambleton, R.K. Situational Leadership: how Xerox managers fine tune managerial styles to employee maturity and task needs. *Management Review*, December 1979, pp. 8–13. Major findings included the following:
3. Values and attitudes can be predicted from behavior, but not vice versa (p. 123).	3. *Task behavior*: the extent to which leaders are likely to organize and define the roles of the members of their group (followers), to explain what activities each is to do and when, where, and how tasks are to be accomplished; characterized by endeavoring to establish well defined patterns of organization, channels of communication, and ways of getting jobs accomplished (pp. 116 & 172).	2.1 As the level of readiness of the follower increases in terms of accomplishing a specific task, the leader should begin to reduce task behavior and increase relationship behavior.	1. Highly effective managers indicate greater knowledge and use of Situational Leadership than less effective managers.
4. Leaders need to be concerned about the impact of leadership style upon human resources: leaders need to develop follower's commitment and competency (p. 124).		2.2 As the readiness level of the follower moves into an above average level, the leader should decrease task behavior and relationship behavior.	2. All managers in the study reported using Situational Leadership at least some of the time. This finding demonstrates that training in this area has substantial on-the-job impact.
5. Successful leaders only influence productivity; successful and effective leaders influence productivity and the internal state or predisposition of an individual or group and thus is attitudinal in nature (p. 129).	4. *Relationship behavior*: the extent to which leaders are likely to maintain personal relationships between themselves and members of their group (followers) by opening up channels of communication, providing socioemotional support, "psycho-	2.21 If the follower's readiness level is low (R1), unable and unwilling, then the appropriate leadership style is "telling,"	3. On the average, managers who apply the model correctly rate their subor-
6. The relationship between the leader and the follower is the key factor; it is the follower who decides whether or not to follow and whether or			

Columns are not numbered for cross reference.

not the leader IS a leader (p. 166).

7. Leaders may need various power bases, depending on the situation (p. 213).

8. An important role of the leader is the development of task-relevant readiness of their followers (p. 229).

9. Leaders need to consistently support only good behavior and improvement, not just any behavior (p. 247).

10. Leaders need to intervene when followers demonstrate less task relevant readiness than previously (p. 249).

11. Leaders need to establish a developmental program for followers that includes establishment of goals, objectives, criteria performance, and leadership style (p. 303).

12. Leaders need to develop strategies to plan, direct, and control change; change is an inevitable danger to maintaining viable, current organizations (p. 333).

13. An organization is an "open social system," that is, all aspects of an organization are interrelated; a change in any one part of it may have an impact on other parts or on the whole organization itself. (p. 361).

logical strokes," and facilitating behaviors (pp. 117 & 172).

5. *Readiness:* How ready a person is to perform a particular task (p. 175).

a. Ability: is the knowledge, experience, and skill that an individual or group brings to a particular task or activity.

b. Willingness: is the extent to which an individual or group has the confidence, commitment, and motivation to accomplish a specific task.

Readiness includes the ability and willingness of people to take responsibility for directing their own behavior; the variables of readiness should be considered only in relation to a specific task to be performed; readiness viewed as a continuum extending from low to high levels of readiness; it includes education and/or experience, and the capacity to set high but attainable goals (achievement motivation) of an individual or group.

6. *Leadership styles* (of communication): Labels of leadership behavior styles useful for quick diagnostic judgments (p. 177). These are as follows:

a. Telling: one-way communication in which the leader defines the roles of the follow-

or high task and low relationship behavior.

2.22 If the follower's readiness level is low to moderate (R2), unable but willing, then the appropriate leadership style is "selling," or high task and high relationship behavior.

2.23 If the follower's readiness level is moderate to high (R3), able but unwilling or insecure, then the appropriate leadership style is "participating," or high relationship and low task behavior.

2.24 If the follower's readiness level is high (R4), able and willing, then the appropriate leadership style is "delegating," or low relationship and low task behavior.

2.3 If a leader has a wide style range, then effectiveness in leadership has a high level of probability, when appropriately applied in a given situation.

2.4 Style adaptability tends to increase the probability of leadership successfullness and effectiveness.

3. If the power bases available to the leader are consistent with the leadership style(s) and appropriate to the readiness level of the followers, then the

dinates' job performance higher than managers who do not. The data in this area are highly supportive of the Hersey-Blanchard model of leadership effectiveness.

4. There is considerable evidence that when Situational Leadership is applied correctly, follower job performance is judged higher; gains in job performance are practically and statistically significant.

In summary, highly effective managers knew more about Situational Leadership and use it more than less effective managers.

c. Angelini, A.L., Hersey, P., & Carcaushansky, S. The situational leadership theory applied to teaching: A research on learning effectiveness, *Group and Organizational Studies,* 7(2), 216–244. Sage Publications, 1982.

d. Numerous dissertations.

2. Applications: Major training tool for Bank of America, Caterpillar, IBM, Mobile Oil, Union 76, and Xerox. Also used in the military services and entrepreneurial companies.

Assumptions	Concepts	Relationship Statements	Evaluation
14. People who work together need a common language (p. 446). 15. Having a common language enables people to give one another feedback and help rationally and unemotionally to affect behavior; also it enables them to recognize that the follower's behavior determines the leadership style to be used with them (p. 447). 16. To lead best is to promote holism; to help people understand and share expectations in their environment; to help people learn to supervise their own behavior and become responsible, self-motivated individuals (p. 447).	ers, and tells them what, how, when, and where to do various tasks. Guiding, directing, or structuring. (S1) b. Selling: While still providing direction, the leader uses two-way communication and socio-emotional support to get the follower(s) to psychologically buy into decisions that have been made. "Why" is added. Explaining, persuading, or clarifying. (S2) c. Participating: While the leader and follower share in decision making, the leader uses two-way communication and facilitating behaviors with followers having task ability and knowledge. Collaborating, facilitating or committing. (S3) d. Delegating: The leader reduces communication while maintaining the relationship, and allows the follower(s) to "run their own show." Observing or monitoring. (S4) 7. *Developmental Cycle:* A leader's attempt to develop their followers at high levels of readiness; the followers can take over much of the responsibility for the day-to-day traditional management functions. A growth cycle (p. 234).	leader will tend to be successful and effective. 3.1 To the same degree that others perceive a leader's power, the leader is enabled to induce compliance or to influence behavior of others. 3.2 If a leader is to avoid an eroding power base and to increase the chances of successfully influencing others' behavior, then the leader needs information about the sources of power he or she is perceived by others as having. 3.3 If a leader communicates the power he or she possesses, then others will tend to perceive it. 3.4 As the readiness level of the follower increases from low (R1) to high (R4), the follower tends to respond to leader influence based on different types of power. 3.41 Low readiness (R1) tends to be influenced by perceived power based on "coercion" and "connection." 3.42 Low to moderate readiness (R2) tends to be influenced by perceived power based on "connection," "reward," and "legitimate."	

3.43 Moderate to high readiness (R3) tends to be influenced by perceived power based on "legitimate," "referent," and "information."

3.44 High readiness (R4) tends to be influenced by perceived power based on "information" and "expertise."

4. If a leader is to break the ineffective cycle and increase task-relevant readiness of followers, then the leader must increase gradually the responsibility delegated to the followers, with a reasonable degree of risk.

4.1 If the leader increases socioemotional relationship or relationship behavior too rapidly, then the followers may view the leader as becoming a "soft touch."

4.2 If the leader rewards as quickly as possible the slightest appropriate behavior exhibited by the individual, then the individual's performance will come closer and closer to the leader's expectations.

5. If the followers begin to behave in a less ready manner for whatever reason, then the leader must intervene to correct inappropriate behaviors with appropriate timing and at the appropriate level on the regressive

8. *Regressive Cycle:* When followers are beginning to behave less ready than they have in the past (p. 249).

9. *Style range:* The extent to which leaders are able to vary their style (p. 271).

10. *Style adaptability:* The degree to which leaders are able to vary their style appropriately to the demands of a given situation (p. 273).

11. *Style profile:* Use of one or combinations of the four leadership styles, i.e., S1, S2, S3, and S4 (p. 286).

12. *Power:* a leader's influence potential; a resource that enables a leader to gain compliance from others (p. 202).

13. *Change:* inevitable in process oriented society and organizations; can be planned or unplanned (p. 333).

14. *Change efforts:* involve attempting to reduce discrepancies between the real (actual) and the ideal (p. 334).

15. *Change cycles:* Change moves from variances in knowledge, attitude, individual behavior, and group or organizational change (p. 339).

16. *Change process:* The process of change occurs in three phases, which are as follows (p. 347);

Assumptions	Concepts	Relationship Statements	Evaluation

Concepts

A. Unfreezing: motivating and making an individual or group ready for change; the breaking down of old mores, customs, and traditions.

B. Changing: identifying and internalizing new patterns of behavior.

C. Refreezing: integrating new behavior patterns into the individuals' personality and ongoing emotional relationships.

Model:

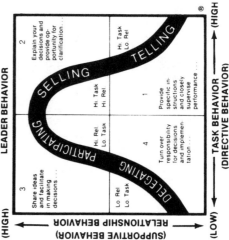

Relationship Statements

cycle at a lower emotional level (i.e., without anger).

5.1 If the behavior is unacceptable to the leader, then the leader needs to make the follower aware of the problem and the follower ultimately is to solve the problem. This is an extensive, temporary intervention by the leader.

5.2 If the behavior is unacceptable to both leader and follower, the follower ultimately is to solve the problems after a period of shared responsibility with the leader. This is a temporary intervention by the leader.

5.3 If the follower's behavior is acceptable to the leader but not to the follower, then the leader needs to be supportive of the follower's efforts to solve his or her own problem. This is a minimal intervention by the leader.

5.4 If the follower's behavior is acceptable and no problem exists, then no intervention on the part of the leader is necessary.

Analysis: B. W. Duldt

Reference: From Hersey, P., & Blanchard, K. *Management of Organizational Behavior: Utilizing Human Resources* (5th ed.). Englewood Cliffs, N. J.: Prentice-Hall, 1988.

Appendix D: DULDT'S THEORY OF HUMANISTIC NURSING COMMUNICATION

Phenomenon Observed: Interpersonal Communication between Nurse and Client, Peers and Colleagues

Assumptions	Concepts	Relationship Statements	Evaluation
Derived from Philosophy:	*Human being:* Man is a living being capable of symbolizing, perceiving the negative, transcending the environment by inventions, ordering the environment, striving for perfection, making choices, and self-reflecting.	1. To the same degree that one receives humanizing communication from others, one will tend to feel recognized and accepted as a human being.	1. *Clearly stated:* This theory is presented in an organized, logical sequence, and is readily understood. Assumptions are stated according to widely recognized academic patterns. Its concepts are extensively defined. The relationship statements are presented in a pattern that covertly implies research designs and statistical analysis. This theory is expected to stimulate more research efforts than the theories of Buber and of Patterson and Zderad.
1. Human beings exist in a "here-and-now" existential context from which there is no escape.			
2. Human beings are continually concerned with such existential elements as: being, becoming, choice, freedom, responsibility, solitude, loneliness, pain, struggle, tragedy, meaning, dread, uncertainty, despair, and death.	**Characteristics:**	a. While applying the nursing process, to the same degree that a nurse is able to use humanizing communication, the client, peer, or colleague will tend to feel recognized and accepted as a human being.	
	1. *Living:* Able to function biologically and physiologically as an animalistic, viable entity.		
	2. *Communicating:* Able to label things and to talk about them when they aren't present.	b. In a given environment, if a critical life situation develops for a client, to the same degree the nurse uses humanizing communication attitudes and patterns while applying the nursing process, the health of the client will tend to move in a positive direction.	2. *Scope:* This theory is applicable to nurse–client interpersonal communication in all areas of nursing. It is also applicable to nurse–peer and nurse–colleague relationships. As a paradigm variation of Buber's "I-Thou" and of Patterson and Zderad's humanistic nursing theory, this theory provides a more readily testable and measurable approach to abstract concepts. It also incorporates the
3. All elements of existential being and the communication imperative are salient issues to be dealt with in critical life situations.	3. *Negativing:* Able to talk about the symbolic negative (−1, no, none, not), make rules (laws regarding the "thou shalt not's"), worry about what may not happen, and consider his or her own nonexistence.		
4. Growth and change arise from within the individual and to a considerable degree depend upon one's choice.	4. *Inventing:* Able to be aware of, know, and do things beyond his or her own immediate environment, to invent things, and to change his relationship to the environment.	2. To the same degree a nurse uses humanizing elements to communicate, that nurse will tend to receive humanizing communications from clients, peers, colleagues, and superiors.	
5. The nurse shares with the client all characteristics of being human.			

Columns are not numbered for cross reference.

Assumptions	Concepts	Relationship Statements	Evaluation

Assumptions

Derived from Communication:

6. Survival is based on one's ability to communicate with others in order to share feelings and facts about the environment and ways of coping.

7. The environment is a "booming, buzzing" world of strange sensations that must be sorted out to determine which are most important; this sorting is achieved through communication with other people.

8. The need to communicate is an innate imperative for human beings.

9. Due to innate fallacies, human beings use and misuse all capabilities, especially the ability to communicate. An example is speaking to a human being as a thing rather than a person.

10. The way in which a person communicates determines what that person becomes.

11. Interpersonal communication is a humanizing factor that is an innate element of the nursing process (assessment, planning, implementation, and evaluation) and of the communication that occurs between nurses and clients, nurses and

Concepts

5. *Ordering:* Able to develop categories and hierarchies according to some value or theme; gives structure and system to one's environment.

6. *Dreaming:* Able to dream of how things could be if all were perfect; expectations, hopes for future.

7. *Choosing:* Able to consider numerous alternatives, implications for the future.

8. *Self-Reflecting:* Able to think about and talk about self, reflect on own behavior and understand self, body, behaviors, etc. Conscious of the existential elements (see assumption 2).

Roles:

Nurse: A human being who practices nursing, intervening through the application of the nursing process to develop a plan of nursing care for a specific client or group of clients. The nurse possesses special educational and licensure credentials as required by society.

Client: A human being who is experiencing a critical life situation, potential or actual. He or she has need of the services of the nurse and is the focus of the nursing process. The client can also be seen to include

Relationship Statements

3. To the same degree that trust, self-disclosure, and feedback occur, humanizing communication or communing also occurs.

4. In the event one tends to experience dehumanizing communication—that is, monological rather than dialogical communication, categorical rather than individualistic, and so on—one tends to move outward (on the model) to the next pattern of interaction. (See figure.)

5. In an interpersonal relationship of trust, self-disclosure, and feedback, to the same degree that dehumanizing communication attitudes are expressed by another, one tends to use assertiveness as a pattern of interaction.

6. To the same degree that assertiveness tends not to reestablish trust, self-disclosure, and feedback, and that dehumanizing communication attitudes continue to be expressed by another, one tends to use confrontation as a pattern of communication.

Evaluation

writings and research of Burke (1966), Jourard (1971), Egan (1970, 1971), Berlo (1960), Patterson & Zderad (1976), Yura & Walsh (1973), Kierkegaard (1957), Maslow (1954), Mead (1934), Rogers & Truax (1971), Sartre (1957), Patton & Giffin (1977), Giffin & Patton (1974), and others.

3. *Applicability:* This theory is realistic in that it recognizes the ways in which nursing and health care systems are dehumanizing to nurses, clients, and others. However, it emphasizes the choice of the nurse in using communication patterns that tend to be humanizing. It is an "is" theory, not a "should" theory. This is also a "state" theory in that it assumes that communication "here and now" can change the future.

4. *Generalizability and agreement with known data:* The theory is derived from a broad base of communication theory and research. It brings together information often taught in nursing curricula and puts it into a cohesive perspective that is intended to be more readily understood and used by nurses.

The theory is unique in that it recognizes the negative, unpleasant encounters nurses often have in clinical practice, and it provides a framework for developing modes of coping with dehumanizing communications.

5. *Research support for the theory.*

a. On trust by K. Giffin (1967). Extensive support from speaker credibility research in the field of speech communication.

b. Jourard (1971), Egan (1970, 1971) on self-disclosure and feedback.

c. Grant (Duldt) (1977) found that anger expressed in the maintenance mode tends to increase group cohesiveness and maintain relationships between nursing task members; the destructive mode of expressing anger tends to destroy relationships, decreasing productivity and group attraction.

d. Duldt (1982) identified the "anger-dismay" syndrome as a complex of behaviors nurses tend to display when receiving destructive-mode anger from others, especially from superiors.

7. To the same degree that confrontation tends not to reestablish trust, self-disclosure, or feedback, and that dehumanizing communication attitudes continue to be expressed by another, one tends to use conflict resolution as a pattern of communication.

8. To the same degree that conflict tends not to reestablish trust, self-disclosure, and feedback, and that dehumanizing communication attitudes continue to be expressed by another, one tends to terminate the relationship by separation.

9. To the same degree that humanizing communication attitudes occur in a relationship, in the event of separation, the relationship can be resumed to the same degree of closeness regardless of the separation.

10. To the same degree that one is aware of one's own choices (and motives) about interaction patterns and attitudes, one is able to develop communication skills and habits that tend to have predictable results in establishing, maintaining, and terminating interpersonal relationships.

the support system of family, friends, and so on.

Peer: A nurse having equal standing or status to another nurse.

Colleague: A member of another profession with whom nurses coordinate and collaborate in the practice of nursing—that is, physicians, administrators, ministers, and members of health care professions and community service agencies.

Nursing: The art and science of positive, humanistic intervention in the changing health states of human beings interacting in the environment of critical life situations. Its elements are communicating, caring, and coaching.

Nursing process: This involves assessment, planning, implementation, and evaluation.

Health: One's state of being, of becoming; of self-awareness. It is indicative of one's adaptation to the environment.

Environment: One's time-space-relationship context.

Critical life situation: A situation in which there is a perceived threat to one's health state, in which one's existential state of being is salient, as in can-

peers, and nurses and professional colleagues.

12. Evaluation of a person's own communication skills is subjective; each individual must make his or her own decisions and choices about communication behavior and choose to change, depending upon his or her ability to utilize feedback.

Derived from Nursing:

13. The purpose of nursing is to intervene to support, maintain, and augment the client's state of health.

14. A human being functions as a unique, whole system responding openly to the environment.

Specific to the Theory:

15. Health, satisfaction and success in a person's life and work—in other words, that person's state of being—is derived from feeling human.

16. Due to the bureaucratic and complex nature of the present health care delivery systems, there is a tendency for clients and professionals to be treated in a dehumanizing manner and to relate to one another in a dehumanizing manner.

17. Humanizing patterns of communication can be learned and can enhance the

Assumptions	Concepts	Relationship Statements	Evaluation
nurse's awareness of and sensitivity to the client's state of being and of becoming. 18. The goal of the humanistic nurse is to break the communication cycle of dehumanizing attitudes and interaction patterns, replacing these with attitudes and patterns that humanize. 19. Interpersonal communication is the means by which the nurse becomes increasingly sensitive to and aware of the client's state of being, of the dynamic relationship between the client and his or her environment, and of the client's potential.	cer, childbirth, accidents, and so on. *Communication:* A dynamic interpersonal process involving continual adaptation and adjustments between two or more human beings engaged in face-to-face interactions during which each person is continually aware of the other(s). A process characterized by being existential in nature, involving an exchange of meaning, concerning facts and feelings, and involving dialogical communing. It contains the following set of attitudes: *Humanizing* *Dehumanizing continuum* Dialogue Monologue Individual Categories Holistic Parts Choice Directives Equality Degradation Positive Regard Disregard Acceptance Judgment Empathy Tolerance Authenticity Role Playing (of feelings) Caring Carelessness Irreplaceability Expendability Intimacy Isolation Coping Helplessness Power Powerlessness Humanistic communication involves an awareness of the unique characteristics of being human.		3. Duldt (1982) found that training workshops in communicating alienating messages, especially anger, decreases feelings of guilt and increases awareness of alienating patterns of communication. Role playing and rehearsal also assist nurses in improving coping. *6. Importance to the Discipline:* Nursing is being described as humanistic by many nurse-authors, but few nurse-theorists have reflected this in their theories of nursing. This theory is not intended to stand alone, but explains in detail only the phenomenon of communication. It is intended to serve with other nursing theories to augment and enhance the realistic applicability of other theories in clinical nursing. For example, the patterns of interactions and the attitudes of this theory would enhance nursing theories involving the nursing process and the communication occurring with its operationalization. Also, the patterns of interaction and attitudes of the nurse are a significant aspect of therapeutic touch theory and would augment this theory as well.

Dehumanizing communication ignores the unique characteristics of being human.

Set of Interaction Patterns of Communication:

1. *Communing:* Dialogical, intimate communication between two or more people; the heart of humanistic communication.

A. *Trust:* One person relying on another, risking potential loss in attempting to achieve a goal, when the outcome is uncertain, and the potential for loss is greater than for gain if the trust is violated.

B. *Self-disclosure:* Risking rejection in telling how one feels, thinks, and so on, regarding "here-and-now" events.

C. *Feedback:* Describing another's behavior, beliefs, and so on, plus giving one's evaluation or feelings.

2. *Assertiveness:* Expressing one's needs, thoughts, feelings, or beliefs in a direct, honest, confident manner while being respectful of others' thoughts, feelings, or beliefs; "asserting with authenticity."

3. *Confronting:* Providing feedback about another plus requesting a change in his or her behavior: "confronting with caring."

Assumptions	Concepts	Relationship Statements	Evaluation
	4. *Conflicting:* Requires a decision over an issue in which there is risk of loss as well as possible gain, in which two or more alternatives can be selected, and in which one's values are involved: "conflicting with dialogue."		
	5. *Separating:* The end of a relationship due to change, choice, or outside commitments: "separation with sadness."		
	Note: Trust, self-disclosure, and feedback represent the center of humanistic communicating—the central tripod.		

Analysis by: Bonnie W. Duldt

References: Reprinted from Duldt, B.W., & Griffin, K. *Theoretical perspectives for nursing.* Boston: Little, Brown, 1985, pp. 248–253; Duldt, B.W., Giffin, K., & Patton, B.R. *Interpersonal communication in nursing: A humanistic approach.* (Philadelphia: Davis, 1984); the present text.

ADDITIONAL REFERENCES

Berlo, D. K. *The process of communication.* San Francisco: Rinehart, 1960.

Burke, K. *Language as symbolic action: Essays on life, literature, and method.* Berkeley: University of California Press, 1966.

Duldt, B. W. Helping nurses to cope with the anger-dismay syndrome. *Nursing Outlook,* 1982, *30,* 168–175.

Egan, G. *Encounter: Group processes for interpersonal growth.* Belmont, Calif.: Brooks/Cole, 1970.

Egan, G. (Ed.). *Encounter groups: Basic readings.* Belmont, Calif.: Brooks/Cole, 1971.

Giffin, K. The contribution of studies of source credibility to a theory of interpersonal trust in the communication process. *Psychological Bulletin,* 1967, *68,* 104–120.

Giffin, K. & Patton, B. R. *Personal communcation in human relations.* Columbus, Ohio: Merrill, 1974.

Grant (Duldt), B. W. *Anger, cohesiveness, and productivity in small task groups.* Doctoral dissertation, University of Kansas, Lawrence, 1977.

Jourard, S. M. *The transparent self* (2nd ed.). New York: Van Nostrand, 1971.

Kierkegaard, S. A. *The concept of dread* (2nd ed.). (Trans. with introduction and notes by W. Lowrie.) Princeton: Princeton University Press, 1957.

Maslow, A. H. *Motivation and personality.* New York: Harper and Brothers, 1954.

Mead, George H. *Mind, self, and society,* (Ed. C. W. Morris), Chicago: University of Chicago Press, 1934.

Patterson, J. G., & Zderad, L. T. *Humanistic nursing.* New York: Wiley, 1976.

Patton B. R. & Giffin, K. *Interpersonal communication in action.* New York: Harper & Row, 1977.

Rogers, C. R. & Truax, C. B. The therapeutic conditions antecedent to change: A theoretical view. In G. Egan (Ed.), *Encounter groups: Basic readings.* Belmont, Calif.: Brooks/Cole, 1971.

Sartre, J. P. *Existentialism and humanism.* (Trans. and with an introduction by P. Mairet.) Brooklyn: Hastings House, 1957.

Yura, H., & Walsh, M. B. *The Nursing process: Assessing, planning, implememting, and evaluating* (2nd ed.), Norwalk, Conn.: Appleton-Century-Crofts, 1973.

Appendix E: COMPARISON OF CASE, FUNCTIONAL, TEAM, AND PRIMARY NURSING AS CONTROL SYSTEMS FOR DELEGATING PATIENT CARE ASSIGNMENTS TO NURSING STAFF ACCORDING TO SELECTED ASPECTS OF CLINICAL NURSING PRACTICE.

Aspect	Case	Functional	Team	Primary
1. Assignments	The nurse contracts with the patient or is assigned by an agency nurse-administrator	Head nurse or nursing coordinator assigns to staff members tasks that fall within their job descriptions	Team leader assigns to team members tasks that fall within their job descriptions	Head nurse or nursing coordinator assigns individual patients to professional nurses, matching the patient's needs to the nurse's skills.
2. Assessment, planning, and evaluation	Related to specific needs of each patient; done by the nurse, often in the patient's home; maximum continuity since nurse usually "lives in"	Related to a specific need of each patient; done by any member of the nursing staff; no continuity	Related to specific needs of each patient; done by the team leader; a limited continuity depending on how long a person remains team leader	Related to specific needs of each patient; done by the primary nurse; maximum continuity, since primary nurse remains throughout patient's stay on hospital unit
3. Implementation	The nurse delivers total care to the patient; may prepare meals, do laundry, and clean	Different members of the nursing staff do tasks for a given patient	Each team member does tasks for all patients, according to job description; the team leader often does medications and charting for the team	Each primary nurse delivers total care to all assigned patients ("For the first time I feel that somebody knows who I am")
4. Documentation	Nurse maintains a record of care given to the degree required to communicate with family and physician	Staff members make notations on only those actions or aspects of care done by them *or* A staff member is assigned to "chart" for a given number of patients; usually no nursing care plan is in evidence	Team leader usually documents care for patients cared for by most, or all, team members; sometimes a team member makes certain entries on patient charts; the team leader documents the nursing care plan	Each primary or associate nurse documents care given to each assigned patient during shift; the primary nurse documents the nursing care plan

5. Reporting at end of shift	No shift reporting; nurse gives report to physician and family as appropriate; reports to "relief nurse" if nurse must take a day off	A "charge" nurse gives report on patients to another charge nurse; most of the information shared is based on reports of other workers	The team leader gives report on the group of patients to the oncoming team; most of the information shared is based on reports of other workers	The primary nurse gives report on each assigned patient to oncoming nurse who will care for the patient; the nurse who reports has interacted directly with all the patients about whom reports are given
6. Responsibility for planning care	The nurse is responsible for planning the nursing care of the patient, from the time the nurse is hired to the time the nurse is dismissed by the patient or family	No one person is responsible for planning unless this is assigned as a functional task to a specific RN for a given period	The team leader is responsible for planning the nursing care for the assigned group of patients	The primary nurse is responsible for planning the nursing care of all primary patients, from the time they are admitted to a nursing unit until they are discharged from that unit
7. Responsibility for providing care	The nurse delivers all nursing care to the patient	Nursing care is delivered in a fragmented manner, with many staff members interacting with the patient as the various tasks are done	As in functional nursing, delivery of nursing care is a "mixed bag"	The primary nurse directly delivers all nursing care to the primary patients when on duty
a. For coordination and outcomes of nursing care	The nurse plans and delivers care to the patient and is answerable to the patient for coordination and outcomes of nursing care	No one nursing staff member is answerable for the coordination and outcomes of nursing care; the head nurse often answers to everyone for the entire staff	The team leader, who plans care but often does not give it, is answerable for the care of each patient in the assigned group and for the coordination and outcomes of nursing care	The primary nurse who plans and delivers the care to each assigned patient is answerable for the coordination and outcomes of nursing care
b. For follow-up on patient problems	The nurse is responsible for follow-up on problems of the patient	Physicians, administrators, and other interdepartmental personnel can rarely pinpoint responsibility for follow-up on problems	The team leader is responsible for follow-up on patient problems, which are often generated by other staff	The primary nurse is responsible for follow-up on problems of assigned patients

Aspect	Case	Functional	Team	Primary
c. "Passing the buck"	Minimal; no one to whom the "buck" can be passed (unless to a member of the household)	"Passing the buck" prevalent	Moderate amount of "buck passing" due to change in staff assignments from day to day	Minimal, if any, "passing the buck," because of constancy of staff assignments to same patients
8. Comprehensiveness of care, in terms of:				
a. Patients' needs	Continuity is maximized in that the same nurse–same patient relationship is maximized. Focus of nursing care may be patient goals rather than nursing actions. Care is usually highly individualized. (However, the nurse could be a "Sarah Gamp")	Not possible; focus of care is on tasks, not on the patient as a unique individual with a broad spectrum of needs and resources	Theoretically, and sometimes actually, possible, since team members are expected to communicate related to patient needs and nursing action to meet those needs; a united approach is the goal; however, plans are often designed with minimal patient and family input, and focus is on nursing action, rather than on patient goals	Inherent in the system, because continuity in same nurse–same patient relationships is maximized; focus of nursing care is on patient goals rather than on nursing action
b. Documentation	Nursing care may be documented, depending on the individual nurse; usually not mandated	Nursing care regimens are rarely documented, so individual approaches are inconsistent	Documented nursing care plans are encouraged but can rarely be demanded, because nursing case load is too large	Documented nursing care plans are mandated and are facilitated by smaller case load of each nurse and by constancy of assignment

	Case	Functional	Team	Primary
9. Communication				
a. between nurses and patients or clients	Patient, family, and significant others can clearly identify the nurse and can share ideas, feelings, and problems freely with this person	Patient, family, and significant others find it difficult to identify a nursing staff member with whom to relate on a continuing basis	Patient, family, and significant others may be confused as to identity of the nursing staff member to whom questions and problems may be directed	Patient, family, and significant others can clearly identify the nurse and can share ideas, feelings, and problems freely with this person
b. Between nurses and staff of other departments	All communications are directed to the nurse. Satisfactory answers may be forthcoming. During waking hours, the nurse is usually near the patient	Physicians, administrators, and interdepartmental staff address questions and problems to nurses or to head nurse on unit, but often satisfactory answers are delayed or are not available	Same as in functional nursing, except team leader rather than head nurse may be consulted	All communications are directed to the primary nurse for each patient. Satisfactory answers are more likely to be forthcoming. Persons may find difficulty in locating specific nurses
c. Between nurses and supervisors	Repetitions of instructions for the patient is usually not necessary because of the single nurse providing care	Instructions often have to be repeated because of changes in staff assignments and lack of consistent documentation of nursing care plans	Same as in functional nursing	Dramatic decrease in repetition of instructions for particular patients due to constancy of assignments and mandatory care plans
10. Cost-effectiveness	Not cost-effective, because: a. Product is of high quality if the nurse is qualified to provide care required	Not cost-effective, because: a. Product (nursing care) is of poor quality owing to fragmentation; this results in many complaints from consumers	Not cost-effective, because: a. Product is of only moderate quality, since expertise in judgment and communication cannot be delegated from the careplanners (team leaders) to the care-givers (team members)	Most likely to be cost-effective, because: a. Product is of high quality since the person most prepared and best equipped to perform does so on a continuing basis for the same patients

Aspect	Case	Functional	Team	Primary
	b. Turnover is minimal if the nurse–patient interactions are satisfactory to both	b. Nursing staff easily becomes frustrated and turnover rate is usually high, thus increasing cost of orientation and of staff development	b. Turnover of nursing staff is moderate but variable	b. Turnover of nursing staff is minimal because of higher level of satisfaction experienced by nurses
	c. Nurses do the job according to the way the patient prefers; patient often views nurse as a personal servant	c. Output from professional nurses is low, since they are not required to perform the full job—the total nursing process—for which they are being paid	c. Same as for functional nursing	c. Professional nurses do the job for which they are being paid; "unproductive" time decreases dramatically

Adapted from Kron, T. The management of patient care: Putting leadership skills to work (5th ed.). Philadelphia: Saunders, 1981, p. 228–232.

Appendix F: THE MOUNT VERNON HOSPITAL NURSING SERVICES
Nursing Clinical Ladder

1. *Philosophy of The Mount Vernon Hospital Clinical Ladder:*
   The Nursing Services of The Mount Vernon Hospital, as a member of the nursing community, is committed to providing opportunities for professional growth and advancement for the nursing staff. By providing these opportunities in the form of a clinical ladder, the Nursing Services will enhance professional practice at The Mount Vernon Hospital and improve nursing care delivery.
2. *Purpose:*
   The purpose of the Nursing Clinical Ladder at The Mount Vernon Hospital is to develop a method for recognition of outstanding expertise and initiative in the professional staff nurse by providing opportunities within nursing for the growth and improvement of professional practice.
3. *Objectives:*
   The establishment of a Nursing Clinical Ladder at The Mount Vernon Hospital will:
   3.1 Improve the quality of patient care by promoting higher levels of nursing practice.
   3.2 Provide for recognition and advancement of the highly qualified and competent professional nurse in patient care activities.
   3.3 Serve as a means for motivating nurses to increase their professional knowledge and skills.
   3.4 Utilize experienced nurses who are educationally prepared in accordance with their level of practice.
   3.5 Increase and maintain job satisfaction for the professional nurse in the clinical setting.
   3.6 Provide explicit expectations for practice that serve as guides for evaluation of performance.

Benefits of a Professionally Oriented Nursing Delivery System

Nursing Services at The Mount Vernon Hospital believes that the health consumer is rightfully entitled to maximum interaction with and direct services from professional registered nurses during the course of any hospitalization.

We also believe that the recognition of and reward to professional nurses who are expert in the management of patients are essential for professional development and job satisfaction.

The motivational and beneficial factors of this professionally oriented and challenging nursing modality have resulted in:
(a) A very high work output of professional registered nurses, in spite of extensive physical stress during recurrent periods of overload census.
(b) Implementation of the complete nursing process by each professional nurse employed here, including patient teaching and discharge planning.
(c) An outstandingly excellent rating of nursing care by patients who present themselves to our hospital for inpatient and/or outpatient care as evidenced by letters and patient surveys.
(d) A high frequency of collaboration between nurses and health care personnel.
(e) Nurses, both during the orientation sessions and after varying periods of employment, expressing a high degree of satisfaction with this nursing care delivery modality which allows them to utilize their clinical knowledge and skills at maximum levels.
(f) Every professional registered nurse on the staff (including administrative nursing personnel) being involved in staff development activities, as teachers and/or learners.
(g) Maximization of contact between hospitalized patients and professional nurses.
(h) Feeling of pride in the nurses' work and the employing hospital, subsequently reducing the rate of turnover.

Title—Primary Nurse I/Primary Nurse II/Primary Nurse III/Primary Nurse IV

The title Primary Staff Nurse I will be designated and defined as the new graduate nurse and will be retained for the first twelve months of employment, provisional to successful completion of Licensure.

The title Primary Staff Nurse II will be retained at The Mount Vernon Hospital and will be defined as the entry level for professional Registered Nurses.

The title Primary Nurse III will be designated and defined as the promotional level for nurses who have satisfactorily completed three (3) months as a Primary Staff Nurse II and met the requirements as outlined for promotion.

The title Primary Nurse IV will be designated and defined as the promotional level for two positions per unit, one with a Clinical Speciality and one with an Administrative Specialty. This title will be assumed by a Primary Nurse III based upon the successful completion of the detailed application process and availability of a position.

Job Description Format

The Job Description and Expected Behaviors for the Primary Staff Nurse I and II at The Mount Vernon Hospital outline the level of practice which is expected of each Primary Nurse in the Hospital.

The Guidelines for Primary Nurse III at The Mount Vernon Hospital will be the criteria on which the nurses' performance is evaluated and which delineate the parameters of professional nursing practice.

The Job Descriptions and Expected Behaviors for the Primary Nurse IV/Clinical Specialty and the Primary Nurse IV/Administrative Specialty outline the levels of practice which are expected of each Primary Nurse IV at The Mount Vernon Hospital.

Eligibility Guidelines for Evaluating Application for Primary Nurse III

1. *Experience*
    1.1. The applicant must have a minimum of 18 months of experience as a registered nurse. The graduate nurse awaiting State Board Examination results may begin his or her 18 months experience with the date of employment.
    1.2. The applicant must have spent the previous three months in the facility where he or she is applying and in the clinical specialty for which he or she is applying.
    1.3. There will be no distinction between A.D., Diploma, or Baccalaureate graduates.
2. *Education*
    2.1. Within the 12 months preceding application, the applicant must have obtained 48 clinical contact hours in continuing education while employed at Mount Vernon Hospital.
        2.1.1. At least 24 of these contact hours must be in the nurse's area on clinical specialty, while the remaining 24 should reflect the applicant's interest in a variety of professional topics and media.
            2.1.1.1. The minimum mandatory hours for attendance at educational programs, i.e. workshops, conferences, in-services, etc. are 30.
        2.1.2. The applicant must have earned at least 8 of the total 48 contact hours by preparing and presenting two (2) one-hour each scheduled, unit- or hospital-wide staff development programs (1 hour presentation = 4 clinical contact hours), or an equivalent time preparing patient education materials. These programs may address a topic in the applicants specialty area or a related topic of professional interest.
        2.1.3. Educational experiences not specifically referred to below will be awarded contact hours as determined by the chairperson of the committee.
        2.1.4. Hours accrued as part of formal education toward a college degree may not be used as clinical contact hours.
    2.2. Contact Hours
        Note: Subject to review by the Chairperson of the Committee of specific program content and assessment by evaluation of the participant's knowledge gained, the following hour values will be awarded eligible individuals at Mount Vernon Hospital. The employee is responsible for maintaining his or her record of Clinical Contact hours. A copy of all program information, attendance, etc., will be kept on the Nursing Unit.
        2.2.1. Unit Staff Development Program—Attendance, 1 hour = 1 Clinical Contact hour. The number of Clinical Contact hours per program should be posted prior to the program. (Excludes Staff meetings.)

2.2.2. Unit Staff Development—Preparation and Presentation, 1 hour = 4 Clinical Contact hours.

2.2.3. Hospital-Wide Staff Development Programs—Attendance, Generally one (1) hour = 1 Clinical Contact hour. The number of Clinical Contact Hours/Program will be posted prior to the program.

2.2.4. Hospital-Wide Staff Development Programs—Preparation and Presentation—1 hour of actual instruction = 4 Clinical Contact hours if done individually; if done as part of a group effort, contact hours will be awarded on an individual basis, depending on the amount of actual participation.

2.2.5. Workshops/Seminars—Number of hours in Attendance = number of Clinical Contact hours.

2.2.6. Special Projects/Research Activities—Clinical Contact hours will be awarded on an individual basis by the Chairperson of the Committee.

Projects or activities must be in writing, with purpose stated, objectives defined, method of implementation outlined, and type of evaluation described prior to initiation of project.

2.2.7. Nursing Journal Articles—reading four pertinent journal articles and evaluating them on the Evaluation/Summary of Nursing Journal Articles form yields one contact hour, not to exceed 4 contact hours (16 journal articles) per year. The Journal Article Evaluation/Summary forms are to be submitted with the Educational Transcript.

2.2.8. Programs which the Primary Nurse presents which are of a repetitive nature (example: Nursing Orientation) will receive 2 contact hours for each hour presented, not to exceed 8 contact hours/year.

2.2.9. Contact hours earned through programmed learning modules may not comprise more than one third of the total contact hours earned. Each is given 4 hours.

2.2.10. Education which is mandatory for employment on a specific unit or at Mount Vernon Hospital cannot be used as contact hours; i.e., CPR Certification, IV Therapy, and new equipment demonstrations by sales representatives.

2.2.11. Optional Activities:

— Committee Work—membership on any committee that is clinically oriented, and the member attends 80% of the meetings = 3 contact hours.

— Community Education—Lectures or presentations to community groups, i.e., scouts, churches, schools, etc = 3 contact hours for 8 hours of presentation.

— Outpatient Education—Number of hours taught = equal number of contact hours.

— Development of Patient Education Packets—Patient education projects that follow approved format = 6 contact hours.

— Patient Classification Monitor—100% of scheduled observations per year = 4 contact hours.

— Quality Assurance Monitor—100% scheduled observations per year = 9 contact hours.

3. *Attendance*

Master time cards will be reviewed.

4. *Attitude*

4.1. Functions well with professional peers, those in supervisory positions, patients, patient's family, physicians, and intradepartmental personnel.

4.2. Professionally serves as a role model to others in areas of moral and ethical character.

4.3. Maintains a professional appearance at work.

4.4. Is realistic about self expectations.

4.5. Evaluates limitations and seeks guidance when necessary.

5. *Leadership*

5.1. Accepts responsibility for his/her own actions regardless of consequences.

     5.2. Handles leadership positions (acts as resource person).

     5.3. Can tolerate unpopular decisions.

     5.4. Exhibits willingness to teach peer group.

     5.5. Accepts constructive criticism, also assists in constructive learning situations.

     5.6. Utilizes variety of approaches in assisting others in problem solving.

6. *Interest*

     6.1. Takes active interest in respective clinical specialty.

     6.2. Is motivated.

     6.3. Demonstrates interest in current developments in his/her own field of endeavor. (Use of Contact hours.)

     6.4. Demonstrates interest in holistic patient care and the effects hospitalization will have on the patient during his stay and after discharge.

7. *Job Knowledge and Skills*

     7.1. Proficient in routine nursing procedures and those applicable to his/her specialty area. (Review criteria established for each individual specialty area.)

     7.2. Demonstrates responsibility and accountability for formulating, documenting and evaluating his/her plan of patient care.

8. *Maintenance of Primary Nurse III*

     8.1. To maintain the status of Primary Nurse III at Mount Vernon Hospital the nurse must obtain 24 Clinical Contact Hours on an annual basis.

          8.1.1. The minimum mandatory hours for attendance at education programs, i.e., workshops, conferences, in-services, etc. are 15.

          8.1.2. Twelve of the total contact hours must be in the nurse's area of clinical specialty, while the remaining twelve hours should reflect a variety of professional interests on the part of the nurse.

          8.1.3. A minimum of four, of the total 24 Contact Hours need to be earned by preparing and presenting 1 one-hour, unit or hospital-wide staff development program addressing a topic of professional interest. An additional 3–5 Contact Hours must be earned from the *Optional Activities List* (see 2.2.11)

9. *Application*

     9.1. Upon meeting the eligibility requirements, the Primary Nurse II will initiate application by submitting her/his Primary Nurse III application form, a copy of his/her Mount Vernon Hospital Education Transcript, and the Education Program Records and Attendance Records from her/his inservice programs, to the Nursing Unit Director of his/her respective unit.

     9.2. The Nursing Unit Director will distribute parts I and III of the Nursing Division Performance Evaluation to the applicant, and part II to the three selected Peer Reviewers from the applicant's Unit.

     9.3. These evaluation forms will be completed and returned to the Nursing Unit Director no later than seven days after receipt.

     9.4. The Nursing Unit Director will complete an evaluation form, and submit all forms to the Chairperson of the Clinical Ladder Committee.

          9.4.1. If an evaluation has been completed in the past year, obtain a copy from the personnel department before submitting required forms to the Committee.

10. *Committee Membership*

     10.1. The Committee Membership will consist of:

          10.1.1. The Education Specialist from the Department of Education to act as Chairperson of the Committee.

          10.1.2. Each Nursing Unit will have a Primary Nurse III or IV representative on the Committee for a minimum of one year.

          10.1.3. If there are no applicants by the 10th of the month the Committee will not meet.

10.1.4. A list of the Committee members will be maintained in the Office of the Assistant Administrator, Director of Nursing Services.

11. *Review*

    11.1. The review process will be as follows:

        11.1.1. The Committee will meet in the third week of each month to review the applications submitted. All applicants should have her/his application complete and to the chairperson by the 10th of the month in order to be reviewed for that month.

        11.1.2. Each member of the Committee will review the completed application and make a recommendation to the Chairperson.

        11.1.3. When the recommendation is unanimously approved, the Chairperson will submit a formal written recommendation for the promotion to the Assistant Administrator, Director of Nursing Services.

12. *Appeal*

    12.1. If the applicant does not feel satisfied with the decision of the Committee in recommending denial of promotion, (s)he may then request a review by the Appeals Committee.

    The Appeals Committee will consist of:

        12.1.1. Assistant Administrator, Director of Nursing Services.

        12.1.2. Director of Employee Relations.

        12.1.3. Administrative Nursing Supervisor for specific shift.

        12.1.4. A registered nurse who is employed in this facility at the *Primary Nurse II* level. This nurse will be chosen by the person making the appeal.

        The decision of this Committee will be considered final but will not preclude the opportunity for re-application in three (3) months.

APPLICATION FOR PRIMARY NURSE III*

DATE: _____

1. Name _____

2. Length of Employment at The Mount Vernon Hospital _____

3. Present Clinical Area _____
    a. Length of Service _____

4. Date Graduated from _____ADN _____Diploma _____BSN _____ MSN

5. Past Clinical Experience including Previous Employment: _____

_____
_____
_____
_____
_____

6. Nursing Division Performance Evaluations
    Required:
    6.1. Self-evaluation form for Primary II parts I and III
    6.2. Three peer evaluations, Part II.
    6.3. Evaluation from Nursing Unit Director.

7. Attach completed copy (do not send original) of The Mount Vernon Hospital Education Transcript.

8. Record of Clinical Contact Hours (attach form).

9. Indicate any activities outside the hospital in which you participate that you would like to have considered in your evaluation.

* APPLICATION AND APPROPRIATE FORMS TO BE SUBMITTED BY THE 10TH OF THE MONTH. THOSE RECEIVED AFTER THE 10TH WILL BE REVIEWED THE FOLLOWING MONTH.

The Mount Vernon Hospital
EDUCATION TRANSCRIPT

Name _____   SS#_____
Last   First   MI

Department _____   Position/Title _____

COURSE TITLE	DATE(S)	HOURS	SPONSOR	CEU CREDITS	COMMENTS
Hospital Orientation			Mount Vernon Hospital		
Nursing Dept. Orientation			Mount Vernon Hospital		

GUIDELINES FOR SELECTION OF PRIMARY NURSE IV

Qualifications for Clinical Primary Nurse IV
1. Current Virginia State Licensure.
2. Twelve (12) months experience as a Primary Nurse III in the same specialty area.
3. Evidence of the required number of clinical contact hours in continuing nursing education.
4. Consistent performance in his/her clinical speciality that exceeds group standards.
5. Bachelor of Science Degree in Nursing or certification in the specialty area or five years experience in an acute care facility.
6. Position subject to yearly review by Nursing Care Manager.

Qualifications for Administrative Primary Nurse IV
1. Current Virginia State Licensure.
2. Twelve (12) months experience as a Primary Nurse III in same specialty area.
3. Evidence of the required number of clinical contact hours in continuing nursing education.
4. Consistent performance in his/her clinical speciality that exceeds group standards.
5. Bachelor of Science Degree in Nursing or within six months of graduation.
6. Position subject to yearly review by Nursing Care Manager.

SELECTION PROCESS FOR CLINICAL AND ADMINISTRATIVE PRIMARY NURSE IV:

1. Personal resume with a letter of intent to the respective Nursing Care Manager.
2. Interview by Search Committee which consists of:—Nursing Care Manager of applicant's unit to chair the Search Committee
   — Nursing Care Manager of another unit.
   — Representative from the supervisory staff in accordance with the shifts worked by the applicant.
   — Chairman of Nursing Clinical Ladder Committee.
   — Two Peer Reviewers from applicants unit.

The final decision will be made by the Nursing Care Manager of the applicant's unit. The applicant, if selected, will be subject to careful annual review by the Nursing Care Manager as well as a three month probationary period.

Salary Adjustment

The Primary Staff Nurse I who successfully completes licensure and has gained one year of clinical experience will receive a salary increase commensurate with moving up one Grade on the wage scale.

Those Primary Nurses achieving Primary Nurse III or IV status will receive a salary adjustment effective the date of promotion. The salary increase will not move the nurse up a Grade on the wage scale. The promotion will not affect the nurse's anniversary date.

Change in Status

Inter-Hospital Transfer

A professional nurse who transfers from another hospital within the Association to The Mount Vernon Hospital and seeks the Primary Nurse III status must meet all criteria as established for that position at The Mount Vernon Hospital.

A professional nurse who transfers from another hospital within the Association to The Mount Vernon Hospital and seeks the Primary Nurse IV level (either Clinical or Administrative) must meet criteria as established for that position at The Mount Vernon Hospital. A transfer Primary Nurse's eligibility for an available level IV position is negotiable between the transferring nurse and the Nursing Care Manager.

Intra-Hospital Transfer

A Primary Nurse III may not transfer to another clinical area within twelve (12) calendar months of her promotion, except at the request of the Nursing Administration.

A Primary Nurse III transferring within the same clinical area will retain her/his Primary Nurse III status. This applies only to intra-hospital transfers between 5A and 3B.

A Primary Nurse III desiring to transfer from one clinical area to another will maintain her/his Primary III status at the discretion of the Director of Nursing Services or her designee. If a nurse reverts to a Primary Nurse II when transferring, she/he will be eligible to reapply for Primary Nurse III in three (3) months, providing all other criteria are met. During this three-month period, she/he will maintain her/his Primary Nurse III salary. If the re-application is denied: the nurse must return to her/his original clinical area if possible, in order to maintain Primary Nurse III status; if the nurse remains in the new clinical area she/he must accept a position and salary as a Primary Staff Nurse II.

A Primary Nurse III returning from Maternity Leave, a Leave of Absence or returning to employment after terminating will be reinstated at the Primary Nurse III level if the absence from the Unit was no more than six months; if she/he has been away for more than six months, he/she must work out a 90 day waiting period before she/he may be reconsidered for a Primary Nurse III position.

Evaluation of the Clinical Ladder

This Committee would like to recommend that a committee be appointed for evaluation of the Clinical Ladder Program, and be tentatively scheduled to meet July 1 of each year. It will consist of three nurses who have attained Primary Nurse IV status, the current Committee, and the Assistant Administrator, Director of Nursing Services.

At the close of each succeeding year the Committee will complete a written evaluation in the form of an annual report and submit this to the Assistant Administrator, Director of Nursing Services.

The Nursing Clinical Ladder was contributed by the Nursing Staff at Mount Vernon Hospital, Alexandria, Virginia. Mount Vernon Hospital is an acute care hospital and affiliate of Fairfax Hospital Systems, a comprehensive health care system serving the mid-Atlantic region.

INDEX

Page numbers followed by *f* refer to figures. Page numbers followed by *t* refer to tables.

Page numbers followed by *f* refer to figures. Page numbers followed by *t* refer to tables.

Page numbers followed by *f* refer to figures. Page numbers followed by *t* refer to tables.

Page numbers followed by *f* refer to figures. Page numbers followed by *t* refer to tables.